Workbook to Accompany

Paramedic Field Care

A COMPLAINT-BASED APPROACH

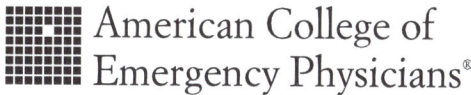
American College of Emergency Physicians®

Contributors:

Jan Auerbach, RN, MSN, EMT-P
Associate Professor for the School of Allied Health
Emergency Medicine Education Program
University of Texas Southwestern Medical Center
Dallas, Texas

Carol Goodykoontz, RN, MS, EMT-P
Associate Professor
Assistant Program Director
Emergency Medicine Education
University of Texas Southwestern Medical Center
Dallas, Texas

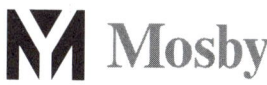 Mosby

St. Louis Baltimore Boston Carlsbad Chicago Minneapolis New York Philadelphia Portland
London Milan Sydney Tokyo Toronto

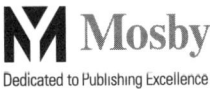

A Times Mirror
Company

Publisher: Don Ladig
Senior Acquisitions Editor: Jennifer Roche
Senior Development Editor: Kellie White and Nancy Peterson
Production Manager: Chris Baumle
Production Editor: Anthony F. Trioli
Manufacturing Supervisor: William A. Winneberger, Jr.
Designer/Compositor: Paul Fennessy
ACEP Developmental Editor: Susan Magee

Copyright © 1998 by The American College of Emergency Physicians

All rights reserved. No part of this publication may be reproduced, stored in a retrieval system, or transmitted, in any form or by any means electronic, mechanical, photocopying, recording, or otherwise, without prior written permission from the publisher.

Permission to photocopy or reproduce solely for internal or personal use is permitted for libraries or other users registered with the Copyright Clearance Center, provided that the base fee of $4.00 per chapter plus $.10 per page is paid directly to the Copyright Clearance Center, 222 Rosewood Drive, Danvers, MA 01923. This consent does not extend to other kinds of copying, such as copying for general distribution, for advertising or promotional purposes, for creating new or collected works, or for resale.

Printed in the United States of America
Composition by Paul Fennessy
Printing/binding by Plus Communications

Mosby–Year Book, Inc.
11830 Westline Industrial Drive
St. Louis, MO 63146

99 00 01 02 03 / 9 8 7 6 5 4 3 2 1

ABOUT THE CONTRIBUTORS

Jan Auerbach, RN, MSN, EMT-P has practiced in emergency nursing and prehospital education since her graduation in 1979 from nursing school. She earned her Master of Science in Nursing Degree from the University of Texas at Arlington and received her paramedic training from the University of Texas Health Science Center at Dallas concurrently in 1986. She has been actively involved in prehospital emergency care through clinical practice, teaching, publishing and research for seventeen years, which earned her the EMS Educator Award from The Bureau of Emergency Management in 1989. Ms. Auerbach is currently an Associate Professor in the School of Allied Health Emergency Medicine Education Program at the University of Texas Southwestern Medical Center in Dallas.

Carol Goodykoontz, RN, MS, EMT-P received a Bachelor of Science degree in nursing from the University of Kentucky in 1973. A move to Phoenix, Arizona launched her interest in EMS. While working in the emergency department, she assisted in the training of the first class of paramedic students for the Phoenix Fire Department. In 1978, she earned a Master's degree in nursing from Texas Women's University and began her ongoing career in paramedic education with the University of Texas Southwestern Medical Center. In 1981, she was promoted to her current position of Assistant Program Director.

Carol has served as a consultant, reviewer, and contributing author to several EMS textbooks. She has been actively involved at the state level in developing certification examinations for EMS personnel and EMS instructor courses. Since 1988, she has served as a site reviewer for the Joint Review Committee of Paramedic Educational Programs. In 1996, she received the finalist award for the Mary Ann Talley Instructor/Coordinator-of-the-Year from the National Associations of EMT's.

DEDICATIONS

For support and encouragement during the development of this book, I feel a deep sense of gratitude to all of the loves of my life.

Jan Auerbach

In memory of my beloved sister, Ann Taylor, whose life and death have had a profound influence on my life. To my husband, Roy, sons Ken and Kevin, and my parents, Jack and Ann, for their ongoing support, love, and belief in me.

Carol Goodykoontz

PREFACE

When the American College of Emergency Physicians (ACEP) set out to develop a new paramedic textbook, its Editorial Board undertook a challenging mission: to prepare paramedic students for the "reality" of prehospital medical practice. The result of this effort is the unique, complaint-based textbook, ***Paramedic Field Care: A Complaint-Based Approach.***

In keeping with the mission of the textbook, this workbook was designed to support and augment the "complaint-based" learning approach by using realistic case presentations. These case presentations require you to *apply* the information presented in the textbook just as you will do when encountering these situations in the real world. We encourage you to complete all workbook chapters because it will assist in your comprehension, retention, and integration of the information presented in the textbook as well as in classroom instruction.

Each chapter begins with **Learning Objectives** that match those in your textbook. These objectives state the expected learning outcomes, that is, what YOU are expected to know and be able to do as a result of reading the corresponding text chapter. The objectives serve as the basis for the questions in each workbook chapter as well as in classroom testing so it is important that you make sure that you understand them.

The first section of each chapter consists of one or more **Case Presentations** followed by corresponding questions. The case presentations appear in boldface print. Each case begins with dispatch information and proceeds through scene assessment, initial assessment, patient management, continued assessment, and finally to case resolution. Changes in the patient's condition, the impact of your interventions, and other factors unfold as you work through the questions. A concerted effort was made to create case presentations that paint a real and accurate picture of the field setting and help you develop a systematic approach to responding to EMS calls and providing patient care.

Each chapter also contains a **General Review Questions** section consisting of questions in a variety of formats that test knowledge that did not lend itself to the case presentations. Multiple-choice, fill-in, short answer, matching, and true/false questions challenge your retention of facts and present questions in a manner similar to traditional examinations.

Several chapters, particularly Chapter 12, also use **illustrations or ECG strips** to test your understanding of a subject area, e.g., interpretation of a cardiac rhythm.

Complete **Answers and Rationale** for all questions are found by chapter number in the back of the workbook. They provide comprehensive information on both the correct and incorrect answers. Each answer is linked to a **Learning Objective** from the chapter or to a **Prerequisite Chapter Objective**. If the answer to a question references a prerequisite chapter objective, this indicates that the content specific to the question is covered in a prior chapter in the textbook or is based on prerequisite knowledge and skills. Inclusion of these types of questions facilitates recall and synthesis of previously learned information.

Admittedly, the variety of question types and the application of information required by the case presentations may prove challenging. However, we are certain that, with careful attention to classroom and lab instruction, careful reading of the textbook, and diligent use of this workbook, you will be well-prepared to face the realities of the paramedic profession that await you.

Jan Auerbach
Carol Goodykoontz

ACKNOWLEDGMENTS

We are grateful to several dedicated individuals whose contributions made this book possible:

Dr. Peter Pons and Debra Cason for providing us with an excellent textbook to work with.

David J. Gurchiek, BS, NREMT-P and John Barron, NREMT-P for their valuable review and comments of this manuscript during its development.

Susan Magee for her unique ability to create order out of confusion. Her vision, support, and sense of humor through this long and tedious process kept us going.

Nancy Peterson for keeping us focused. Her suggestions, along with those of the external reviewers, contributed to the clarity and continuity of the workbook. Her wisdom and sensitivity were invaluable.

Terri Staines, Brenda Holcomb, Denise Fechner, and Carla Goldberg for the countless hours spent typing, retyping, mailing, faxing, and supporting this project. We thank each of them for their perseverance.

Our students, peers, family members, and numerous others for their patience and understanding which allowed us to bring this project to fruition.

CONTENTS

QUESTIONS

Section 1 The Paramedic and EMS
- Chapter 1   Overview of the EMS System 1
- Chapter 2   Roles and Responsibilites 9
- Chapter 3   The EMS Call 12
- Chapter 4   Medical Accountability 17
- Chapter 5   Legal Accountability 21

Section 2 Foundations for Practice
- Chapter 6   Medical Terminology 27
- Chapter 7   Basic Body Systems 34
- Chapter 8   Principles of Pathophysiology 43
- Chapter 9   Shock 51
- Chapter 10 Infection Control 59
- Chapter 11 General Pharmacology 64
- Chapter 11a Appendix: Prehospital Medications 73
- Chapter 12 Basic Rhythm Interpretation 83
- Chapter 13 Interpersonal Communications Skills 93
- Chapter 14 Communication and Documentation 97

Section 3A Scene and Patient Assessment
- Chapter 15 Scene Assessment, Safety, and Control 103
- Chapter 16 Mechanism of Injury 108

Section 3B Assessment of the Critical Patient
- Chapter 17 Initial Assessment 115
- Chapter 18 The Patient With Airway and Breathing Compromise 121
- Chapter 19 The Patient Without a Pulse 130
- Chapter 20 The Patient With Compromised Circulation 138
- Chapter 21 The Critical Trauma Patient 146
- Chapter 22 The Critical Pediatric Patient 153

Section 3C Continued Patient Assessment
- Chapter 23 Clinical Significance of Vital Signs 163
- Chapter 24 Focused and Continued Assessment 169
- Chapter 25 Pediatric Assessment 175
- Chapter 26 Geriatric Assessment 181

Section 4A Patient Presentations—Medical
- Chapter 27 Dyspnea 190
- Chapter 28 Nontraumatic Bleeding 197
- Chapter 29 Syncope 203
- Chapter 30 Altered Mental Status 209
- Chapter 31 Chest Pain 215

Section 4A Patient Presentations—Medical (continued)

Chapter 32	Palpitations and Dysrhythmias	221
Chapter 33	Headache	229
Chapter 34	Weak, Dizzy, and Malaise	236
Chapter 35	Diabetic Emergencies	241
Chapter 36	Abdominal, Genitourinary, and Back Pain	249
Chapter 37	Pregnancy and Childbirth	257
Chapter 38	Fever	265
Chapter 39	Eye, Ear, Nose, and Throat Complaints—Medical	273
Chapter 40	Nontraumatic Extremity Complaints	279
Chapter 41	Poisoning and Overdose	285
Chapter 42	Drugs of Abuse	294
Chapter 43	Environmental Emergencies	300
Chapter 44	Aquatic Emergencies	308
Chapter 45	Behavioral Emergencies	314

Section 4B Patient Presentations—Trauma

Chapter 46	Truncal Trauma	322
Chapter 47	Head, Eyes, Ears, Nose, Mouth, and Throat Trauma	329
Chapter 48	Orthopedic Injuries	338
Chapter 49	Burn Injuries	342

Section 5 Special Situations

Chapter 50	General Principles of Rescue	350
Chapter 51	Multiple-Casualty Incidents and Disasters	356
Chapter 52	Hazardous Materials and Radiation Incidents	361
Chapter 53	Air Medical Services	368
Chapter 54	Rural EMS	371
Chapter 55	Specialized Adjuncts for Therapy	376
Chapter 56	Issues of Personal Violence	382
Chapter 57	Death and Dying	389
Chapter 58	Stress and Stress Management	395

ANSWERS 401

ILLUSTRATION CREDITS 519

Questions

Section 1

THE PARAMEDIC AND EMS

1. Overview of the EMS System
2. Roles and Responsibilites
3. The EMS Call
4. Medical Accountability
5. Legal Accountability

Chapter 1

Overview of the EMS System

OBJECTIVES

1. Explain the development of EMS in the United States, including important legislative and other developments.
2. Identify the five stages of the EMS system from a patient's perspective.
3. List the 15 components of an EMS system.
4. Explain the relationship between medical direction and the quality of prehospital health care provided within an EMS system.
5. List the different funding mechanisms in EMS.
6. Outline the role of regulatory agencies in EMS systems.
7. Describe the use of standards in EMS, including the various mechanisms for certification and licensure.
8. Define the terms *mutual aid* and *reciprocity*.
9. Explain the need for system planning and identify five system goals.
10. Identify various EMS system participants and standards.
11. Describe the four components of EMS Communications.
12. Describe the role of research in EMS.

CASE PRESENTATION #1 (QUESTIONS 1–8)

You are dispatched to a rural area outside your city to care for a choking baby. Your unit's response time will be at least 15 minutes. A first responder unit, which is less than 5 minutes away, has already been dispatched. The dispatcher tells you that the baby is not breathing, and that the mother has been given pre-arrival instructions.

1. Providing pre-arrival instructions:
    a. is prerequisite to becoming a certified dispatcher.
    b. is a component capability only in 911 systems.
    c. requires specialized training in emergency medical dispatch (EMD).
    d. is standard practice for all dispatchers.

Sending a first responder unit is an example of a tiered response in an emergency medical services (EMS) system.

2. What type of training is required for dispatchers in a tiered system?

3. How does a tiered response benefit both the patient and the EMS system? Briefly discuss your response.

The first responder unit is on the scene; unit members radio to tell you that cardiopulmonary resuscitation (CPR) is in progress. Both first responders are Basic Emergency Medical Technicians (EMTs).

4. Once you arrive on the scene, the most important information that you must obtain from the first responders is:
   a. the age and approximate weight of the patient.
   b. the condition of the patient upon arrival of the first responders at the scene.
   c. information about what the patient choked on.
   d. the patient's medical history.

5. As an advanced life support (ALS) provider, what procedures can you perform that may potentially benefit the patient?

You contact medical direction and are advised to follow your pediatric cardiac arrest protocol.

6. Medical direction of an EMS system is the responsibility of the:
   a. EMS division chief.
   b. EMS medical director.
   c. hospital that provides off-line medical direction.
   d. senior paramedic in the department.

7. What are treatment protocols; who oversees them in an EMS system?

This call is outside your service delivery area. Your department has established "mutual aid" agreements with the county.

8. Briefly explain how and why this is important for the provision of patient care during the prehospital phase.

CASE PRESENTATION #2 (QUESTIONS 9–10)   MED LEGAL

You are dispatched to a local hospital for an emergency transfer. The patient is an elderly man who appears to have had a stroke. He is being transferred because his physician is located at another hospital. His vital signs are unstable, and he is receiving medications that are not included in your local protocols. The patient's vital signs are as follows: blood pressure (BP) 200/130; pulse 64; respirations 28 and shallow.

9. Are you directly responsible for the care of this patient during the transfer? Briefly explain your response.

10. Should medical personnel (physician/nurse) from the transferring hospital accompany you? Why or why not?

CASE PRESENTATION #3 (QUESTIONS 11–13)

You are dispatched to a motor vehicle collision. Several cars are involved, and after surveying the scene, you request three additional ambulances. On further evaluation as triage officer, you determine that there are eight patients: two critically injured, four with serious injuries, and two patients with minor injuries. You change your request to four additional ambulances, if they are available. When the additional ambulances arrive at the scene, the critical patients are directed to them.

11. The critical patients should go to a Level _____ trauma facility, if one is available.

12. What is a trauma center?

13. How does an established trauma system enhance patient care in the prehospital setting?

GENERAL REVIEW QUESTIONS

14. List the five stages of care provided within the EMS system, from a patient's perspective.

(a)

(b)

(c)

(d)

(e)

15. Discuss the findings and significance of the "White Paper" in terms of the development of EMS.

16. The National Highway Traffic Safety Administration (NHTSA) is responsible for:

17. List the 15 components of an effective EMS system.

For each of the following statements (18–22), circle the correct response, True or False. Briefly explain your answer.

18. Funding mechanisms in EMS are limited to general tax revenues and direct payment by the patient.

TRUE   **FALSE**

Briefly explain your answer: _____

19. EMS activities (e.g., certification/licensure of personnel and vehicles, facility designation) are governed by state law.

TRUE   **FALSE**

Briefly explain your answer: _____

20. In many states, ambulances must conform to federal department of transportation (DOT) standards for ambulance construction.

TRUE   **FALSE**

Briefly explain your answer: _____

21. COBRA requires that an emergency facility that is transferring a patient must accurately document and communicate the need for transfer to the receiving facility.

TRUE   **FALSE**

Briefly explain your answer: _____

_____

22. A paramedic who is nationally registered (NREMT-P) is automatically guaranteed reciprocity to practice in other states.

TRUE   **FALSE**

Briefly explain your answer: _____

_____

23. Briefly discuss the importance of a systems approach to EMS.

24. What is REMSO?

25. System coordination and organization at the state level are most often led by: _____.

26. Certification or licensure of EMS personnel is required in all states. This is usually regulated by the:
    a. hospital that provides on-line medical direction.
    b. local EMS division chief executive officers (CEOs).
    c. national registry for EMTs and paramedics.
    d. state health department or EMS office.

27. What are the five elements that should be considered and coordinated within an EMS during system planning?

28. Briefly describe the following four components of EMS communications:

System access: _____

_____

Dispatch centers: _____

_____

Trained dispatchers: _____
_____

Dispatch and medical communications systems: _____
_____

29. Describe the role of research in EMS.

Answers to questions from chapter 1 can be found on page 402.

Chapter 2

Roles and Responsibilities

OBJECTIVES

1. Apply the principles of the EMT Code of Ethics to specific patient care situations.
2. Discuss the impact of the White Paper on EMS.
3. Describe the differences among the education and training of an EMT-Basic, EMT-Intermediate, and EMT-Paramedic.
4. List eight major functions of the paramedic and the tasks associated with each function.
5. Describe the benefits of continuing education.
6. Identify three national EMS organizations that promote the advancement of prehospital emergency care.
7. Define the terms *certification, licensure,* and *reciprocity.*
8. State the major purpose of a national registry agency in EMS.

CASE PRESENTATION #1

You are dispatched to the scene of an accident [collision] involving a pedestrian who was struck by a motorcycle. Upon arrival, you learn that the pedestrian is a crying 5-year-old boy with a possible upper extremity fracture. The 26-year-old driver appears dazed and confused with only minor abrasions to his forehead. Police on the scene inform you that the driver is legally intoxicated and was not wearing a helmet.

1. Identify your responsibility to these patients according to the EMT Code of Ethics.
    a. You are not responsible for caring for the cyclist. Because he is legally intoxicated, his care is the responsibility of the police.
    b. You are not responsible for caring for the cyclist because he is not seriously injured.
    c. You are responsible for caring for both the cyclist and the young child because they both have sustained injuries.
    d. You are responsible only for care of the young child because he was an innocent pedestrian who was struck by an intoxicated cyclist.
    e. None of the above is correct.

Case Presentation #2

You are dispatched to evaluate the condition of an injured person at a homeless shelter. The patient is a 60-year-old woman who fell earlier in the day and is now complaining of mild discomfort to her hip when she walks. She is an illegal alien and has no means of paying for your services.

2. Briefly describe your responsibility to this patient, according to the EMT Code of Ethics.
   a. You are not responsible for this patient's care because the patient's injury is not life-threatening and she is unable to pay for the services provided by your system.
   b. You are responsible for the patient's care regardless of her circumstances.
   c. You are not responsible for her care. She has no means of paying for the services; therefore, the shelter is responsible for her care.
   d. You are not responsible for her care because she is an illegal alien and, therefore, is not entitled to health care services.
   e. None of the above is correct.

General Review Questions

Match the description in Column 1 with the appropriate level of licensure in Column 2.

Column 1

3. ____ Trained to perform select advanced skills according to local protocols
4. ____ Trained to perform noninvasive procedures
5. ____ Trained to perform invasive procedures and to administer medications (extensive list)

Column 2

a. EMT-Basic
b. EMT-Intermediate
c. EMT-Paramedic

Match the task listed in Column 1 with the corresponding category of paramedic function in Column 2. Some tasks may fall into more than one category of function.

Column 1

6. ____ Assessing the scene
7. ____ Transferring patients
8. ____ Writing prehospital care reports
9. ____ Reading professional journals
10. ____ Attending professional conferences
11. ____ Talking with patients, peers, and physicians
12. ____ Coordinating patient care with other EMS personnel on the scene
13. ____ Considering possible on-scene problems and needs
14. ____ Learning medical protocols
15. ____ Assessing the patient's condition
16. ____ Immobilizing the trauma patient

Column 2

a. Preparation
b. Activation
c. Evaluation
d. Stabilization
e. Communication
f. Transportation
g. Documentation
h. Education

17. After making the decision to transport a trauma patient, the paramedic should perform what procedures?

18. Briefly describe the impact of the White Paper on the EMS system.

19. Identify three national EMS organizations.

    (a)

    (b)

    (c)

20. State the major purpose of a national registry agency in EMS.

Match the term in Column 1 with its correct definition in Column 2.

	Column 1	**Column 2**
21. ____	Certification	a. Means by which patient care can be provided under the supervision and license of a physician
22. ____	Licensure	b. Granting of licensure or certification for comparable licensure or certification by another agency
23. ____	Reciprocity	c. Recognition that an individual has met predetermined standards
		d. Granting of permission to engage in a profession or occupation

24. Identify two benefits of continuing education.

    (a)

    (b)

Answers to questions from chapter 2 can be found on page 404.

Chapter 3

The EMS Call

OBJECTIVES

1. Describe the role of the public in the EMS system.
2. Describe the main functions of dispatch.
3. Identify vital information needed from dispatch in order to prepare for patient care.
4. Identify the key factors that should be assessed when evaluating the scene.
5. Given a set of patient situations, identify appropriate transport decisions.
6. Describe the appropriate transfer of responsibility for patient care in the receiving emergency department.
7. Describe prerun and postrun activities.

CASE PRESENTATION #1 (QUESTIONS 1–7)

You receive a call about a possible heart attack victim in a residential neighborhood. The dispatcher informs you that the only information she was able to obtain from the hysterical caller is that the patient is unconscious, not breathing, and has no pulse. Repeated efforts by dispatch to reestablish contact with the caller have been unsuccessful.

1. Based on the information that dispatch was able to obtain from the caller, what is the appropriate level of EMS response that should be sent to provide appropriate care for this patient?

2. If the dispatcher had been able to reestablish contact with the caller, what lifesaving instructions could have been given to improve this patient's outcome?

3. List six aspects of care that you should consider while en route to the scene so that you will be prepared for this patient and situation.

   (a)

   (b)

   (c)

   (d)

   (e)

   (f)

You and your partner arrive at the scene approximately two minutes after the First Responders. You find them performing CPR on the patient on the front lawn, where she was found. The patient's daughter meets you screaming, "My mother is dying, do something!"

4. Who should control the scene now? Explain why.

5. In dealing with this patient's daughter, you should:
   a. be aggressive in telling her to calm down because her behavior is interfering with her mother's care.
   b. call for police assistance so that she can be arrested.
   c. remember that the daughter is under tremendous stress and must be dealt with gently.
   d. tell her to wait in the cab of the ambulance until she is told otherwise by emergency personnel.

Despite treatment delivered at the scene, the patient's condition remains unchanged. On the basis of your protocols and in conjunction with medical direction, you begin a transport with lights and sirens to the hospital of approximately 10 minutes. You arrive at the emergency department (ED), where you transfer care of the patient to the nurses and physician.

6. Which of the following would *not* be an accepted part of a typical patient transfer process?
   a. You provide written and verbal reports of the patient's condition to the admitting clerk.
   b. You provide an opportunity for the nurse or physician to further question you about the patient's condition.
   c. You remain at the hospital until the physician has performed an initial assessment of the patient's condition, if you are not needed on another call.
   d. You turn over all patient valuables and personal effects to the ED staff.

7. What additional postrun procedures should you follow after transfer of this patient is complete and before you begin your next call?

CASE PRESENTATION #2 (QUESTIONS 8-13)

You are dispatched to the scene of a possible natural gas leak in a warehouse. The dispatcher has no information regarding whether there are patients involved in the incident.

8. What additional support personnel should be sent by dispatch to the scene?

9. Should you begin searching for patients who may have been overcome by fumes, so that early assessment and treatment can be initiated? Why or why not?

On arrival, you determine that only one patient has been removed from the building and taken away from the hot zone. The patient is an unconscious 25-year-old woman who was overcome by gas fumes. She shows no signs of respiratory distress, and her vital signs are stable.

10. At what point should you initiate treatment for this patient?

11. In choosing a hospital destination for this patient, which of the following are important considerations?
    a. the capabilities of the receiving hospital
    b. the effect of the transport time on the patient's condition
    c. the ability of the patient to pay for hospital services
    d. a and b
    e. a, b, and c

Immediately after receiving a high concentration of oxygen, the patient begins to respond to verbal questioning. Her vital signs and overall condition are still stable at this time. She is requesting to go to a hospital that is approximately 10 minutes away.

12. Should you request a helicopter for transport of this patient? Why or why not?

13. Which of the following is not necessary in the postrun review of this patient call?
    a. discussing the review in an informal, nonthreatening manner
    b. discussing what was done well
    c. discussing what could be improved on
    d. listening to your partner's ideas
    e. taking extensive written notes

General Review Questions

14. Determine to which hospital (**X, Y,** or **Z**) each patient (**a** through **e**) should be transported. Indicate by filling in the appropriate letter. Distance to the hospital is not a consideration.

    X. Hospital X is a 900-bed hospital affiliated with the medical school. It is a Level I trauma center with a helipad on the roof. It is capable of providing comprehensive emergency and surgical care 24 hours a day.

    Y. Hospital Y is a 100-bed hospital with 24-hour physician coverage only in the ED and coronary care unit. X-ray and laboratory facilities also operate 24 hours a day. Personnel can be activated at all times for special cardiac procedures.

    Z. Hospital Z is a 50-bed hospital with no coronary care unit. The ED is staffed 24 hours a day with physician assistants who can call staff physicians as needed for consults. X-ray and laboratory facilities are open from 7 a.m. to 7 p.m. Technicians are on call after 7 p.m.; if needed, they are available within 10 minutes response time.

    a. _____ A 21-year-old man with second- and third-degree burns over 40% of his body resulting from a house fire

    b. _____ A 30-year-old woman who is complaining of abdominal pain after being involved in a motor vehicle collision

    c. _____ A 16-month-old boy who has had an earache for 2 days

    d. _____ A 52-year-old patient who is complaining of acute onset of chest pain and nausea

    e. _____ A 13-year-old patient who needs a tetanus booster after sustaining a superficial laceration

15. List the main functions of emergency dispatch.

16. Identify the two areas of public education in which EMS should be involved to maximize prehospital patient care.

    (a)

    (b)

17. What information is not vital to obtain from those telephoning for emergency medical assistance?
    a. nature of the complaint
    b. location of the incident
    c. specific details of the complaint
    d. scene accessibility

18. The use of air transport is considered when which of the following would be of benefit to the patient?
    a. faster access to poorly accessible or remote areas
    b. faster transport to an appropriate facility
    c. higher level of care at a distant facility
    d. a and b
    e. a, b, and c

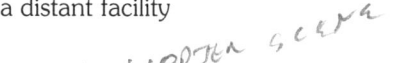
SEE HELICOPTER SCENE RESPONSE

19. Identify five key items that should be assessed during evaluation of the scene.

(a)

(b)

(c)

(d)

(e)

Answers to questions from chapter 3 can be found on page 405.

Chapter 4

Medical Accountability

OBJECTIVES

1. Describe the concept of delegated practice.
2. Describe the off-line and on-line responsibilities of a physician EMS medical director.
3. Compare and contrast prospective, concurrent, and retrospective medical direction.
4. Discuss the role of medical direction in prehospital education, evaluation, policy and protocol development, and operational issues.
5. Define the term *protocol* and identify appropriate areas to consider in the development of medical protocols.
6. Explain why hospital categorization (designation) and destination policies are important to an EMS system.
7. Discuss the role of the quality assurance and quality improvement processes in the EMS system.
8. Describe the role of field EMS providers in EMS research.

CASE PRESENTATION #1 (QUESTIONS 1–4)   *GOOD*

You are dispatched to the scene of a motor vehicle collision. While you are en route, dispatch informs you that five vehicles are involved and that two other ambulances have also been dispatched. Your unit is the last to arrive. As you approach the scene, a traffic officer directs you to a patient who has been ejected from the vehicle and is unconscious. Because your EMS system handles a high volume of trauma cases, you have been trained extensively in trauma care and you have received certification in Basic Trauma Life Support. You recently attended a recertification class. You quickly review your system's protocols as you approach the patient.

1. The medical director of your EMS system is actively involved in both managing the system and directing personnel. Identify at least two activities in this case presentation that illustrate prospective medical direction.

    (a)

    (b)

Your assessment of the patient reveals a possible closed head injury, rib fractures with absent breath sounds on the right, and bilateral fractured femurs. The patient's vital signs include the following: BP 210/100; pulse 50; respirations 4 and shallow. After assessing the patient's airway, you decide to intubate, which is part of the standing orders in your trauma protocol.

2. Standing orders in medical protocols are:
   a. followed only when medical direction cannot be contacted.
   b. decided on a case-by-case basis by the ALS provider after arrival on the scene.
   c. established for the system by the EMS medical director.
   d. utilized only in large urban EMS systems.

You further stabilize your patient and prepare for transport. Your protocol states that you should contact on-line medical direction for destination advice. On contacting on-line medical direction, you are told which trauma facility is available and you are prepared for transport of the patient to that destination.

3. How does this illustrate prospective medical direction?

4. Medical protocols form the backbone of care rendered by the EMS provider; they require multiple sources of input to be effective. Briefly discuss this concept as it relates to this case presentation.

CASE PRESENTATION #2 (QUESTIONS 5-7)

You are dispatched to a private residence to help a patient who is experiencing breathing difficulty. On arrival at the scene, you find a 68-year-old man sitting at the breakfast table. He is conscious and alert, but in obvious respiratory distress. Medical history reveals that he is a long-time smoker with chronic shortness of breath. His vital signs are as follows: BP 170/100; pulse 130; respirations 40 and labored. His skin is pale, and you note significant swelling in his ankles and lower legs. The patient has a history of chronic obstructive pulmonary disease (COPD), and you assume this to be the cause of his deteriorating condition. You contact on-line medical direction to report your findings; you advise that you are administering low-concentration oxygen. While en route to the hospital, the patient's respiratory distress worsens; however, the patient is conscious when you arrive at the emergency department.

5. In the ED, the patient is given medication for his pulmonary edema, which has occurred secondary to heart failure. What assessment could you have performed while the patient was in your care that might have pointed to this condition and indicated the need for different treatment?
   a. breath sounds
   b. capillary refill
   c. size and reaction of pupils
   d. strength of extremities

The medical director calls you during your next shift to inform you that this patient was admitted with acute pulmonary edema, secondary to congestive heart failure (CHF). While discussing the case, you realize that your assessment was incomplete; you are appreciative of the feedback and follow-up information that were provided to you concerning this patient.

6. How does this situation illustrate principles of medical accountability?

The medical director has discovered three similar cases in which there were incomplete assessments of patients with congestive heart failure. He has contacted the coordinator of paramedic continuing education to discuss methods of reviewing, in an upcoming class, appropriate assessment procedures to be followed in the treatment of patients with congestive heart failure.

7. This is an example of: prospective, retrospective, or both types of medical direction. (Circle your answer.) Explain your response.

GENERAL REVIEW QUESTIONS

8. Paramedics are given authority to provide patient care under the legal concept of:
   a. delegated practice.
   b. Good Samaritan law.
   c. medical extension.
   d. paramedic independent practice.

9. While you are answering a call to assist a patient with a possible heart attack, the EMS medical director arrives on the scene to assist you in patient care and to accompany you to the hospital. This is an example of which type of medical direction?
   a. concurrent
   b. on-line
   c. prospective
   d. retrospective
   e. both a and b

10. Who bears the ultimate responsibility for patient care?
   a. the EMS administrator
   b. the hospital administrator
   c. the EMS medical director
   d. prehospital care personnel

11. Destination policies are important to the function of an EMS because they:
   a. allow the prehospital provider to make independent transport decisions.
   b. allow hospitals to dictate the location to which patients should be transported.
   c. assist in providing guaranteed revenue for the EMS.
   d. equally distribute patient load among area medical facilities.

Match the definition in Column 1 with its correct term in Column 2.

Column 1

12. ____ A written procedure used by prehospital providers for treating and/or evaluating a clinical condition

13. ____ Review of medical care at the time it is rendered

14. ____ Direct voice communication between a field unit team and a physician or designee for the purpose of providing appropriate medical care to an emergency patient

15. ____ The medical oversight of EMS patient care that occurs before and after patient care

Column 2

a. Concurrent medical direction
b. Off-line medical direction
c. On-line medical direction
d. Protocol
e. Good Samaritan law

16. Medical direction is best defined as a system of physicians who:
    a. have minimal standing orders and strict protocols.
    b. review run reports monthly and oversee the dispatch center.
    c. provide at least three people for leadership to local EMS providers and the system.
    d. provide quality assurance that ensures professional and public accountability for medical care in the prehospital setting.

17. Medical directors should be involved in the development of both _____ protocols and _____ policies.

18. The overall goal of quality improvement is to:
    a. collect data for the EMS.
    b. evaluate the performance of prehospital personnel.
    c. identify personnel who consistently make errors.
    d. improve the quality of patient care.

19. Briefly describe the importance of research for the effective function of an EMS system; include a discussion of the paramedic's role in the research process.

Answers to questions from chapter 4 can be found on page 406.

Chapter 5

Legal Accountability

OBJECTIVES

1. Describe the basic structure of the legal system in the United States.
2. Define negligence and recognize the four elements that must be proved in order to recover damages.
3. Explain *standard of care* as it pertains to prehospital care.
4. Identify statutory provisions pertinent to the paramedic.
5. Describe the paramedic's responsibilities in using and protecting a patient's medical information.
6. Differentiate among express consent, implied consent, and involuntary consent.
7. Define abandonment as it relates to prehospital care.
8. Identify legal issues in the nontransport patient encounter.
9. Explain the principles of use of force and use of restraints.
10. Identify factors affecting resuscitation decisions in the prehospital setting.
11. Describe the paramedic's professional responsibilities related to preservation of evidence at a crime or accident scene.

CASE PRESENTATION #1 (QUESTIONS 1–6)

You are dispatched to a private residence for treatment of a pediatric patient. The caller claims the child is crying for no apparent reason. On arrival, you are met by an anxious teenaged girl. She called for an ambulance because the 2-year-old she is babysitting "won't stop crying" and she is not sure why. As you approach the patient in his crib, you note that he appears to be in severe pain.

1. Your primary concern as you prepare to examine this patient is to:
   a. relieve his pain.
   b. decrease his emotional stress.
   c. identify any life-threatening conditions.
   d. confirm any suspicions of child abuse.

2. The patient's ABCs are intact. When performing your assessment, you should apply which of the following principles?
   a. Explain each procedure thoroughly.
   b. Do not separate him from the babysitter.
   c. Examine any injuries or painful areas first.
   d. Conduct a detailed physical examination from toe to head.

Your physical assessment reveals an edematous, deformed elbow and bruises to the child's lower extremities. You become suspicious when the babysitter tells you that she now remembers the patient falling from his crib earlier. The child's vital signs are: BP 86 palpable; pulse 140; respirations 30. The babysitter tells you that she has been unable to locate the parents and that they are not expected to return for several hours. As you splint the patient's elbow and prepare to transport, your partner expresses some reservations about treating a minor without parental consent.

3. You are operating under which of the following general principles of consent?
    a. Good Samaritan
    b. involuntary consent
    c. implied consent
    d. guardian consent

While en route to the hospital, the patient becomes increasingly irritable and attempts several times to remove his elbow splint. His overall condition is unchanged on arrival at the emergency department. You turn the patient over to the hospital staff and prepare for your next call.

4. Would it have been appropriate to restrain the patient from removing his elbow splint? Why, or why not?

5. Are you obligated to report your suspicions of child abuse to the hospital staff? Why, or why not?

As you are walking back to your ambulance, you run into a friend in the parking lot. During your conversation, you mention that you have just transported a victim of child abuse to the emergency department.

6. Was it appropriate for you to share this information with your friend? Why, or why not?

CASE PRESENTATION #2 (QUESTIONS 7-13)

You are dispatched to a motor vehicle collision involving a truck that collided head-on into a light pole in icy road conditions. The condition of the single patient is unknown at this time. On arrival at the scene, you discover that the driver of the vehicle is sitting on the side of the road and appears to be in no acute distress. As you approach him for questioning, you note that he has facial abrasions and a hematoma to his forehead. He quickly tells you that he is not injured and does not want to go to the hospital.

7. Does this patient have the right to refuse treatment? Why, or why not?

8. If you attempt to transport this patient against his will, he could charge you with:
   a. battery.
   b. false imprisonment.
   c. tort.
   d. a and b

9. You advise the patient of the risks and consequences of refusing treatment. This is known as:
   a. abandonment.
   b. informed consent.
   c. informed refusal.
   d. probable cause.

10. List two additional actions that you should take before terminating the patient encounter.

   (a)

   (b)

You perform a physical examination, which reveals bruising to the chest and abdomen. Breath sounds are clear, and the abdomen is soft and nontender. The patient displays no sensory or motor deficits. Pupils are equal and reactive. Skin is dry with normal capillary refill. Vital signs include: BP 110/60; pulse 112 and regular; respirations 20. As you are documenting your observations while still on the scene, the patient begins to experience back and neck pain and decides he will go with you after all.

11. Refusing to transport the patient now could be considered:
   a. informed refusal.
   b. abandonment.
   c. probable cause.
   d. stare decisis.

Before transporting this patient, you apply a cervical collar, administer oxygen, initiate a precautionary intravenous (IV) solution, and connect him to the electrocardiogram (ECG) monitor, which indicates sinus tachycardia. The patient's condition remains unchanged en route to the hospital. When you arrive in the ED, the nurses criticize you for not immobilizing the patient properly.

12. The accepting physician informs you and your partner that this improper immobilization could be grounds for negligence. Explain why, and list four elements required to prove negligence.

   (a)

   (b)

   (c)

   (d)

13. Did you comply with the standard of care in immobilizing this patient? Why, or why not?

GENERAL REVIEW QUESTIONS

Match the legal concept in column 1 with its appropriate description in column 2.

Column 1

14. _____ Criminal law
15. _____ Civil law
16. _____ Administrative law
17. _____ Good Samaritan
18. _____ Common law

Column 2

a. A private law between two persons or parties
b. Conduct or offenses that have been classified legally as "public wrongs" or crimes "against the state"
c. Statutes of immunity
d. The government's authority to enforce rules, regulations, and pertinent statutes of governmental agencies
e. If allowed, it relieves governmental employees from liability for certain types of negligent acts
f. Law derived from the evolution of society's acceptance of customs or norms

Fill in the blanks with the type of consent under which you would be operating in each of the following patient situations.

19. _____ A 21-year-old woman is unconscious after having had a seizure in a restaurant.

20. _____ A 35-year-old man is arrested after an accident for driving without a driver's license. He has a laceration to his wrist that requires sutures, but he refuses to cooperate with you.

21. _____ A 55-year-old man calls you to take him to the hospital because he has severe chest pain.

22. _____ A 5-year-old girl is unconscious after having struck her head on playground equipment. The child's parents are unavailable.

23. Circle the letter in front of each patient situation in which it would be inappropriate to withhold resuscitation efforts, according to the American Heart Association guidelines.
   a. A middle-aged homeless man is found in an alley with no vital signs; dependent lividity and rigor mortis are evident.
   b. A 16-year-old youth has been decapitated in a motor vehicle collision.
   c. A 58-year-old woman has a history of cancer, and a neighbor finds her at home in cardiac arrest.

24. Most states have statutes that mandate reporting what five types of patient cases?

(a)

(b)

(c)

(d)

(e)

25. List four questions that you should ask yourself when considering the appropriateness of restraints.

(a)

(b)

(c)

(d)

26. Provide three simple guidelines that are important for you to follow when preserving evidence at a crime scene.

(a)

(b)

(c)

27. What should be the basis of a paramedic's decision to withhold or stop resuscitation procedures?

Answers to questions from chapter 5 can be found on page 407.

Section 2

Foundations for Practice

CHAPTERS

6. Medical Terminology
7. Basic Body Systems
8. Principles of Pathophysiology
9. Shock
10. Infection Control
11. General Pharmacology
11a. Appendix: Prehospital Medications
12. Basic Rhythm Interpretation
13. Interpersonal Communications Skills
14. Communication and Documentation

Chapter 6

Medical Terminology

OBJECTIVES

1. Identify and define commonly used prefixes, root words, suffixes, and abbreviations.
2. Describe standard anatomic position.
3. Identify the imaginary planes and lines of the body and the relationships of body structures to these lines.
4. Describe anatomic relationships in the extremities.
5. Describe the various positions of the body at rest.
6. Describe movements of the body and extremities.
7. Recognize and use common terminology related to specific body systems and their diseases.

GENERAL REVIEW QUESTIONS

Match the term in Column 1 that refers to direction and position with its correct definition in Column 2.

Column 1

1. _____ Proximal
2. _____ Distal
3. _____ Supine
4. _____ Prone
5. _____ Lateral recumbent
6. _____ Semi-Fowler's
7. _____ Trendelenburg

Column 2

a. Lying supine with the head elevated
b. Away from the trunk
c. Lying face up
d. Lying on either the right or the left side
e. Nearer to the trunk
f. Lying face down
g. Lying supine with the head lower than the trunk
h. Lying supine with the legs elevated thirty degrees

Label Figure 6-1, which refers to movement, by filling in the blank next to each label with the corresponding letter in the drawing.

8. _____ Pronation
9. _____ Adduction
10. _____ Extension
11. _____ Supination
12. _____ Flexion
13. _____ Abduction

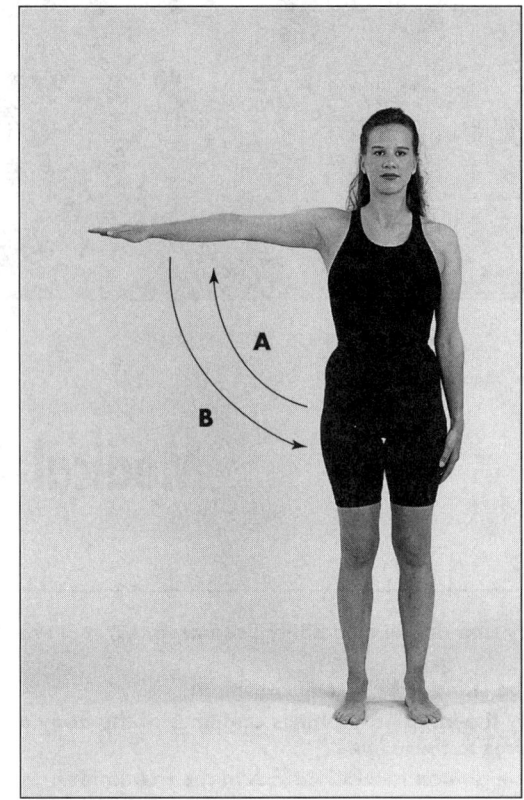

Figure 6-1

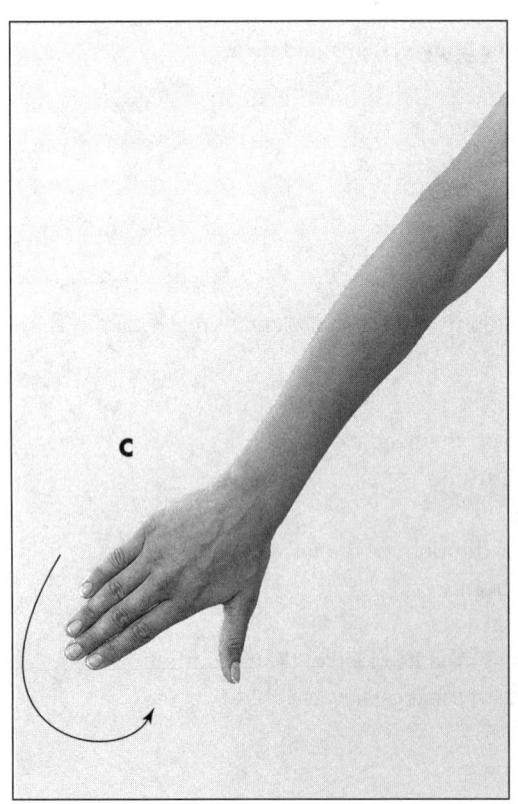

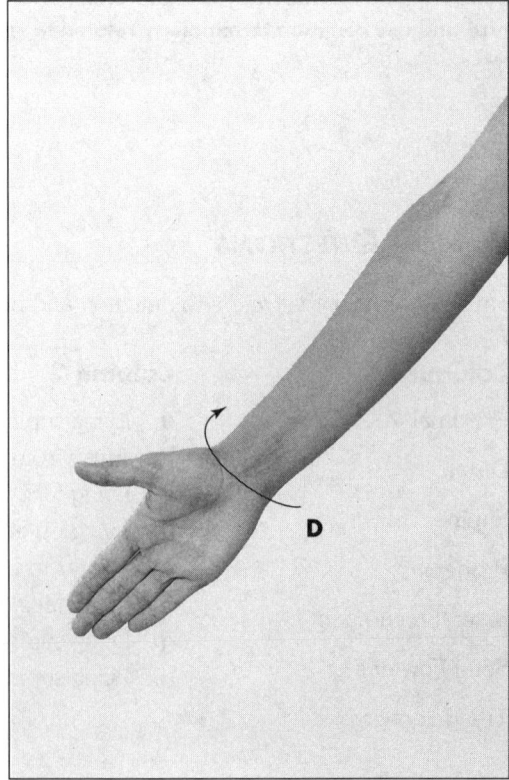

Figure 6-1 *(continued)*

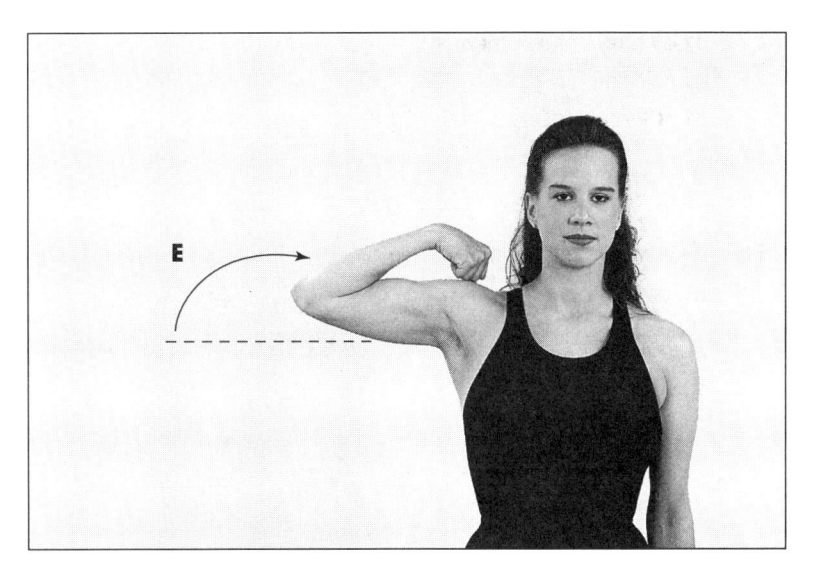

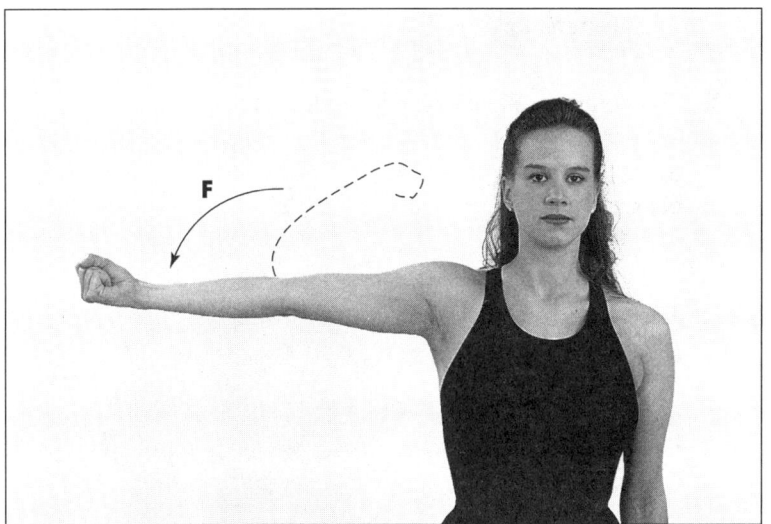

14. The prefix "dys" means:
    a. against or opposed to.
    b. difficult or painful.
    c. inside or within.
    d. slow or sluggish.

15. The prefix "hypo" means:
    a. above or excessive.
    b. below or deficient.
    c. many or too much.
    d. without or none.

16. The prefix "supra" means:
    a. fast.
    b. behind.
    c. above.
    d. around.

17. The suffix "emia" means:
    a. blood.
    b. pain.
    c. state.
    d. too much.

18. The suffix "genic" means:
    a. surgical removal.
    b. causing or denoting origin.
    c. excessive flow.
    d. through.

19. The suffix "itis" means:
    a. pain.
    b. paralysis.
    c. condition.
    d. inflammation.

20. The common abbreviation for history is:
    a. HR.
    b. HTN.
    c. h.
    d. Hx.

21. The common abbreviation for immediately is:
    a. SVT.
    b. STAT.
    c. tach.
    d. IM.

22. The common abbreviation PRN means:
    a. as needed.
    b. every day.
    c. every hour.
    d. twice a day.

Match each word in Column 1 with its correct definition in Column 2.

Column 1

23. _____ Tachycardia (tachy + cardi)
24. _____ Dyspnea (dys + pnea)
25. _____ Dysuria (dys + uri)
26. _____ Hemorrhage (hemo + rrhage)
27. _____ Hemiplegia (hemi + plegia)

Column 2

a. Excessive flow of blood
b. Fast heart rate
c. Paralysis in one half of the body
d. Difficulty breathing
e. Difficult or painful urination

Name the disease process indicated by each abbreviation.

28. AMI _____

29. CA _____

30. CHF _____

31. COPD _____

32. CVA _____

33. DM _____

34. HTN _____

35. TIA _____

36. TB _____

Fill in the blanks with the common abbreviations for each of the following terms.

37. ethyl alcohol _____

38. drops _____

39. fracture _____

40. at bedtime _____

41. intracranial pressure _____

42. laceration _____

43. obstetric _____

44. after _____

45. unconscious _____

46. Rewrite the following paragraph using as many accepted medical abbreviations as possible.

    You are dispatched to a private residence to care for an elderly woman who passed out prior to your arrival. On physical examination, she is awake, alert, and oriented to person, place, and time. Her chief complaint is bilateral hip pain, although she can move all extremities with ease. Her pupils are equal and reactive to light; vital signs are within normal limits, except for a blood pressure reading of 200/110. She has a history of hypertension, but takes no medications. In addition to providing spinal stabilization, you administer the following treatment procedures before transport to the emergency department by mobile intensive care unit: oxygen at 4 liters per minute with a nasal cannula; electrocardiogram monitoring; intravenous line with normal saline solution at a to-keep-open rate.

47. Rewrite the following paragraph using the appropriate medical terminology for the boldface words or phrases.

You are dispatched to a park to evaluate a 52-year-old man who is having **difficulty breathing** after having been stung by a bee. He also complains of **difficulty swallowing** and that his **throat is closing off**. You note that the patient has a **bluish discoloration around the mouth** and a **fast heart rate**. His medical history includes **surgical removal of tonsils** and a heart problem for which he takes **a drug that prevents disturbances in cardiac rhythm**. After receiving treatment for an allergic reaction, the patient is **without symptoms**.

_____
_____
_____
_____
_____
_____
_____
_____
_____
_____

48. Refer to Figure 6-2 on the following page to answer the following questions below.
  a. Describe the position of the wound at point A.

  b. Describe the position of the wound at point B.

  c. Describe the position of the wound at point C.

  d. Mark an "X" on the diagram corresponding to a point that is about 2 finger breadths inferior and 2 finger breadths lateral to the umbilicus on the right.

  e. Mark a "Y" on the diagram corresponding to a point on the anterolateral surface of the distal left thigh.

  f. Mark a "Z" on the diagram corresponding to a point on the medial aspect of the right leg that is 2 fingerbreadths inferior to the knee.

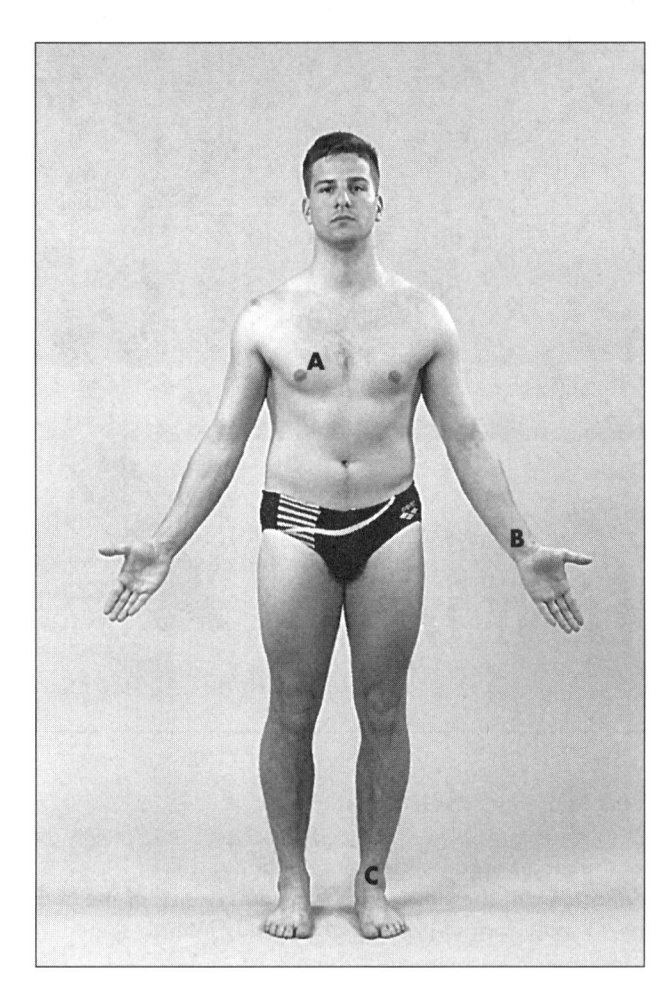

Figure 6-2

Answers to questions from chapter 6 can be found on page 408.

Chapter 7

Basic Body Systems

OBJECTIVES

1. List the four major tissue types.
2. Describe the unique characteristics of each of the four major tissue types.
3. List the 11 major organ systems of the body.
4. Identify the key anatomic structures in each of the major organ systems of the body.
5. Describe the functions of the major anatomic structures of the eleven major organ systems of the body.
6. Describe how major anatomic structures of the 11 major organ systems of the body interact to perform the specified functions of the system.

CASE PRESENTATION #1 (QUESTIONS 1-8)

You are dispatched to a park to care for a patient who is experiencing severe dyspnea. On arrival, you find a teenaged boy who is obviously struggling to breathe. His friend tells you that the patient is having an asthma attack and does not have his medication with him. As you expose the patient's chest to auscultate breath sounds, you note retractions of the muscles between his ribs and at his neck. His wheezing is worse when he exhales. As you administer a high concentration of oxygen with a nonrebreather mask, your partner measures his vital signs, which are: BP 128/88; pulse 112 and bounding; respirations 26 and labored.

1. Would you expect this patient's hemoglobin to have a high or low saturation of oxygen? Explain your response.

2. Given this patient's condition, is his expiration primarily an active or passive process? Explain your response.

3. Which accessory respiratory muscles are being used in an attempt to increase the inflow of air to this patient's lungs? List an assessment finding to support your answer.

4. Which nervous system has been activated to assist this patient in compensating for his condition? List an assessment finding to support your answer.

5. Without adequate oxygen at this patient's tissue level, energy may be obtained from what type of metabolism? Is this efficient or inefficient? Explain your response.

You establish an IV and contact medical direction. After hearing your report, the physician orders you to administer epinephrine 0.3 mg subcutaneously to your patient. Within minutes of administration of this drug, the patient's breathing improves. On reassessment, his wheezing and muscle retractions are almost completely gone. His vital signs are now: BP 122/80; pulse 112; respirations 18 and of normal quality. The patient remains stable while en route to the hospital, and he has no signs or symptoms of respiratory distress upon arrival to the emergency department.

6. Explain how epinephrine improved this patient's breathing.

7. Was the response that was created by the epinephrine an adrenergic or a cholinergic one?

8. Why is this patient's pulse rate still slightly elevated?

Case Presentation #2 (Questions 9–11)

You are dispatched to a construction site where a worker has fallen approximately 20 feet. On arrival, you find an unconscious 25-year-old man lying face down on the ground. He has a pulse and respirations.

9. Should you exercise any precautions when turning this patient? Explain your response.

The patient is turned, and spinal immobilization is accomplished. Your crew continues to prepare him for transport. They administer oxygen with a nonrebreather mask and establish an IV while you and your partner assess for any life-threatening injuries. The patient's vital signs are: BP 160/90; pulse 60; respirations 16 and uncompromised. You note a large hematoma to his forehead and clear fluid leaking from the patient's nose.

10. Is it significant that clear fluid is leaking from the patient's nose? Explain your response.

No additional injuries are found, and the patient appears stable at this time. While you are en route to the hospital, your partner tells you that the patient moved his leg slightly when his knee was accidentally tapped by the stretcher restraint buckle. Therefore, the patient cannot possibly have a spinal cord injury.

11. Is your partner's determination of a lack of spinal cord injury correct? Explain your response.

The patient is delivered to the emergency department with his condition unchanged.

CASE PRESENTATION #3 (QUESTIONS 12–16)

On a rainy day, you are dispatched to the scene of a motor vehicle collision involving a single automobile. While you are en route, dispatch informs you that the police are on the scene and report that the only patient is the driver, a 55-year-old man who is still in the driver's seat of the vehicle. The patient claims to have lost control of the vehicle on the wet pavement; he crashed into a sign pole at approximately 50 miles per hour.

12. Based on the information provided to you by dispatch, what can you conclude at this point about the scene and the patient?

As you approach the scene, you note significant damage to the front of the vehicle. The patient is alert but appears pale and anxious. He is complaining of severe pain in the right thigh, midway between the hip and knee, and mild discomfort to the anterior chest, which he attributes to the pressure of the seatbelt. He denies any respiratory difficulty or loss of consciousness.

13. Based on the patient's described location of pain, what bone structure in the lower extremity could be injured?

14. Based on the discomfort that he describes in his anterior chest and the mechanism of injury, what highly vascular internal organs could be injured?

Your partner quickly cuts the patient's shirt and trousers while you measure his vital signs. The patient has gross swelling of the right upper leg and slight bruising of the anterior chest over the right nipple area. No crepitus or obvious deformities are noted, and breath sounds are clear. Vital signs are: B/P 90/60; pulse 118 and regular; respirations 20 and unlabored. Treatment during and after extrication includes spinal immobilization with a pneumatic anti-shock garment (PASG) on the long board, oxygen administered via a nonrebreather mask, a 16-gauge IV tube with isotonic fluid, and application of a traction splint to the right leg. Upon arrival at the emergency department, the patient is in stable condition. In the emergency department, as part of this patient's management, the nurse inserts a catheter into the bladder to allow measurement of urine output.

15. Why is it important to measure this patient's urinary output?

16. With normal hydration and circulation, what would be a "normal" quantity of urine output for this patient?

General Review Questions

17. List the 11 major body systems.

    (a)

    (b)

    (c)

    (d)

    (e)

    (f)

    (g)

    (h)

    (i)

    (j)

    (k)

18. List the key structures of the:

    (a) central nervous system

    (b) peripheral nervous system

19. Complete the following sentences regarding the components of blood.

    Approximately 50% of the total blood volume is made up of a watery, colorless fluid known as (a)_____. (b)_____ are the most common blood cells. They transport (c)_____, an iron compound that carries oxygen from the lungs to the cells, and carbon dioxide from the cells to the lungs for removal. Lymphocytes, neutrophils, and macrophages are types of (d)_____; they represent the main line of defense against invading organisms. (e)_____, the body's smallest cells, aid in blood clot formation.

20. Describe the physical processes of inhalation and exhalation.

    (a) Inhalation:

    (b) Exhalation:

21. Describe the function of the lymphatic system.

22. Describe how hormones secreted by endocrine glands reach their target organs.

23. For each of the following hormones, list the primary target tissue and one action the hormone may have on that target site.

Hormone   **Target**   **Action**

   a. antidiuretic hormone

   b. oxytocin

   c. parathyroid

   d. epinephrine

   e. aldosterone

   f. insulin

   g. glucagon

24. Place in order the structures through which inspired air passes in the respiratory system.

   _____ **a.** bronchioles

   _____ **b.** trachea

   _____ **c.** larynx

   _____ **d.** alveoli

   _____ **e.** lungs

   _____ **f.** pharynx

   _____ **g.** bronchi

25. Place in order the structures through which ingested food passes in the digestive tract.

   _____ **a.** esophagus

   _____ **b.** large intestine

   _____ **c.** cardiac sphincter

   _____ **d.** small intestine

   _____ **e.** rectum

   _____ **f.** stomach

   _____ **g.** mouth

   _____ **h.** pyloric valve

Match each cranial nerve in Column 1 with the description of its function in Column 2.

Column 1

26. ____ Olfactory
27. ____ Optic
28. ____ Trigeminal
29. ____ Vestibulocochlear
30. ____ Vagus

Column 2

a. Hearing and balance
b. Sensory to face and teeth
c. Vision
d. Smell
e. Parasympathetic to viscera of thorax and abdomen
f. Motor to tongue muscles

Match each tissue type in Column 1 with the description of its function in Column 2.

Column 1

31. ____ Epithelial
32. ____ Muscle
33. ____ Connective
34. ____ Nervous

Column 2

a. Ability to tightly join together to form surfaces
b. Assists in regulating acid-base balance
c. Functions primarily to protect, connect, and support
d. Characterized by its contractile abilities
e. Responsible for message formation and transmission

35. The only organs that are completely encased in bone for protection are the:
    a. liver and spleen.
    b. kidneys and spleen.
    c. brain and spinal cord.
    d. heart and lungs.

36. Exchange of oxygen and carbon dioxide takes place within the:
    a. diaphragm.
    b. bronchioles.
    c. lymphocytes.
    d. alveoli.

37. Which of the following statements about the heart is true?
    a. The heart has its own electrical system.
    b. Heart sounds are produced by opening of the heart valves.
    c. The somatic nervous system helps to regulate heart rate.
    d. The right side is the heart's most heavily muscled side.

38. Which of the following systems assist in regulating the acid-base balance of the body?
    a. heart and urinary
    b. lymphatic and digestive
    c. integumentary and respiratory
    d. urinary and respiratory

39. Which of the following statements about the sympathetic nervous system is true?
    a. uses acetylcholine as a neurotransmitter
    b. creates a cholinergic response
    c. opposes an adrenergic response
    d. acts as a stress response division

40. Label the major structures of the central nervous system pictured in Figure 7-1 by filling in the blank next to the corresponding letter.

a. _____

b. _____

c. _____

d. _____

e. _____

f. _____

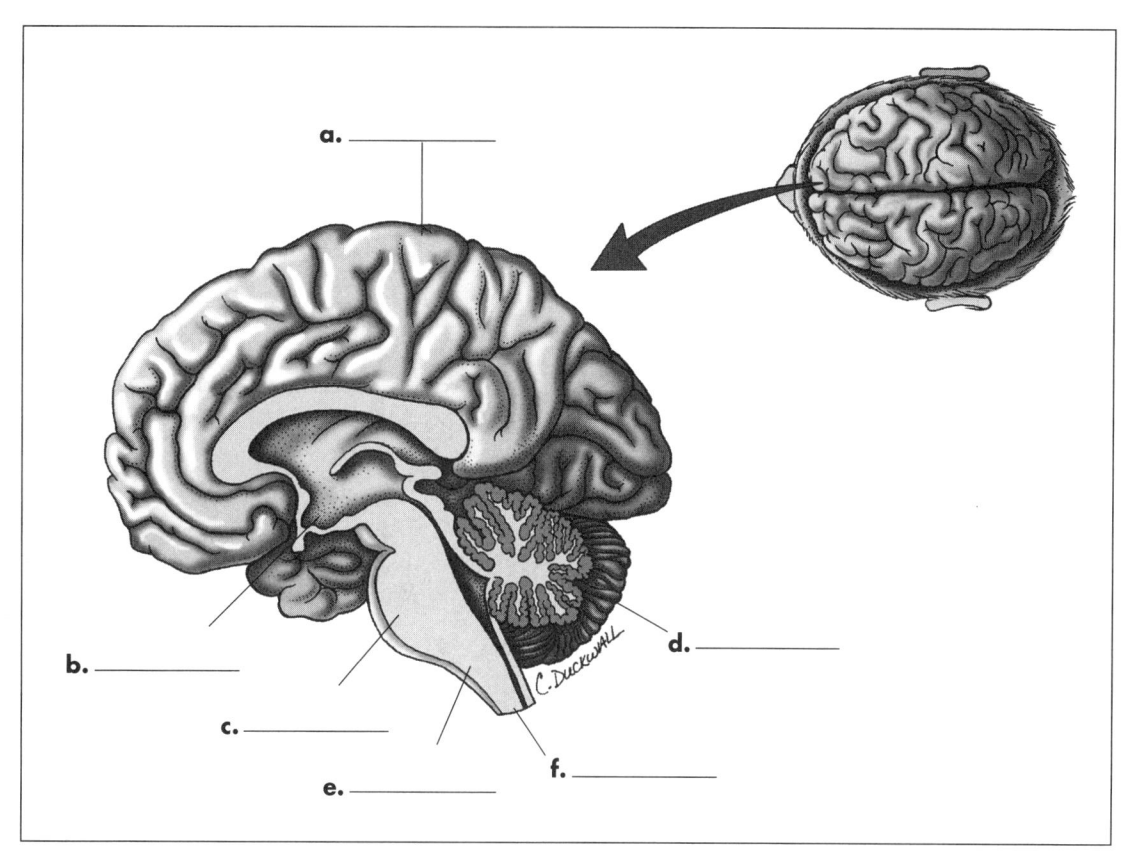

Figure 7-1 _____

41. Label the bones of the body identified in Figure 7-2 by filling in the blank next to the corresponding letter.

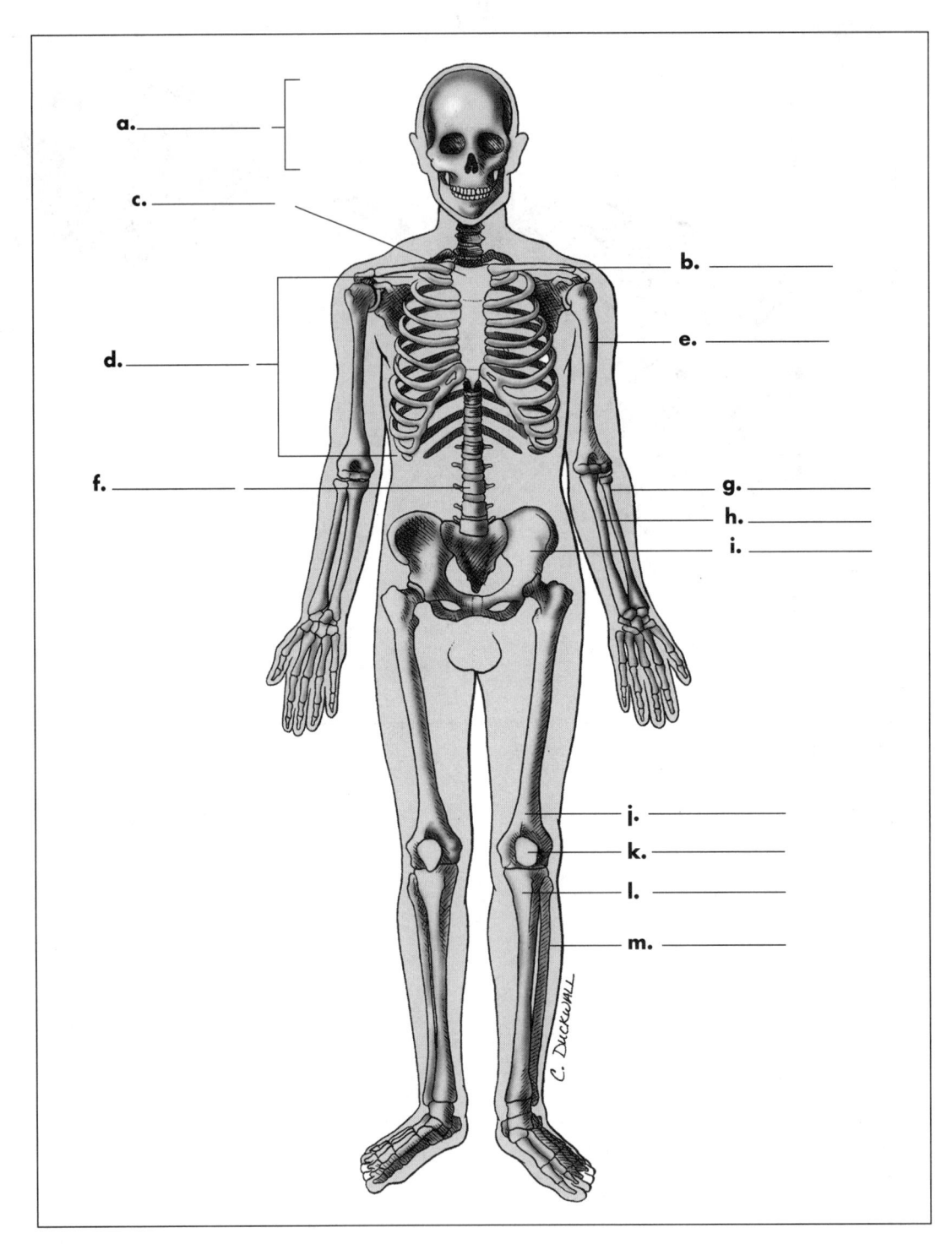

a. _____
b. _____
c. _____
d. _____
e. _____
f. _____
g. _____
h. _____
i. _____
j. _____
k. _____
l. _____
m. _____

Figure 7-2 _____

Answers to questions from chapter 7 can be found on page 410.

Chapter 8

Principles of Pathophysiology

OBJECTIVES

1. Explain the primary function of the following:
   a. Plasma
   b. Plasma proteins
   c. Electrolytes
   d. Red blood cells
   e. White blood cells
   f. Platelets
   g. Spleen
2. Describe five key functions of blood.
3. Define *hemoglobin* and *hematocrit,* and describe their relationship to red blood cells.
4. State the normal blood volume for the average adult patient.
5. Explain the purpose and function of the lymphatic system.
6. Identify the universal donor and recipient.
7. Discuss the significance of the Rh factor in terms of blood typing and pregnancy.
8. Identify the average percentage of total body water for an adult.
9. Describe the following terms in relationship to total body water:
   a. Intracellular
   b. Extracellular
   c. Interstitial
   d. Intravascular
10. Correlate body fluid composition to the conditions of dehydration and overhydration.
11. List signs and symptoms for dehydration and overhydration.
12. Define the major functions of the following electrolytes:
    a. Sodium
    b. Calcium
    c. Potassium
    d. Magnesium
13. Define the terms *osmosis* and *diffusion* and explain the role of each process in human fluid dynamics.
14. Define the following and describe their relationship to body fluid balance:
    a. Crystalloid
    b. Colloid
    c. Hypertonic
    d. Hypotonic
    e. Isotonic
15. Discuss the purpose of IV therapy in the prehospital setting.
16. Discuss the composition and rationale for use for the following IV fluids:
    a. 5% dextrose in water
    b. Ringer's lactate
    c. Normal saline
17. Define *normal body pH range, metabolism, acidosis,* and *alkalosis.*
18. Explain the importance of acid-base balance in the body.
19. Briefly describe the mechanism of action for the following acid-base compensatory mechanisms:
    a. Bicarbonate–carbonic acid
    b. Respiratory
    c. Kidney

(continues)

20. Identify the most important aspect of prehospital care that can positively affect acid-base imbalances.
21. Discuss the pathophysiology and the common causes of the following:
    a. Respiratory acidosis   c. Metabolic acidosis
    b. Respiratory alkalosis   d. Metabolic alkalosis
22. Describe the purpose and function of the autonomic nervous system.
23. Identify circumstances when the autonomic nervous system is activated.
24. Describe the two branches of the autonomic nervous system in terms of their specific effects and the target organs they mediate.
25. Describe the effects of the following receptor sites on the heart, veins, lungs, skin, and pupils:
    a. Alpha
    b. Beta 1
    c. Beta 2

CASE PRESENTATION #1 (QUESTIONS 1–8)

You are dispatched to an apartment complex for treatment of a patient for possible overdose. The patient is a 22-year-old man who is lying on the living room floor. His roommate tells you that the patient "shot up too much heroin" about 20 minutes ago. The patient is unconscious and responds minimally to physical stimuli.

1. After opening and checking his airway, your next assessment priority is to:
   a. check for pinpoint pupils.
   b. evaluate rate of respiration.
   c. obtain a palpated blood pressure reading.
   d. look for needle tracks.

Further information reveals that the patient has been a drug user for a couple of years; he has been hospitalized on three occasions. Vital signs are: BP 106/60; pulse 64 and regular; respirations 6 and shallow. You begin to assist ventilations.

2. With his clinical presentation, you suspect that the patient is most likely in:
   a. respiratory acidosis.
   b. respiratory alkalosis.
   c. metabolic acidosis.
   d. metabolic alkalosis.

3. Briefly explain the rationale for your answer to Question #2.

4. At this point in your assessment, would you suspect his pH to be low or high? Briefly explain your response.

5. Given this patient's acid-base derangement, which buffer system responds within minutes?

6. Which buffer system is the "back-up"? How long before it is effective?

7. In the prehospital setting, what is the most immediate and beneficial treatment measure you can provide to correct this acid-base abnormality?
   a. Assist his respirations.
   b. Administer sodium bicarbonate.
   c. Monitor his oxygen level with pulse oximetry.
   d. Rapidly administer IV fluids.

You deliver the patient safely to the emergency department in stable condition. Upon arrival, the patient's blood gases are drawn. You and your partner remain in the emergency department until the results of the arterial blood gases are available.

8. How could information from this test result be beneficial to you?

CASE PRESENTATION #2 (QUESTIONS 9–16)

You respond to a possible heart attack call. On arrival at the scene, you are met at the door by an anxious, middle-aged woman. She leads you to the dining room where her husband is seated at the table. He is conscious and alert and is complaining of substernal chest pain and breathing difficulty. His skin is pale and moist. Vital signs are: BP 152/60; pulse 110, rapid and weak; respirations 28 and shallow.

9. Your first assessment priority is to:
   a. administer oxygen.
   b. check for allergies.
   c. prepare him for transport.
   d. obtain a medical history.

As you further evaluate the patient, he denies any vomiting, diarrhea, or melena; no trauma is present. You suspect that he is having a heart attack.

10. In a time of stress, the body compensates by activating the _____ nervous system.

11. The nervous system in Answer #10 is divided into two branches: the sympathetic and the parasympathetic. Based on this patient's presentation, most likely, which branch has been stimulated? Explain your answer.

12. Given this patient's presentation (signs and symptoms) listed in Column 1, circle the appropriate receptor site(s) in Column 2 that is/are being stimulated.

    Column 1
    a. increased heart rate
    b. increased respiratory rate
    c. sweating
    d. increased blood pressure

    Column 2
    beta or alpha
    beta 1 or beta 2
    alpha or beta
    alpha, beta, or both

Medical history reveals that the patient has a history of heart problems and takes several medications, including potassium supplements.

13. Why was this supplement prescribed for the patient? Briefly explain the effect of potassium on the heart.

You contact medical direction and give your report. You start an IV and prepare the patient for transport.

14. Based on the information you have obtained, does this patient need fluid replacement? Why or why not?

15. What type of IV solution is indicated for this patient?

16. Is this a crystalloid or a colloid solution?

Case Presentation #3 (Questions 17-20)

You are dispatched to a medical emergency. The patient is an elderly woman who is complaining of having vomited blood for the past 2 hours. Conscious and alert, she tells you she has a long history of ulcers and alcohol abuse. She is pale, sweaty, and dizzy when she stands. Her vital signs are: BP 84/60; pulse 120 and weak; respirations 24.

17. Based on this initial information, you suspect that this patient is underhydrated or overhydrated and does or does not need fluid replacement. (Circle the correct answers.)

18. Is she likely to be acidotic or alkalotic? Explain your response.

19. What type of IV fluid would be appropriate, and why?

20. What do her vital signs and skin signs indicate in terms of autonomic nervous system influence? Briefly explain.

General Review Questions

21. Formed elements in the blood serve essential functions. Briefly describe their chief functions in the following categories:
    (a) respiratory:
    (b) nutritional:
    (c) regulatory:
    (d) excretory:
    (e) protective:

Match the term in Column 1 with its correct definition in Column 2.

Column 1

22. _____ Hemoglobin
23. _____ Electrolytes
24. _____ Plasma proteins
25. _____ Platelets
26. _____ Red blood cells
27. _____ White blood cells
28. _____ Hematocrit

Column 2

a. The percentage of red blood cells (RBCs) in whole blood
b. Essential for blood coagulation and control of bleeding
c. Defend the body against infection; remove debris
d. The most abundant in blood; primarily responsible for tissue oxygenation
e. Function as antibodies and clotting factors and move water in the circulation
f. Enables RBCs to carry 100 times more oxygen
g. Charged particles located in the plasma (e.g., sodium, potassium)
h. Blood cell production
i. Initiate nerve impulses

29. What is the function of the spleen?

30. An average blood volume for a 70-kg adult is approximately:
   a. 4000 milliliters.
   b. 5000 milliliters.
   c. 8000 milliliters.
   d. 7000 milliliters.

31. Lymphoid organs serve as a link between _____ and the _____ system.

32. Briefly describe two functions of the lymphatic system:

   (a)

   (b)

33. The blood type that can be donated to anyone is:
   a. A.
   b. B.
   c. AB.
   d. O.

34. Briefly discuss the significance of Rh-positive babies being born to Rh-negative mothers.

35. The approximate percentage of water in the adult human body is:
   a. 30%–40%.
   b. 40%–50%.
   c. 56%–60%.
   d. 55%–70%.

36. Fill in the following blanks:

Most of the body's weight is composed of fluid (total body water). Two thirds is inside the cells and is called **(a)** _____ fluid. About one third is outside the cells and is called **(b)** _____ fluid. This latter fluid is divided among two components: **(c)** _____ space (between the cells) and the **(d)** _____ space (inside the blood vessels).

37. Which fluid imbalance occurs more frequently?
   (a) dehydration
   (b) overhydration
Briefly explain your response: _____
_____
_____

38. Briefly discuss the major functions of the following electrolytes:

   (a) sodium

   (b) potassium

   (c) calcium

   (d) magnesium

39. The chief intracellular cation is:
   a. calcium.
   b. magnesium.
   c. potassium.
   d. sodium.

Match each term from Column 1 with its corresponding description in Column 2.

Column 1
40. _____ Hypotonic
41. _____ Isotonic
42. _____ Hypertonic
43. _____ Osmosis
44. _____ Diffusion

Column 2
a. Movement of water from an area of lesser concentration to one of greater concentration
b. A solution with a lower concentration of particles than fluid
c. Movement of particles from a solution of greater concentration to one of lesser concentration
d. A solution that is considered equal in concentration of both particles and fluid
e. A solution with a higher concentration of particles than fluid

Match each of the following conditions in Column 1 with its corresponding type of hydration imbalance (a or b) and the appropriate IV fluid to be administered for treatment of the condition (c, d, or e), both of which are listed in Column 2. There may be more than one answer for each condition.

Column 1
45. _____ Diarrhea
46. _____ Heart failure; pulmonary edema
47. _____ Fever
48. _____ Increased sweating
49. _____ Excessive water intake
50. _____ Burns

Column 2
a. Overhydration
b. Dehydration
c. Normal saline (NS)
d. Ringer's lactate (RL)
e. 5% Dextrose in water (D5W)

51. The normal body pH range is _____

52. The primary buffer that maintains acid-base balance in the body is the:
   a. bicarbonate–carbonic acid system.
   b. kidneys.
   c. respiratory system.
   d. none of the above

53. The acid-base abnormality most often seen in the prehospital setting is:
   a. metabolic acidosis.
   b. metabolic alkalosis.
   c. respiratory acidosis.
   d. respiratory alkalosis.

Identify the acid-base derangement that would be suspected in the following patient presentations:

54. _____ A 42-year-old man who has a severe head injury; respirations 6 and shallow

55. _____ A 26-year-old diabetic patient with fruity breath and vomiting; blood sugar >250; respirations 32 per minute, deep and labored

56. _____ A 26-year-old woman who is very upset because her boyfriend left her; she is hyperventilating; respirations 36 and shallow

57. _____ A 64-year-old man in cardiac arrest

58. The most important sign of an acid-base disturbance in a patient is:
   a. blood pressure variance.
   b. pulse abnormality.
   c. respiratory status.
   d. All are equally important.

59. The principal nerve of the parasympathetic system is the _____. Its primary effect is to _____ (slow/speed) the heart rate.

60. Listed below is the mnemonic for the beta effects on the heart. State what each letter represents.

   C–

   A–

   R–

   D–

   I–

   O–

Answers to questions from chapter 8 can be found on page 413.

Chapter 9

Shock

Objectives

1. Describe the components necessary for normal tissue perfusion.
2. Describe the functions of the precapillary sphincters and the vascular system.
3. Define the following terms:
   a. Afterload
   b. Aldosterone
   c. Baroreceptors
   d. Capacitance vessels
   e. Preload
4. Discuss factors that affect peripheral vascular resistance.
5. Define and discuss the significance of the Frank Starling Law.
6. Define and describe the overall clinical picture of shock.
7. Discuss factors that affect compensation for shock in the elderly and pediatric age groups.
8. Identify patients and/or conditions that are at high risk for the development of shock.
9. Identify the most useful method to assess for the presence of shock in the prehospital setting.
10. Discuss the basic pathophysiology, signs and symptoms, and complications of early shock and late shock (progressive, irreversible).
11. Discuss the compensatory mechanism of shock exerted by the autonomic nervous system.
12. Discuss why blood pressure can be normal in early shock.
13. Describe assessment and management for shock in the prehospital setting.
14. Describe the types of shock (cardiogenic, hypovolemic, distributive) in terms of pathophysiology, causes, specific signs and symptoms, complications, and general management.
15. Identify factors that can affect the body's ability to compensate for shock.

Case Presentation #1 (Questions 1-8)

You are dispatched to an auto/pedestrian incident at rush hour. On arrival at the scene, you find a woman lying face down next to the curbside. Bystanders report that the patient was crossing the street when a car, which was traveling approximately 40 miles per hour, struck her. The car that struck her has fled the scene.

1. After determining that it is safe to approach the patient, your first priority is to:
   a. assess her airway status.
   b. check for obvious bleeding.
   c. get a description of the car that struck her.
   d. look for a medical identification bracelet.

While protecting her cervical spine, you log roll the patient so that you can examine her. She is conscious, moaning, and complaining of severe abdominal pain. She has multiple abrasions on her face, neck, and arms. During your initial assessment, you note that she has contusions and a large scrape on her abdomen. Her chest is rising equally, and it is clear bilaterally. She is moving all four extremities, and no obvious fractures or major external injuries are evident. Her skin is slightly pale, and she is complaining about being thirsty.

2. Given this initial information, could this patient be in shock? Explain your answer.

Vital signs are as follows: BP 122/74; pulse 130 and weak; respirations 24. You ask the engine crew on the scene for assistance in getting equipment so that you can prepare the patient for transport. With spinal immobilization equipment in place, she is quickly moved.

3. What do her vital signs indicate, in terms of the possibility of shock?

4. When shock occurs, the body attempts to compensate by activating the:
   a. autonomic nervous system.
   b. central nervous system.
   c. reticuloactivating system.
   d. voluntary nervous system.

Once the patient is in the ambulance, you quickly hook up an ECG monitor, apply oxygen, call medical direction, and prepare for transport.

5. While en route to the hospital, you should start an IV of:
   a. 5% dextrose in water.
   b. 0.45% normal saline.
   c. 0.9% normal saline.
   d. Ringer's lactate.
   e. Either c or d.

6. The patient's condition remains unchanged en route to the hospital. You suspect that she is in what type of shock?
   a. cardiogenic
   b. early (compensated)
   c. hypovolemic
   d. late (progressive)
   e. both b and c.

7. Why would her blood pressure be normal if she is in shock, as you suspect?

8. Is the type of shock that this patient is in more common than other types of shock? Explain your response.

CASE PRESENTATION #2 (QUESTIONS 9–15)

In the middle of a hot summer afternoon, you are dispatched to a private residence for treatment of a possibly unconscious person. Upon arrival, you are met by a woman who leads you to the backyard. Her husband is lying on his side by the pool. She reports that while her husband was cleaning the pool, he suddenly grabbed his chest and fell over. You quickly assess for ABCs and find that they are intact. The patient is minimally responsive to verbal stimuli.

9. As you apply oxygen, what initial question would be the most important to ask the patient's wife?
    a. Did he complain of any chest pain before his collapse?
    b. Does he have any major medical problems?
    c. Has he ever had a heart attack?
    d. Is he allergic to any medications or other substances?
    e. Is he taking any medications currently?

You continue your assessment of the patient. The patient's vital signs are: BP 74/50; pulse 64 and weak; respirations 14 and labored. The patient is diaphoretic, and you note that he has cyanosis around his mouth, nail beds, and feet.

10. Does his condition indicate early or late shock? Explain your response.

His wife tells you that her husband had been complaining of chest pain earlier in the day but refused to go to the hospital. He did have a heart attack 7 years ago, and his health has been good since that time. Just before he collapsed, he told her that the pain was like the pain he felt when he had had his first attack; he told her to call 9-1-1 immediately.

11. What type of shock is this patient most likely experiencing? Briefly explain the pathophysiology of this type of shock.

12. For assessment of this type of shock, there are two distinctive characteristics that you should seek during physical examination. What are they?

    (a)

    (b)

13. Based on your knowledge of this patient's clinical condition, you would suspect that he is in:
    a. metabolic acidosis.
    b. metabolic alkalosis.
    c. respiratory acidosis.
    d. none of the above.

You prepare for transport. You have administered oxygen, you have begun ECG monitoring, an IV has been established, and you have placed the patient in a position of comfort.

14. Should the IV rate be fast or slow? Explain your rationale.

15. While you are en route to the hospital, you should observe for what potential problems?

CASE PRESENTATION #3 (QUESTIONS 16–20)

You are dispatched for a medical emergency in a school yard. On arrival at the scene, you find a 15-year-old boy sitting beside the tennis court. He is conscious and is complaining of breathing difficulty. He tells you that he was retrieving a tennis ball from the grass, and when he reached down to get the ball, he got stung by several ants. He has a history of allergy to ants. You note that he is using accessory muscles to breathe, has obvious stridor, and is extremely anxious.

16. What is your most immediate concern regarding this patient's condition?

Further examination reveals a generalized rash, itching, and swollen eyelids. The patient is feeling faint. Vital signs are as follows: BP 100/70; pulse 126; respirations 36 and labored.

17. Based on the assessment findings, what do you suspect the patient is experiencing?
    a. acute asthma
    b. anaphylactic shock
    c. heat exhaustion
    d. neurogenic shock
    e. vasovagal episode

You quickly administer oxygen, monitor the patient, start an IV, and prepare for transport. The patient remains alert, but he is in significant respiratory distress.

18. You anticipate that the first drug to be administered to this patient will be:
    a. Benadryl.
    b. dopamine.
    c. epinephrine.
    d. steroids.

19. Is his condition life-threatening? Explain your response.

His parents cannot be reached for consent to take him to the hospital. School officials are concerned about this because they cannot locate the pre-signed release form for consent in case of an emergency, which his parents submitted on the first day of school.

20. What should you do? Explain your answer.

General Review Questions

21. For adequate tissue perfusion to occur, which of the following is/are necessary? Circle all that apply.
    a. adequate blood volume
    b. functioning heart
    c. intact blood vessels
    d. lungs
    e. all of the above

22. Define chemoreceptors and describe their function.

23. The vascular system regulates blood flow, thus controlling two main factors. What are they?

(a)

(b)

24. The capacitance vessels are the:
   a. arteries.
   b. arterioles.
   c. capillaries.
   d. venules.

25. Given that all the patients listed below present with signs and symptoms of shock, which patient is most likely to be in septic shock?
   a. a 48-year-old man who fell from a tree and has bilateral fractured femurs
   b. a 26-year-old woman who has been stung by a bee and is very short of breath
   c. a 56-year-old man with chest pain, rales, and hypotension
   d. a 43-year-old woman who has had vomiting and diarrhea for 3 days
   e. a 62-year-old man who has an in-dwelling Foley catheter; temperature: 102° F

26. Precapillary sphincters help to:

(a)

(b)

27. Factors that affect peripheral vascular resistance include: (Circle all that apply.)
   a. diameter of the blood vessels.
   b. length of the blood vessels.
   c. parasympathetic influence.
   d. capillary sphincter opening and closing.
   e. viscosity of the blood.

Match the term in Column 1 with its correct definition in Column 2.

Column 1

28. ____ Afterload
29. ____ Preload
30. ____ Cardiac output
31. ____ Frank Starling law
32. ____ Baroreceptors
33. ____ Perfusion
34. ____ Aldosterone

Column 2

a. The stretch of the myocardial fiber at end diastole
b. The volume of blood expelled by the heart in one full minute (heart rate stroke volume)
c. Pressure-sensitive nerve endings in the walls of the atria of the heart, the venae cavae, the aortic arch, and the carotid sinus
d. A hormone released by the pituitary to help conserve water in the kidney
e. Conserves sodium in the kidney and further helps to conserve body fluid
f. Adequate oxygenation and nourishment provided to the body tissues by the blood
g. Known as the "washout phenomena"
h. Means that the more the ventricular wall is stretched, the stronger the contraction becomes
i. The load or resistance against which the left ventricle must eject its volume of blood during contraction

35. Describe the differences in compensatory mechanisms for shock in the following populations:

   (a) Elderly patients:

   (b) Pediatric patients:

36. Identify patients who are at high risk for developing shock, as compared with the average population.

37. During field care, the most useful method for evaluating for the presence of shock is:
   a. recording of blood pressure readings.
   b. consideration of only high-risk patients.
   c. estimation of the percent of blood loss.
   d. determination of general signs and symptoms.

38. Which of the following is not a sign or symptom of early (compensated) shock?
   a. cyanosis
   b. pale skin
   c. rapid respirations
   d. tachycardia

39. Briefly discuss the complications that ensue with the development of progressive and irreversible shock.

40. The most important intervention a prehospital care provider can make in terms of mortality in shock cases is:
   a. differentiating the type of shock present.
   b. early recognition and treatment of the condition.
   c. rapid administration of IV fluids.
   d. providing vasopressor therapy.

41. Which type of shock typically is accompanied by a slow pulse?
   a. anaphylactic
   b. cardiogenic
   c. hypovolemic
   d. neurogenic
   e. septic

42. Which of the following could cause hypovolemic shock in an adult patient?
    a. burns
    b. gastrointestinal bleeding
    c. closed head injury
    d. myocardial infarction
    e. a and b
    f. a, b, and c

43. What is mechanical or obstructive shock? Name two typical causes.

44. Neurogenic shock results from one of two causes. Briefly discuss each of them.

    (a)

    (b)

45. The pathophysiology of anaphylaxis is summarized by a discussion of its effects, including increased capillary dilation, permeability, and smooth muscle constriction. Briefly discuss how this is manifested in the patient, and why it can be life-threatening.

46. Factors that can affect the body's ability to compensate for shock include:

    (a)

    (b)

    (c)

Answers to questions from chapter 9 can be found on page 415.

Chapter 10

Infection Control

OBJECTIVES

1. Define the following terms:
   a. Antibody
   b. Antigen
   c. Carrier
   d. Host
   e. Host resistance
   f. Incubation period
   g. Microorganism
   h. Pathogen
   i. Seroconversion
   j. Virulence
   k. Window phase
2. Differentiate between a communicable disease and an infectious disease.
3. Differentiate between direct and indirect transmission of a communicable disease.
4. Describe the hazards to paramedics posed by communicable diseases.
5. List common signs and symptoms, high-risk groups, mode(s) of transmission, and precautions specific for tuberculosis, hepatitis B, and acquired immunodeficiency syndrome.
6. Describe Universal Precautions and Body Substance Isolation as they apply to prehospital use.
7. Define legal issues related to treatment or transport of patients with a communicable disease.
8. Identify the precautions that prehospital personnel should take to protect themselves from communicable diseases.
9. Describe the goal, proper selection, use, and disposal of personal protective equipment.

CASE PRESENTATION #1 (QUESTIONS 1-3)

You are dispatched to a private residence for an unknown medical emergency. On arrival, you find a 36-year-old woman who tells you that she has been diagnosed with hepatitis B. She is complaining of nausea and has vomited twice today. You quickly determine that the patient has no immediate threats to her life and her vital signs are stable. You administer oxygen via nasal cannula, initiate a precautionary IV, and prepare the patient for transport.

1. Which of the following statements is false regarding why you should be especially careful when disposing of this patient's contaminated IV needle?
   a. Hepatitis B is easily spread by infected blood.
   b. Hepatitis B cannot be transmitted by a needlestick.
   c. Chronic hepatitis may be a lifelong disability.
   d. Paramedics have died as a result of occupationally acquired hepatitis B infection.

2. Should you have recapped the IV needle before placing it in the sharps container? Explain why or why not.

When you deliver the patient to the emergency department, she is in stable condition. You prepare for your next call. You dispose of the oxygen delivery device used by the patient, change the linen on the stretcher, and wash your hands.

3. List additional protection that you should have against this specific communicable disease (as required by the Occupational Safety and Health Administration [OSHA]).

CASE PRESENTATION #2 (QUESTIONS 4–7)

Your patient is a 55-year-old man who has been living in a homeless shelter for the past six months. He is complaining of night sweats and a productive cough. He does not appear to be in acute distress; his vital signs are B/P 130/84; pulse 92; respirations 20. After the patient informs you that he had a positive tuberculosis (TB) skin test two weeks ago, your partner is hesitant to perform a physical examination of the patient.

4. Under the Americans with Disabilities Act, failure to provide care for this patient may constitute
   _____.

5. The best way that you and your partner can be protected from possible infection is by:
   a. wearing gloves.
   b. placing a mask on the patient.
   c. wearing a mask.
   d. getting vaccinated.
   e. All of the above.

6. Transport of this patient should be done with the ambulance ventilation at _____ settings.

The patient's condition is unchanged on arrival to the emergency department. You provide a thorough report of history and physical findings to the physician who accepts the patient. Before leaving the emergency department, you also tell the physician that you are concerned about possible exposure to a communicable disease during treatment of this patient. The physician reassures you that you will be notified if the patient is confirmed to have TB.

7. Under the Ryan White Act, the hospital is required to notify you:
   a. automatically.
   b. within 48 hours of disease determination.
   c. only if the patient has an airborne transmissible disease.
   d. All of the above.

GENERAL REVIEW QUESTIONS

Match each of the terms in Column 1 with its correct definition in Column 2.

Column 1

8. ____ Communicable disease
9. ____ Antigen
10. ____ Carrier
11. ____ Host
12. ____ Microorganism
13. ____ Pathogen
14. ____ Virulence
15. ____ Host resistance
16. ____ Antibody
17. ____ Infectious disease

Column 2

a. A microorganism capable of causing disease in a suitable host
b. A person or animal capable of supporting or harboring another organism
c. A protein produced by the body to provide immunity against a specific antigen, pathogen, or other foreign substance
d. Any disease caused by a pathogen or an etiologic agent
e. The growth of an organism within a suitable host
f. A person who harbors a pathogen, but who currently has no symptoms of disease
g. A substance or pathogen that the body recognizes as foreign, thereby causing activation of the immune system
h. The relative strength of a pathogen, or its ability to produce disease
i. The ability of the exposed individual to withstand infection
j. Any disease that can be spread from person to person
k. A life form, such as a bacterium, virus, fungus, or parasite, that is too small to be seen with the unaided eye

For each of the following statements (18–23), circle the correct response, True or False. Briefly explain your answer.

18. Many victims with communicable diseases are completely asymptomatic.

    TRUE   **FALSE**

    Briefly explain your answer: _____

19. Most patient care equipment can be disinfected with soap and water.

    TRUE   **FALSE**

    Briefly explain your answer: _____

20. Linen should be changed after each patient use only if it is contaminated with body fluids.

    TRUE   **FALSE**

    Briefly explain your answer: _____

21. Work uniforms should be laundered at home for effective decontamination.

    TRUE   **FALSE**

    Briefly explain your answer: _____
    _____
    _____

22. TB bacteria usually can be killed with a weak solution of bleach and water.

    TRUE   **FALSE**

    Briefly explain your answer: _____
    _____

23. Under Body Substance Isolation (BSI), only blood is considered potentially infectious.

    TRUE   **FALSE**

    Briefly explain your answer: _____
    _____

24. The paramedic should be tested on an annual basis for which of the following communicable diseases?
    a. human immunodeficiency virus (HIV)
    b. TB
    c. hepatitis B
    d. tetanus
    e. all of the above

25. Which group of people are at high risk for contracting tuberculosis? (Circle all that apply.)
    a. alcoholics
    b. nursing home patients
    c. HIV victims
    d. infants

26. The personal protective equipment (PPE) that is recommended to be used by paramedics during emergency childbirth is:
    a. gown, disposable gloves, protective eyewear, and mask
    b. disposable gloves and mask
    c. disposable gloves only
    d. gown, disposable gloves, and mask

Complete each sentence with the correct answer.

27. The time interval between exposure to a communicable disease and the development of symptoms is known as the _____ _____.

28. The time between exposure to a disease and the development of measurable antibodies is termed the _____ _____.

29. A person who develops antibodies after disease exposure is said to have _____.

30. _____ transmission occurs when exposure is from person to person.

31. _____ transmission of a communicable disease occurs when exposure is via a contaminated object.

32. List three common sense rules that you should follow to minimize the risk of acquiring a communicable disease.

(a)

(b)

(c)

33. State the purpose of personal protective equipment.

34. List the five infectious diseases that pose the greatest risk to paramedics and the mode of transmission for each.

(a)

(b)

(c)

(d)

(e)

35. In addition to receiving a hepatitis B vaccination, paramedics should be immunized against what six diseases?

(a)

(b)

(c)

(d)

(e)

(f)

36. List three modes of transmission of AIDS.

(a)

(b)

(c)

Answers to questions from chapter 10 can be found on page 418.

Chapter 11

General Pharmacology

OBJECTIVES

1. Describe differences in generic and trade names of medications.
2. Explain the role of government agencies (FDA, DEA) and the laws that affect drug administration in prehospital care.
3. Describe how drugs are absorbed, distributed, metabolized, and eliminated.
4. Discuss therapeutic effects and processes that affect abosrption and distribution of drugs.
5. Define the following terms:
   a. Receptor
   b. Target tissue
   c. Drug agonist
   d. Drug antagonist
   e. Dose response
   f. Therapeutic window.
6. Describe how drug effects are related to the autonomic nervous system.
7. Define the following terms:
   a. Contraindication
   b. Dependence
   c. Hypersensitivity
   d. Idiosyncrasy
   e. Indication
   f. Precaution
   g. Side Effects
   h. Therapeutic Action
   i. Tolerance
   j. Toxicity
8. Describe the five "patient rights" of drug administration.
9. Identify the units of measurement and common abbreviations used in the metric system.
10. Convert units of measurement utilized in the metric system.
11. Given a dosage of medication to be administered and how it is supplied, calculate the correct amount to administer.
12. Given a patient's weight in pounds and a dosage of medication in mg/kg, calculate the volume of a drug to be administered.
13. Given a scenario with a macro- (regular) or microdrip infusion set, calculate the IV drip rate per minute.
14. Given an amount of medication and solution for an intravenous infusion, calculate the IV drip rate per minute.
15. Describe the routes of drug administration used in prehospital care and compare their rates of absorption.
16. Describe the therapeutic action, uses, and side effects of general drug categories.
17. List specific examples of drugs in each category.

Case Presentation #1 (Questions 1-6)

You are dispatched to an apartment complex for a medical emergency. You are met by a 25-year-old man who tells you that his girlfriend has overdosed on pain pills. Initial assessment reveals that the patient is semiconscious, and she arouses to verbal commands. Her vital signs are: BP 92/60; pulse 70; respirations 8 and shallow. Her boyfriend tells you she has taken six tablets from a prescription that contained ten tablets. The prescription was filled two hours before the emergency call.

1. The first priority in care is to:
   a. assist respirations.
   b. induce vomiting.
   c. obtain additional information on her drug history.
   d. start an IV.

2. Her altered level of consciousness and respiratory depression indicate an excessive amount of a drug in her system. This condition is called drug _____.

Upon questioning, her boyfriend provides the following information: The patient has a long history of drug abuse, including heroin, pain pills, and sleeping pills. He says it takes more and more pills to satisfy her, and that she uses drugs daily to function on the job.

3. Taking increased amounts of a drug to get the same results and to satisfy physiologic need is called:
   a. contraindication.
   b. idiosyncrasy.
   c. potentiation.
   d. tolerance.

4. Physiologic need for a drug to function adequately is called:
   a. dependence.
   b. hypersensitivity.
   c. therapeutic action.
   d. overdose.

In the patient's bathroom, you find other pill bottles containing Darvon®, Percodan®, and Vicodin®.

5. These drugs are classified as:
   a. antidepressants.
   b. antipsychotics.
   c. narcotic analgesics.
   d. sedatives/hypnotics.

During transport to the hospital, her respiratory status improves. However, she is euphoric, giddy, and nauseated.

6. These symptoms are the expected _____ _____ of the drug classification _____ _____.

General Review Questions

7. Describe the difference between generic and trade drug names.

8. Testing and marketing of prescription drugs is controlled by:
   a. the Department of Labor.
   b. the Department of Transportation (DOT).
   c. the Food and Drug Administration (FDA).
   d. the State Health Department.

9. What is the role of the Drug Enforcement Agency (DEA), and how does it regulate controlled substances?

Fill in the following blanks:

10. The purpose of administering a drug is to create a **(a)** _____ at a **(b)** _____. All drugs go through a process to accomplish this: entering into the body and the bloodstream by **(c)** _____; movement through the bloodstream to a target organ, which is **(d)** _____; production of a desired drug effect or chemical breakdown, which is called **(e)** _____; and removal from the body, which is **(f)** _____.

11. Briefly discuss factors that affect drug:

    (a) absorption:

    (b) distribution:

Define the following terms related to the mechanism of drug action:

12. Receptor: _____

13. Drug agonist: _____

14. Drug antagonist: _____

15. Dose response: _____

16. Therapeutic window: _____

17. What is the "lock and key" theory, and how is it related to the autonomic nervous system?

What is the role of the following organs in metabolism and elimination?

18. liver: _____

19. kidney: _____

Match the term in Column 1 with its correct definition in Column 2.

Column 1

20. _____ Indication
21. _____ Contraindication
22. _____ Therapeutic action
23. _____ Potentiation
24. _____ Precaution
25. _____ Hypersensitivity
26. _____ Idiosyncratic reaction

Column 2

a. Enhancement of a drug by another one administered
b. Desired effect or beneficial action of a drug
c. Information about the handling of a drug that will prevent adverse effects
d. Indication that a drug should not be administered
e. An undesirable side effect that occurs with routine therapeutic dose
f. Specific use of a drug
g. A side effect regarded as harmful to the patient
h. Unexpected adverse drug effects that are peculiar to an individual
i. Psychological or physiologic need for a drug to function adequately
j. Action of increased intensity after administration of several doses of a drug
k. Allergic reaction to a medication, not related to dosage

27. The metric system is based on units of _____.

28. The primary unit of volume in the metric system is the _____.

29. The primary unit of length in the metric system is the _____.

30. The primary unit of mass in the metric system is the _____.

Match the prefix in Column 1 with its correct equivalent in Column 2.

Column 1
31. ____ kilo
32. ____ deci
33. ____ centi
34. ____ milli
35. ____ micro

Column 2
a. 1/1,000,000 or 0.000001
b. 1/10 or 0.1
c. 1/1000 or 0.001
d. 1/100 or 0.01
e. 1000
f. 1/10,000 or 0.0001

Convert the following units to the units indicated.

36. 1 gram = ____ mg
37. 1 mL = ____ cc
38. 2 gm = ____ mg
39. 65 L = ____ mL
40. .75 L = ____ mL
41. 1000 mL = ____ liters
42. 1 kg = ____ pounds
43. 65 mL = ____ L
44. 256 gm = ____ mg
45. 45 mg = ____ gm

Calculate the following drug dosages.

46. The physician orders 6 mg of a drug. It is supplied 10 mg/2 mL. How many mL should be administered?

47. The physician orders 25 mg of a drug. It is supplied 50 mg/1 mL. How many mL should be administered?

48. The physician orders 75 mg of a drug. It is supplied 100 mg/10 mL. How many mL should be given?

49. The physician orders epinephrine 1:1000 for a pediatric patient who weighs 50 pounds. The drug is supplied 1 mg/1 mL. Dose = .01 mg/kg. How much should you administer?

50. You wish to administer an IV drip at 150 mL/hour. The tubing delivers 15 drops/mL. How many drops/minute should the IV run?

51. You wish to administer an IV drip to run at 250 mL/hour. The tubing delivers 10 drops/mL. How many drops/minute should the IV run?

52. You wish to administer an IV of Ringer's lactate 1000 mL to infuse at an 8-hour rate. The tubing delivers 10 drops/mL. How many drops/minute should the IV run?

For questions 53 and 54, use the following formula to calculate the dopamine drip.

$$\frac{(\text{Pt's weight in kg}) \times (\text{Dr's mcg/kg/min order}) \times 60}{\text{Your mixture of mcg/cc}} = \text{gtts/min}$$

Remember: 1000 mcg = 1 mg

Example: You are ordered to run a dopamine drip at 8 mcg/kg/min. Your patient weighs 121 lbs. You mix 400 mg in 500 mL D5W. How many gtts/min do you run your IV?

    Pt's weight = 55 kg

    Dr's order = 8 mcg/kg/min

    Your mixture = 400 mg/500 mL

            ↓

        .8 mg/1 mL

            ↓

        800 mcg/mL

Formula:

$$\frac{55 \times 8 \times 60}{800} = 33 \text{ gtts/min}$$

53. The physician orders a dopamine drip to run at 5 mcg/kg/min. Your patient weighs 154 lbs. You mix 200 mg in 500 mL of D5W. How many gtts/min do you run your IV?

54. You have a dopamine drip concentration of 800 mcg/mL. Your minidrip is running at 40 gtts/min on your 75-kg patient. How many mcg/kg/min is this patient receiving?

Match the route of administration in Column 1 with its correct definition in Column 2.

Column 1

55. ____ Oral
56. ____ Topical/Dermal
57. ____ Inhaled
58. ____ Intravenous
59. ____ Intraosseous
60. ____ Endotracheal
61. ____ Subcutaneous
62. ____ Intramuscular
63. ____ Sublingual

Column 2

a. Absorbed via the lungs
b. Injected superficially into skin
c. Injection into bone marrow
d. Administered by mouth
e. Local application to skin
f. Administered directly into vein
g. Administered under the tongue
h. Administered directly into the lungs via an airway device
i. Administered deep into the muscle

64. The fastest route of drug administration is _____, and the slowest route of drug administration is _____.

Fill in the following blanks:

65. The physician orders you to give Valium® 5 mg to a patient who is actively seizing. The first step you should take is to **(a)** _____. Once you have done this, you prepare to give the medicine. You should be sure that it is the RIGHT **(b)** _____ and the RIGHT **(c)** _____. To check the dosage, you should first check the **(d)** _____ on the box or container. **(e)** _____ the correct amount of drug, based on how it is supplied. Reverify the correct **(f)** _____, **(g)** _____, and dose. Review any special **(h)** _____ or **(i)** _____ that you must be alert for; then administer the drug.

CASE PRESENTATION #2 (QUESTIONS 66–70)

You are dispatched to a possible victim of a heart attack. Upon arrival at 11:30 a.m., you find an elderly patient. He is conscious and is complaining of nausea, fatigue, and feeling weak and dizzy. His symptoms began about 1½ hours ago. He states that he took his medication right after breakfast at 6:30 a.m. Upon further questioning, the patient tells you that he has mistakenly taken two Digoxin® tablets, instead of one, for the past two days. His medical history reveals that he had an acute myocardial infarction 6 years ago; he also has congestive heart failure and hypertension. He takes the following medications: Digoxin, Lasix®, Inderal®, and Mexitil®. His vital signs are: B/P 86/50; pulse 45; respirations 20.

66. From his signs and symptoms, you suspect he could be suffering from _____ toxicity. Briefly explain your answer.

67. Mexitil® is prescribed for control of:
    a. coronary artery disease.
    b. high blood pressure.
    c. migraine headache.
    d. ventricular dysrhythmias.

68. Inderal® is classified as a(n):
    a. antidysrhythmic.
    b. beta blocker.
    c. calcium channel blocker.
    d. coronary vasodilator.

69. The therapeutic action of Digoxin is that it:
    a. dilates the coronary arteries.
    b. increases the force of myocardial contractions.
    c. increases the heart rate.
    d. minimizes blood clots.
    e. removes excess fluid from the body.

70. Lasix® is classified as a **(a)** _____. The therapeutic goal of this group of drugs is to **(b)** _____. For this patient, it has probably been prescribed to control his **(c)** _____ and **(d)** _____.

GENERAL REVIEW QUESTIONS

Define the therapeutic action and list one example of each of the following:

71. Beta blockers:

72. Calcium channel blockers:

73. Coronary vasodilators:

74. Thrombolytics:

75. Vasodilators:

76. Antidepressants may be used for: (Circle all that apply.)
   a. chronic depression.
   b. eating disorders.
   c. panic disorders.
   d. psychotic behavior.
   e. seizure disorders.

77. The therapeutic action of major tranquilizers is to:
   a. alter pain response.
   b. induce sleep.
   c. modify thought processes in the brain.
   d. treat depression.

78. Which of the following are classified as sedative/hypnotic drugs?
   1. Dalmane®
   2. Mellaril®
   3. Seconal®
   4. Valium®
   5. Xanax®
      a. 1, 2, and 3
      b. 1, 2, and 5
      c. 2, 3, and 5
      d. all except 2
      e. all of the above

Match the drug category in Column 1 with its therapeutic action in Column 2.

Column 1

79. _____ Anticoagulant
80. _____ Antihistamine
81. _____ Antidiarrheal
82. _____ Antiinflammatory
83. _____ Antisecretory
84. _____ Diabetic medication
85. _____ Antituberculosis
86. _____ Lipid lowering
87. _____ Antiemetic
88. _____ Bronchodilator
89. _____ Anticonvulsant
90. _____ Antibacterial
91. _____ Skeletal muscle relaxant

Column 2

a. Reduces tonic muscle activity
b. Inhibits nausea and vomiting
c. Helps regulate insulin in the body
d. Lowers blood cholesterol
e. Dilates the bronchi
f. Destroys bacteria causing tuberculosis
g. Increases blood clotting time
h. Reduces inflammation and swelling
i. Reduces the effect of histamine
j. Inhibits seizure activity in motor cortex
k. Inhibits gastrointestinal motility
l. Inhibits secretion from the gastrointestinal tract
m. Destroys bacteria

Answers to questions from chapter 11 can be found on page 419.

Chapter 11a

Appendix: Prehospital Medications

OBJECTIVES

1. Identify common trade names for the medications listed below.
2. Describe class, therapeutic action, mechanism, indications, contraindications, adverse reactions, drug interactions, how supplied, their usual adult and pediatric dosage, and other considerations for the medications listed below.
3. Given a description of patients with different clinical findings, identify which of the drugs below is indicated in their treatment.

Activated charcoal	Lorazepam
Adenosine	Magnesium sulfate
Albuterol	Mannitol
Aminophylline	Meperidine
Aspirin	Morphine sulfate
Atropine sulfate	Naloxone
Bretylium tosylate	Nitroglycerin
Calcium chloride	Nitrous oxide
Cyanide antidote kit	Norepinephrine
Dextrose	Oxygen
Diazepam	Oxytocin
Diphenhydramine	Procainamide
Dobutamine	Proparacaine
Dopamine	Propranolol
Droperidol	Racemic epinephrine
Epinephrine	Sodium bicarbonate
Flumazenil	Steroids
Furosemide	Streptokinase
Glucagon	Succinylcholine
Ipecac (syrup of)	Thiamine
Isoproterenol	Tissue plasminogen activator
Labetolol	Verapamil
Lidocaine	

Case Presentation #1 (Questions 1-14)

While you are eating lunch at the fire station, a middle-aged woman walks in and tells you that she thinks her husband, who is behind her, is having a heart attack. She says that, about 5 minutes ago, while they were driving to the neighborhood grocery, he began experiencing severe chest pain that is radiating to his left arm. He is pale and diaphoretic and appears to be very uncomfortable. Your crew quickly springs into action. The patient's vital signs are: BP 172/100; pulse 110 and regular; respirations 16 and unlabored.

1. What are your treatment priorities for this patient at this time? Explain why.

The patient is placed onto a stretcher in the ambulance and is given oxygen at 10 L/min via nonrebreather mask. The monitor leads are attached, and an IV line is established at a keep open rate. One 325-mg aspirin tablet is administered by mouth. The wife reports that the only medication her husband is taking is Procardia®; she asks if you gave the aspirin to help relieve his pain.

2. What is the rationale for administering aspirin to this patient?

3. What is the class and therapeutic action of Procardia®?

As you are attaching leads to obtain a 12-lead ECG, the patient says that his pain is getting worse. You have standing orders to administer sublingual nitroglycerin for chest pain that is suspected to be of myocardial origin. You give the patient sublingually one 0.4-mg tablet.

4. Was it safe to administer nitroglycerin to this patient under your standing orders? Why, or why not?

5. In addition to providing pain relief, what is the clinical goal of administering nitroglycerin to this patient?

6. In addition to hypotension, what other potential adverse reactions might be seen in this patient after you administer the nitroglycerin?

While you are contacting medical direction, your partner reassesses the patient. The patient's BP is now 160/90. The 12-lead ECG indicates an ST elevation in two anterior leads. The patient's pain is not relieved after administration of the dose of nitroglycerin.

7. What is the maximum number of times that you may repeat the dose of nitroglycerin for this patient with the goal of relieving his pain?

8. Why would treatment with dopamine be preferred to the use of norepinephrine if this patient becomes hypotensive?

Given this patient's history, examination findings, and ECG reading, the medical direction physician informs you that he is a candidate for thrombolytic therapy; you are instructed to begin transport to the hospital immediately. Your ETA is 7 minutes. The patient's pain has not been relieved with the repeated use of nitroglycerin. This is the only analgesic you carry on the ambulance other than Nitronox®. While en route, the patient states, "I feel like I am going to die."

9. Is there significance to this patient's statement that he feels he is going to die? Explain your response.

10. Would it be appropriate to request Nitronox® for this patient's pain? If so, how would it be administered?

11. What common narcotic analgesic medication most likely will be administered to this patient on arrival at the emergency department? By what route will it be provided?

Although his pain is unrelieved, the patient remains stable while en route. As you are transporting him from the ambulance into the emergency department, you notice multifocal PVCs across the ECG monitor.

12. What two antiarrhythmic drugs may be indicated for this patient's ventricular ectopy? In what order would they be given if both had to be administered?

As you are moving the patient from the ambulance stretcher to the hospital bed in the emergency department, he becomes unconscious. The monitor now shows ventricular fibrillation. The patient has no palpable pulse and is not breathing. Because the nurse is assisting the physician to defibrillate the patient, she asks you to grab 1 mg of epinephrine from the crash cart. You open the cart to find 1 mg epinephrine supplied in 1-ml, 1:1000 and 10-ml, 1:10,000 concentrations.

13. Which epinephrine concentration is indicated for this patient?

Because the emergency department is extremely busy and short on staff, you stay and assist with CPR on this patient. After 8 minutes of aggressive advanced cardiac life support (ACLS) therapy, the patient converts to a normal sinus rhythm and regains a pulse. As you are preparing to leave, you hear the attending physician tell the nurse to cancel the streptokinase (Streptase®) medication order from the pharmacy.

14. In your opinion, why did he cancel this medication order?

CASE PRESENTATION #2 (QUESTIONS 15–20)

You respond to an "unconscious person" call downtown. On arrival, you find a man lying behind a trash dumpster; there are multiple empty wine bottles scattered about the scene. He appears to be about 30 years old, is unkempt, and smells of urine and alcohol. A quick assessment for life threats reveals an intact airway and pulse. There are also no obvious signs of trauma. His pupils are pinpoint, and he is unresponsive to a verbal or painful stimulus. As your partner administers high- flow oxygen, you obtain the following vital signs: BP 94/60; pulse 74 and regular; respirations 14 and shallow. His rapid glucose determination is 80. You note multiple scarred tracts along the veins in his arms as you prepare to initiate an IV of Ringer's lactate. Your partner connects him to the cardiac monitor, which reads normal sinus rhythm.

15. Based on your assessment findings, what two medications may be indicated? Give the correct initial dosage of each.

After treatment, the patient awakens. He is belligerent and uncooperative. He admits to having a long history of heavy drinking and drug abuse, and he has been hospitalized multiple times with delirium tremens.

16. What medication should be given to this patient as soon as possible after administration of IV glucose? Explain why.

You call medical direction to give a report. The physician orders you to administer Ativan® 2 mg slow IV push to your patient before beginning transport. Your ETA is 20 minutes.

17. In your opinion, why did the physician order Ativan® rather than Valium®?

18. After you administer Ativan®, for what adverse reactions should you be alert for in this patient?

19. Is this patient at a higher risk for developing adverse reactions from Ativan®? Explain why, or why not.

20. Should you transport this patient with lights and sirens? Explain why or why not.

The patient is more cooperative after receiving the Ativan®, and he remains calm and stable while en route to the hospital. He is admitted to the emergency department for observation.

Case Presentation #3 (Question 21-25)

You are dispatched to an elementary school playground for a patient who is having an allergic reaction. On arrival, you find a 6-year-old girl who is sitting next to the slide and crying. Her skin is flushed, and she has obvious swelling to her face, especially around the eyes. Her teacher tells you that the patient was stung by a bee approximately 10 minutes before you arrived.

21. How will you assess for airway patency in this child?

22. What is your initial management priority?

The patient is in no respiratory distress; breath sounds are clear bilaterally. She is complaining of itching at the site of the bee sting on her right arm. You remove the stinger from her skin. Her vital signs are: BP 94/50; pulse 100; respirations 20 and uncompromised. She weighs approximately 40 kg. You contact medical direction for orders.

23. List the two medications that are indicated for this child. Provide the order in which they should be given, as well as the dosage and route of administration.

24. What additional actions might medical direction order for the purpose of retarding the absorption of the antigen from the site of the bee sting?

25. If this patient had presented with a severe allergic or anaphylactic reaction and you had a long transport time, what additional medication might medical direction have ordered? Explain why.

The patient responds favorably to the treatment rendered and is transported without delay to the local emergency department for evaluation.

General Review Questions

Match the medication in Column 2 with the condition for which it is indicated in Column 1.

Column 1	Column 2
26. _____ Metabolic acidosis	a. Adenosine
27. _____ Cardiogenic shock	b. Oxytocin
28. _____ Acute pulmonary edema	c. Albuterol
29. _____ Post delivery of the placenta	d. Dopamine
30. _____ Eclampsia	e. Magnesium sulfate
31. _____ Asthmatic attack	f. Sodium bicarbonate
32. _____ Unstable PSVT	g. Meperidine
33. _____ Cerebral edema from head trauma	h. Mannitol
	i. Morphine sulfate

For each of the following statements (34–39), provide the medication (by generic name) that is indicated in the particular patient situation described. All patients have stable vital signs.

34. A 25-year-old who took a half-bottle of aspirin 10 minutes ago. She is awake and alert.

    Medication:

35. A 55-year-old farmer who feels dizzy after fertilizing his crops all day. He is salivating heavily and has a pulse rate of 40 per minute.

    Medication:

36. An 8-year-old who was bitten by a spider while playing in a basement. He is extremely restless and is complaining of abdominal pain.

    Medication:

37. A 65-year-old who thinks she may have taken too many Elavil® tablets. She is drowsy. Her ECG shows sinus rhythm with a wide QRS complex.

    Medication:

38. A 66-year-old with depressed respirations after receiving morphine sulfate for chest pain.

    Medication:

39. An 18-year-old who became unconscious after shooting heroin with his friends.

    Medication:

For each of the following statements (40–43), identify the correct pediatric dose (mg/kg) and route of administration for each of the medications listed after the situation for which it is indicated.

40. A 3-year-old who is in asystole. You successfully intubated the patient, but you are unable to establish IV access.

Atropine

Dose: _____

Route: _____

41. A 4-year-old with mild wheezing caused by an acute asthma attack.

Albuterol

Dose: _____

Route: _____

42. A 6-year-old who is very drowsy after he accidentally ingested six of his mother's narcotic headache medication tablets.

Naloxone

Dose: _____

Route: _____

43. A 5-year-old who is in status epilepticus. IV access was established before the onset of seizure activity.

Diazepam

Dose: _____

Route: _____

44. Which of the following medications may be given by endotracheal route?
   a. diazepam
   b. naloxone
   c. lidocaine
   d. b and c
   e. a, b, and c

45. Narcan® reverses the side effects of which of the following medications?
   a. Demerol®
   b. nitrous oxide
   c. morphine sulfate
   d. a and c
   e. b and c

46. Which of the following factors should be considered when you are determining the initial dose of Lasix® for a particular patient?

   a. the amount of patient distress
   b. patient weight
   c. the amount of Lasix® that has been taken as an outpatient
   d. a and b
   e. a, b, and c

47. An insoluble precipitate forms when this drug is mixed with sodium bicarbonate.

   a. potassium
   b. calcium
   c. glucagon
   d. Mannitol®
   e. Labetolol®

48. Which of the following medications is an adjunct to endotracheal intubation but has limited use in the prehospital setting?

   a. diazepam
   b. succinylcholine
   c. albuterol
   d. Ventolin®
   d. steroids

49. What is the maximum dose of atropine IV push that should be given to a 13-year-old with pulseless electrical activity?

   a. 0.5 mg
   b. 0.3 mg
   c. 0.1 mg
   d. 1.0 mg
   e. 3.0 mg

50. You are treating a 33-year-old woman whose only complaint is chest palpitations. She is in ventricular tachycardia at a rate of 210 per minute. Her blood pressure is 120/84. Which of the following medications is the most appropriate for this patient to receive?

   a. procainamide
   b. lidocaine
   c. adenosine
   d. isoproterenol
   e. bretylium tosylate

51. You are treating a 2-year-old who is in mild respiratory distress with the croup. Which of the following medications is the most appropriate for this patient to receive?

   a. epinephrine
   b. albuterol
   c. aminophylline
   d. racemic epinephrine
   e. isoproterenol

52. You are treating a 25-year-old woman who is in active labor and is screaming for pain relief. Which of the following medications is the most appropriate for this patient to receive?
    a. nitrous oxide
    b. oxytocin
    c. morphine sulfate
    d. magnesium sulfate
    e. succinylcholine

53. You are treating a 22-year-old who is requesting pain relief for his eye. He thinks he got a piece of sawdust in it while he was working in his woodshop. Which of the following medications is the most appropriate one for this patient to receive?
    a. steroids
    b. Proparacaine®
    c. lidocaine
    d. Meperidine®
    e. nitrous oxide

Answers to questions from chapter 11a can be found on page 423.

Chapter 12

Basic Rhythm Interpretation

OBJECTIVES

1. Describe the normal electrical activity in the heart.
2. Describe the relationship between the electrical activity in the heart and the electrocardiogram.
3. Define the standard leads and special monitor leads.
4. Describe the five basic blocks to determine rhythm.
5. Describe the major methods to determine rate of rhythm.
6. Describe the six different patterns of rhythm.
7. Describe and explain aberrant conduction.
8. Describe the three relationships where the atrium can cause the ventricle to fire.
9. Define the four sites that can originate an impulse to the heart.
10. Define and describe the four rhythms that begin in the sinus node.
11. Define and describe the three types of premature complexes.
12. Define and describe atrial fibrillation and atrial flutter.
13. Define and describe the four variations of block in the AV node.
14. Describe the function of pacemakers and implanted defibrillators.
15. Describe the four different rhythms that must be associated with a cardiac arrest.

CASE PRESENTATION #1 (QUESTIONS 1–4)

You are dispatched to a retirement center for a "possible stroke" victim. The patient is a 67-year-old man who is complaining of lightheadedness. His symptoms began suddenly about 15 minutes ago while he was playing dominoes with a friend. He denies any significant medical history. On examination, he appears pale and diaphoretic. His pulse is slow, regular, and weak; respirations are 22 and normal; blood pressure is 80/60. You administer high-concentration oxygen, establish an IV of D5W TKO, and connect the patient to the cardiac monitor. You immediately recognize that this patient has an atrioventricular (AV) heart block. (See Figure 12-1.)

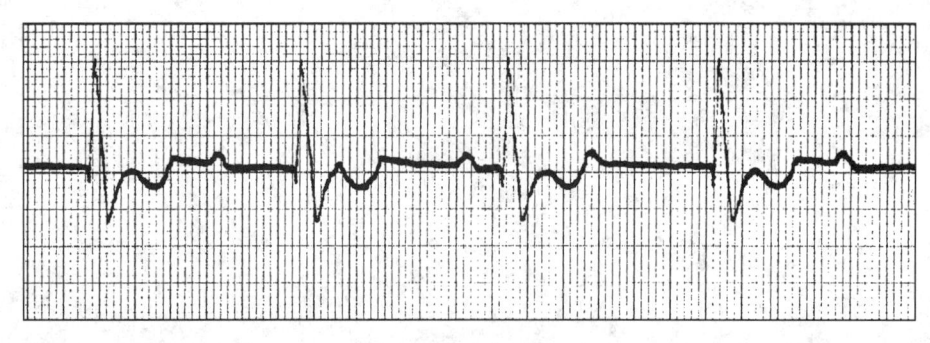

Figure 12-1

1. What degree of AV block is indicated by this patient's ECG?

2. List the five basic steps that can be followed to determine this patient's rhythm.

    (a)

    (b)

    (c)

    (d)

    (e)

3. What is the significance of the QRS complexes in this patient's ECG rhythm?

You contact medical direction and are ordered to administer atropine in an effort to increase the patient's heart rate and blood pressure. When your patient does not respond to multiple doses of atropine, medical direction orders you to begin pacing. You set the transcutaneous pacemaker rate at 70 and gradually increase the current to obtain electrical capture.

4. What changes on this patient's ECG will indicate electrical capture?

The patient appears more alert. His pulse has increased to 70, and his blood pressure is now 112/70. Your expected time of arrival (ETA) at the hospital is 5 minutes. The patient's condition is unchanged on arrival at the emergency department. You later learn that he had surgery for implantation of a permanent artificial pacemaker and is doing well in the cardiovascular intensive care unit.

CASE PRESENTATION #2 (QUESTIONS 5–10)

You are dispatched to a grocery store where you find a 70-year-old woman complaining of severe chest pain that is radiating down her left arm. The pain began suddenly just minutes ago while she was shopping. The patient is anxious and confused at moments, which makes it difficult for you to obtain a history. Physical examination reveals the following: Skin is pale and cool; pulse is weak and regular; respirations are 24 and shallow, with minimal basilar crackles auscultated; and BP is 88/50.

5. Most likely, what is this patient experiencing?
   a. anaphylaxis
   b. acute asthma
   c. cardiogenic shock
   d. pneumonia

You administer high-concentration oxygen, establish an IV, place the patient on the cardiac monitor using a modified lead II, and contact medical direction.

6. Explain why you used a modified lead II to monitor this patient.

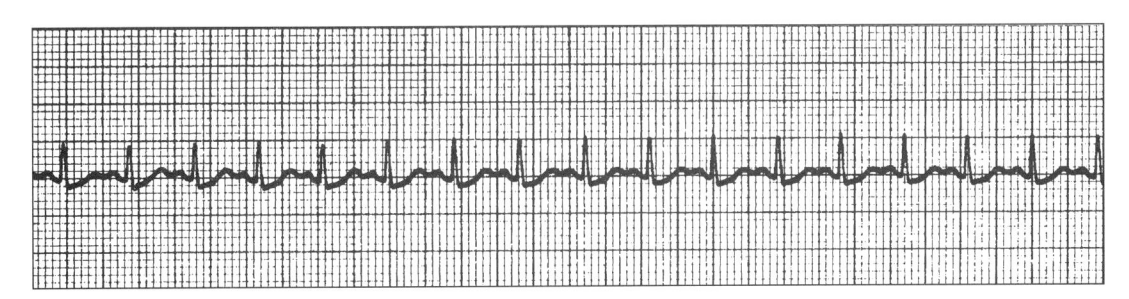

Figure 12-2

7. What is your interpretation of the patient's ECG rhythm (shown in Figure 12-2)?
   Interpretation:
   (a) Rate:
   (b) Pattern:
   (c) QRS width:
   (d) Atrial activity:
   (e) Relationship:

8. Which of the following medications would you expect medical direction to order for this patient?
   a. atropine
   b. dopamine
   c. epinephrine
   d. nitroglycerin

While en route to the hospital, you notice the following change on the ECG monitor. (See Figure 12-3.) Your patient is still awake.

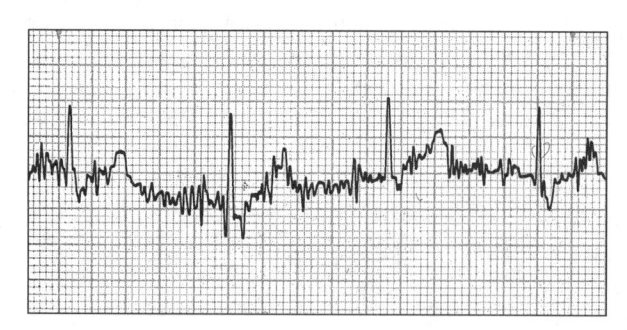

Figure 12-3

9. Which of the following is *not* a possible reason for the change in this patient's ECG?
   a. amplifier problem
   b. disconnected electrode
   c. movement
   d. ventricular fibrillation

The patient is delivered to the emergency department in stable condition. Her blood pressure is now 110/70. The physician orders a 12-lead ECG. Because the emergency department is extremely busy, you stay long enough to assist the nurse with this procedure.

10. Describe where you will attach the electrodes on this patient to obtain a 12-lead ECG.

Case Presentation #3 (Questions 11–14)

While off-duty, you are working out with weights at the local YMCA. Suddenly, a middle-aged man collapses on the indoor jogging track. You rush to his side and determine that he is in full cardiac arrest. A local physician comes to your aid with a pocket mask that he keeps in his locker. You both begin CPR and direct a bystander to call 9-1-1.

11. List the names of four possible rhythms that you might see if this patient were connected to a cardiac monitor.

   (a)

   (b)

   (c)

   (d)

Within minutes, the fire rescue EMTs arrive. They attach an automatic electrical device (AED) and deliver three shocks. After the third shock, the patient regains a pulse and spontaneous respirations. As the EMTs are measuring vital signs and applying high-concentration oxygen, the paramedics arrive. Vital signs are: pulse 68 and slightly irregular; BP 92/60; respirations 12 and shallow. The paramedics establish an IV and connect the patient to the cardiac monitor.

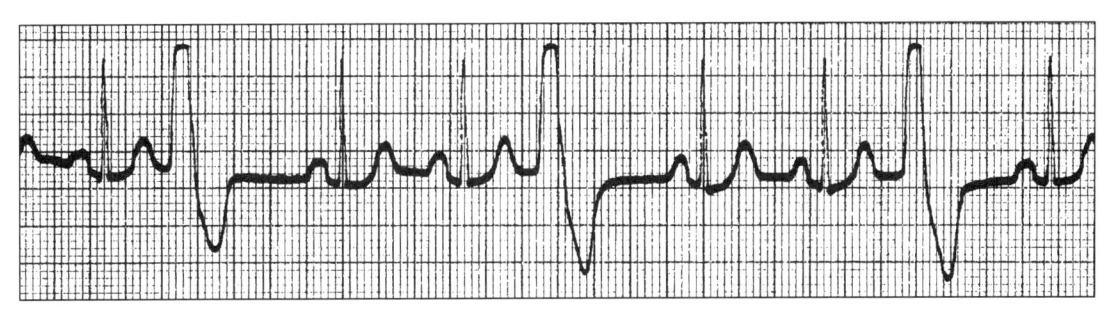

Figure 12-4

12. Identify the ectopic beats in this patient's ECG rhythm (see Figure 12-4), and describe their characteristics.

13. What drug can you expect the paramedics to administer to this patient? Explain your response.

You assist the EMTs with crowd control as the paramedics load the patient into the ambulance. He is transported to the closest hospital, which is 4 minutes away. After you report to work the next day, you inquire about this patient's outcome. You learn that he is stable in the Coronary Care Unit after receiving thrombolytic therapy.

14. What prehospital events of the day before most likely led to this patient's survival?

GENERAL REVIEW QUESTIONS

Rearrange the following components of the conduction system by placing them in the actual order of normal conduction through the heart.

15. ____
16. ____
17. ____
18. ____
19. ____
20. ____

a. Purkinje fibers
b. Sinoatrial (SA) node
c. Atrioventricular (AV) node
d. Internodal pathways
e. Bundle of His
f. Right and left bundle branches

Identify the four major sites of origin of an impulse in the heart and give their inherent rates per minute.

Sites **Rates**

21. _____ _____

22. _____ _____

23. _____ _____

24. _____ _____

Match the ECG component in Column 1 with the statement in Column 2 that best describes it.

Column 1

25. _____ QRS complex
26. _____ P wave
27. _____ T wave
28. _____ U wave
29. _____ PR segment

Column 2

a. Ventricular repolarization
b. Ventricular depolarization
c. Atrial depolarization
d. Part of final repolarization of ventricles
e. Atrial depolarization and delay in the AV node
f. Delay in the ventricles

Calculate heart rate for the following ECGs:

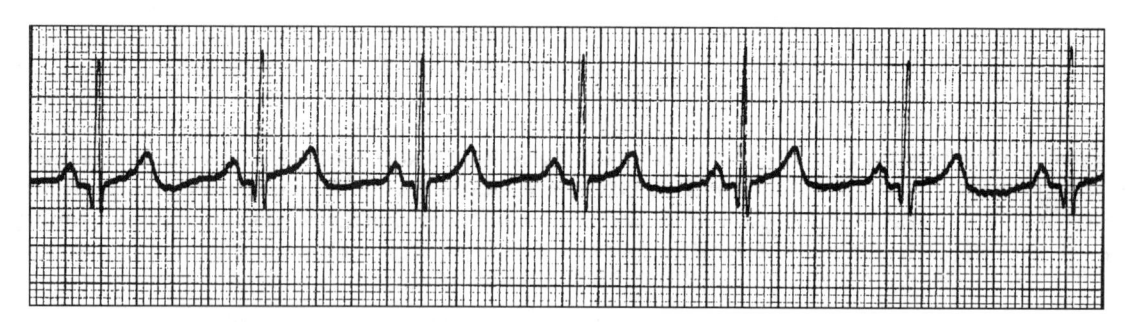

Figure 12-5 _____

30. Use 6-second method.   Rate: _____

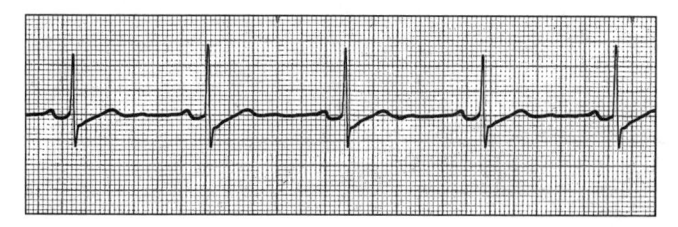

Figure 12-6 _____

31. Use small box method.   Rate: _____

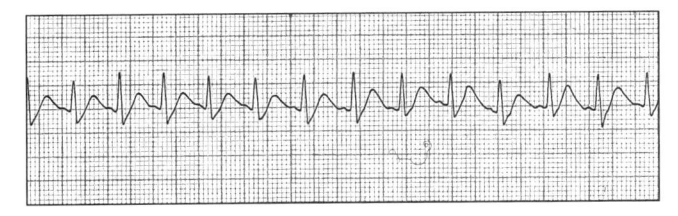

Figure 12-7

32. Use large box method.   Rate: _____

Match each rhythm in Column 1 with its corresponding description in Column 2.

Column 1

33. _____ Atrial fibrillation
34. _____ Sinus arrhythmia
35. _____ Atrial flutter
36. _____ Paroxysmal supraventricular tachycardia
37. _____ Premature junctional complex
38. _____ First-degree heart block
39. _____ Second-degree fixed AV block
40. _____ Bundle branch block

Column 2

a. Starts with a positive P wave and appears early
b. Normal rhythm with a rate that varies with respirations
c. Regular rhythm that begins in the AV node
d. Atrial pattern is a result of chaotic firing of the atrial muscle.
e. Sudden onset of tachycardia with a narrow QRS
f. PR interval that conducts may be normal or prolonged, but is constant.
g. PR interval of >.20 is constant with every beat.
h. Atrial activity causing a wide, >.12- second, QRS
i. Pattern of atrial activity is sawtoothed in appearance.

41. What is the name for the ability of cardiac cells to transmit an electrical impulse?
   a. automaticity
   b. conductivity
   c. depolarization
   d. excitability

42. What is the term for the ability of cardiac cells to initiate electrical discharges on their own, then recharge?
   a. automaticity
   b. contractibility
   c. excitability
   d. repolarization

43. When cardiac cells are stimulated by an electrical current, they electrically discharge or:
   a. depolarize.
   b. polarize.
   c. retract.
   d. repolarize.

44. Place the electrodes in the appropriate place on Figure 12-8 for each of the leads indicated by marking a (+) for positive and a (-) for negative.

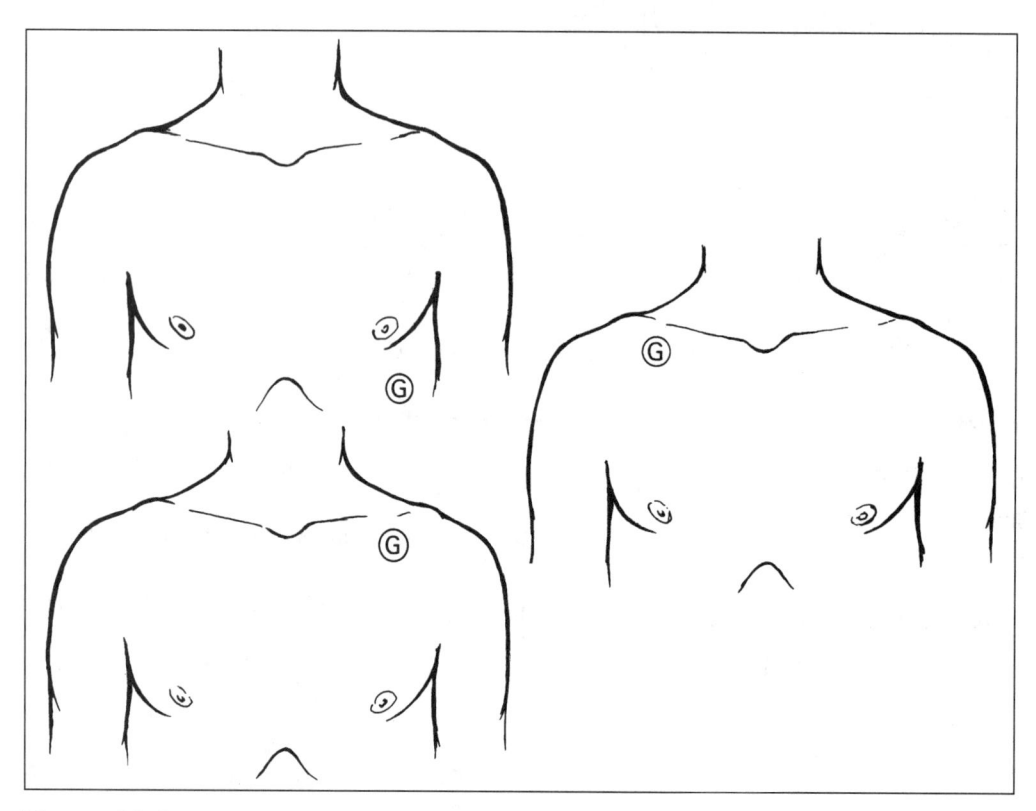

Figure 12-8 _____

Interpret each of the following ECGs:

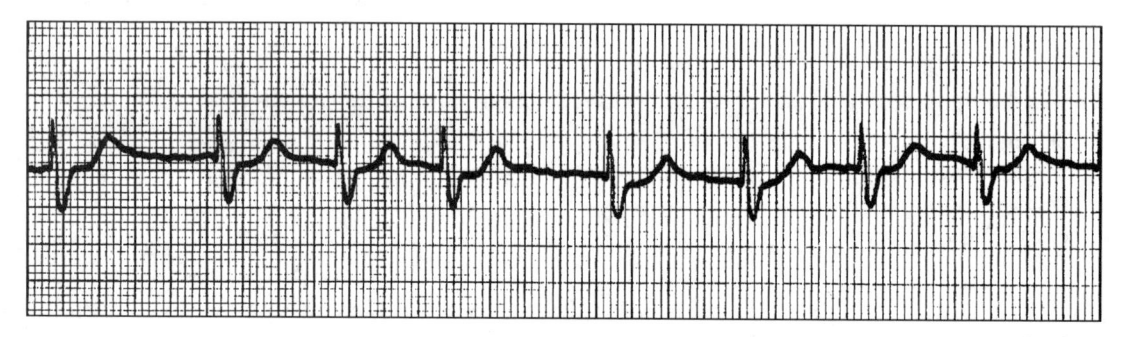

Figure 12-9 _____

45. _____

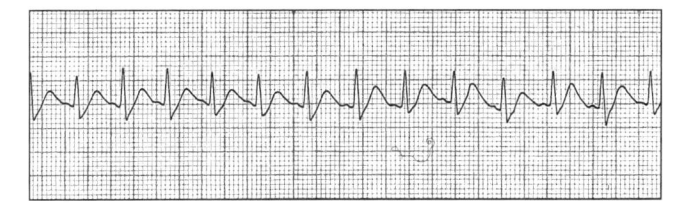

Figure 12-10

46. _____

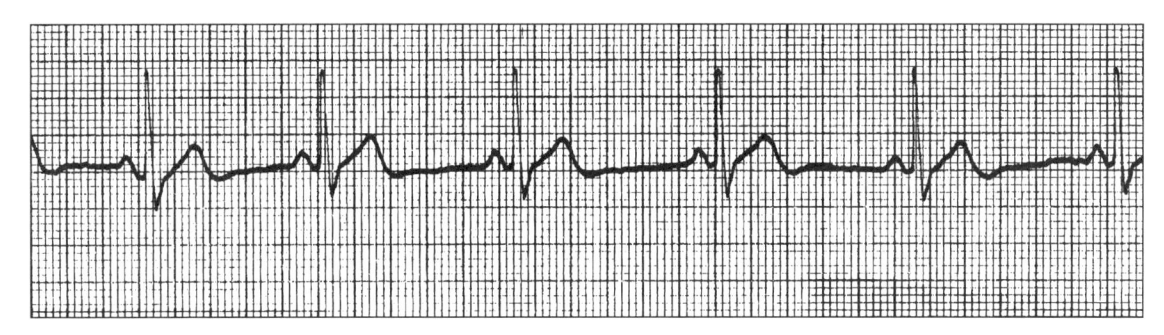

Figure 12-11

47. _____

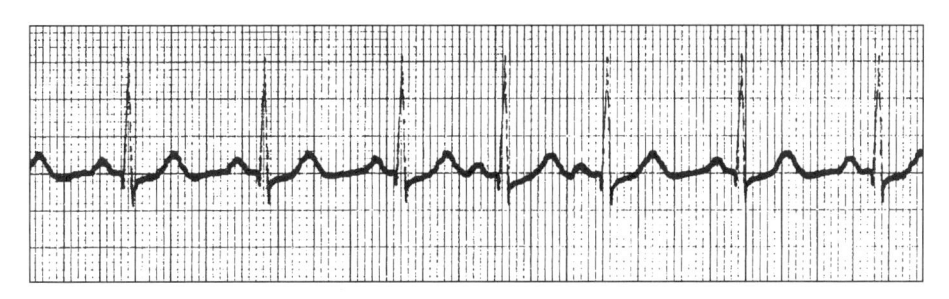

Figure 12-12

48. _____

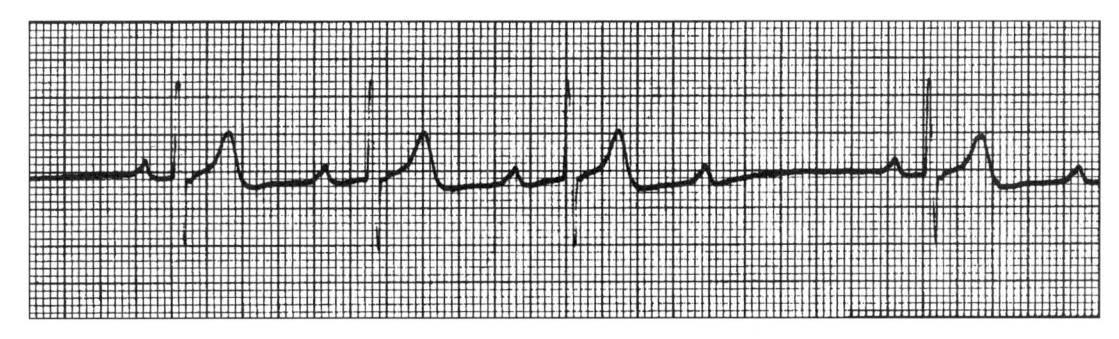

Figure 12-13

49. _____

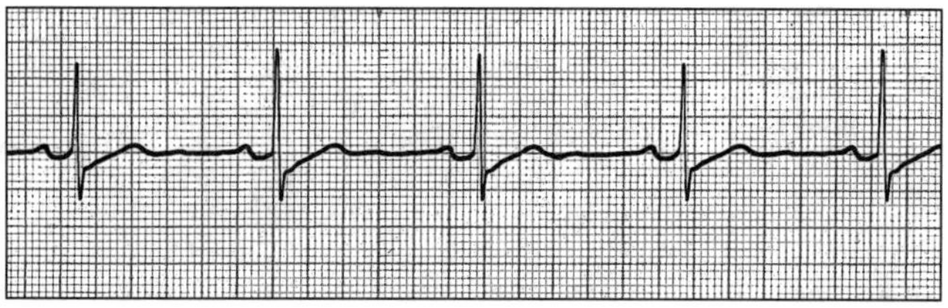

Figure 12-14 _____

50. _____

Answers to questions from chapter 12 can be found on page 425.

Chapter 13

Interpersonal Communication Skills

OBJECTIVES

1. Describe the importance of effective interpersonal communication skills.
2. Describe the three coping mechanisms that people may exhibit in response to stress.
3. Describe how the following factors can enhance or inhibit communication in an emergency situation:
   a. Introductions and first impressions
   b. Voice dynamics
   c. Eye contact
   d. Facial expression
   e. Body stance and posture
   f. Positioning
   g. Touching
   h. Good listening
4. Describe specific tactics for establishing trust and rapport.
5. Explain special communication techniques to employ when dealing with the following types of patients:
   a. Pediatric according to age range
   b. Geriatric
   c. Mentally impaired
   d. Foreign language speaking
   e. Hearing impaired
   f. Obstinate or potentially volatile persons
6. Discuss appropriate communication methods to use with families and bystanders.
7. Discuss the need for effective communication with professional colleagues.

CASE PRESENTATION #1 (QUESTIONS 1–3)

You are dispatched to a private residence for treatment of a man who is having a possible heart attack. Upon arrival, you find a 65-year-old man sitting on his bed. He is awake and alert and appears extremely frightened. His wife is standing by him and is sobbing hysterically.

1. The first step for establishing rapport in this situation is to:
   a. tell the patient to calm down and that you are in control.
   b. tell the wife to go into the other room.
   c. introduce yourself and tell the patient that you are there to help him.
   d. take the patient's vital signs and check the ECG monitor.

2. Briefly describe other key techniques for enhancing communication and fostering the patient's trust.

3. The wife is very upset and continues to cry. The best way for you to assist her is by doing all of the following EXCEPT:
    a. Keep her informed about the situation.
    b. Explain what you are doing for her husband and why you are doing it.
    c. Tell her to calm down so you can take care of her husband.
    d. Reassure her that you will be getting him to the hospital as soon as possible.

Case Presentation #2 (Questions 4-6)

You are dispatched to a scene involving a possible overdose. On arrival, you note that there are several people gathered in a crowded living room. The patient is shouting for you to "get out," that she doesn't want or need your help. Her friends are trying to calm her down.

4. Your first action in this situation should be to:
    a. tell her friends to leave the room.
    b. tell the patient to sit down and be quiet.
    c. ensure that the scene is safe.
    d. check for empty pill bottles.

5. To increase cooperation and defuse this situation, you should (circle all that apply):
    a. raise your voice above the level of the patient's to gain control.
    b. try to determine why the patient is upset and angry.
    c. get close to the patient and tell her to sit down so that you can examine her.
    d. be aware of how your posture and presence are affecting the situation.

6. Some of the patient's friends at the scene are very upset that she has allegedly taken several pills "to kill herself." You have managed successfully to establish rapport with the patient. To assist with "crowd control," you should do all of the following EXCEPT:
    a. Keep them informed and relate to them as needed.
    b. Try to determine who is the crowd "leader" and employ his or her help.
    c. Consider letting one of the friends stay close by the patient to provide reassurance.
    d. Tell the friends that they will have to leave the room so that you can attend to the patient.

General Review Questions

7. Match each of the terms in Column 1 with its BEST definition in Column 2.

   Column 1
   a. _____ Regression
   b. _____ Depression
   c. _____ Aggression

   Column 2
   1. Striking out verbally or physically against threats
   2. Closing from within and withdrawing from others
   3. Using behaviors that worked in earlier stages of development

Complete each sentence with the BEST answer:

8. Voice elements facilitate effective communication. The crucial elements include:

   (a) _____, (b) _____, (c) _____, and (d) _____.

9. Describe the benefits of good listening in interpersonal communication.

List two specific guiding principles that can help when one is dealing with the following age groups:

10. Infants

    (a)

    (b)

11. 9 to 17 months of age

    (a)

    (b)

12. 18 to 24 months of age

    (a)

    (b)

13. 2 to 3 years of age

    (a)

    (b)

14. 4 to 5 years of age

    (a)

    (b)

15. 6 to 12 years of age

    (a)

    (b)

16. Adolescents

    (a)

    (b)

17. When establishing rapport with geriatric patients, it is important to:
    a. use the patient's formal name (e.g., Mrs. Jones).
    b. speak slowly to the patient.
    c. enunciate words very clearly.
    d. demonstrate respect during the interview.
    e. all of the above.

18. Briefly discuss communication techniques to employ when dealing with a foreign language–speaking patient who is accompanied by an interpreter.

19. When communicating with hearing impaired patients, you should do all of the following EXCEPT:
    a. Ask the patient what will work best.
    b. Use sign language, if someone who knows it is available.
    c. Talk louder to the patient to enhance understanding.
    d. Use note writing in certain circumstances.
    e. Provide a well-lit area, if lip reading is being used.

20. List three reasons why professional communication with colleagues is important for the paramedic.

Answers to questions from chapter 13 can be found on page 427.

Chapter 14

Communication and Documentation

OBJECTIVES

1. Describe the overall significance of accurate communication of patient data in the prehospital setting.
2. Describe the two types of verbal reports and the goals and purposes of each.
3. List and discuss three general principles that should be utilized when presenting patient data.
4. Define "SOAP" format, and describe its use in communication of patient data.
5. Describe pertinent findings (positive and negative) and their importance in the verbal report.
6. Given a patient scenario, list the 11 components of a standard radio report and the order of presentation.
7. Discuss the techniques that contribute to effective radio communication.
8. List the purposes of the patient care report (PCR).
9. List and describe the components to include on a PCR.
10. Describe three important characteristics of a PCR.
11. Discuss three major pitfalls associated with the preparation of PCRs.
12. List 10 cases in the prehospital setting that are more likely to result in an inquiry or litigation.

CASE PRESENTATION #1 (QUESTIONS 1–14)

Your unit, Unit 1, is dispatched to the residence of a 68-year-old man with chest pain. Upon arrival, you find the patient alert and sitting in a chair in the living room. He states that the pain started approximately 30 minutes ago while he was reading a book. He describes the pain as a "squeezing" sensation in the center of his chest and says it is the "worst pain I've ever had in my life." He denies having pain anywhere else and tells you he has taken three nitroglycerin tablets without any relief. He feels very nauseated but is not short of breath. On physical examination, you find the following: skin is pale and diaphoretic; B/P is 84/60; pulse is 56 and weak; respirations are measured at 20. Medical history reveals that the patient has had hypertension for 15 years and he had a heart attack 5 years ago. The patient has no known allergies and currently is taking Isordil® and Catapres®.

After placing the patient on oxygen and applying the ECG monitor, you prepare him for transport. You establish an IV D5W TKO. ECG rhythm reveals sinus bradycardia. You retake his vital signs and find the following: B/P 94/60; pulse 62; respirations 20. The patient states that his pain is less intense now, and he is not feeling as nauseated. You are approximately 10 minutes away from St. Joseph's Medical Center.

Complete the following verbal report to on-line medical direction (OLMD).

1. Description of the scene: _____
   _____

2. Level of consciousness, age, and sex of the patient: _____

3. Chief complaint: _____

4. Vital signs: _____

5. Brief history of the present illness: _____
   _____

6. SAMPLE history S=

   A=

   M=

   P=

   L=

   E=

7. Associated signs and symptoms: _____
   _____

8. Physical examination findings: _____
   _____

9. Treatment provided before contact is made with OLMD: _____
   _____

10. Results of treatment: _____
    _____

11. Estimated time to arrival and destination: _____

12. List two significant "negative" findings that should be included in the verbal report, regarding the history and physical examination.

    (a)

    (b)

13. Write a concise, complete radio report that communicates the appropriate patient information to OLMD.

14. Document the patient's situation, using the SOAP format:

    S: _____

    _____

    _____

    O: _____

    _____

    A: _____

    _____

    P: _____

    _____

General Review Questions

15. The goal of radio reporting is to provide OLMD with a _____ image of the patient and his situation.

16. List six techniques that you can employ to enhance effective radio communication.

    (a)

    (b)

    (c)

    (d)

    (e)

    (f)

17. List three actions that you should avoid when transmitting via radio.

    (a)

    (b)

    (c)

18. Aside from documentation of patient care information, there are three other primary purposes of a patient care report (PCR). List and briefly explain each one.

    (a)

    (b)

    (c)

19. Describe the components of treatment data included on a PCR.

20. Failure to provide adequate document information on the PCR could: (Circle all that apply.)
    a. be appropriate in certain circumstances.
    b. be reviewed as poor patient care.
    c. contribute to a court's decision to award in favor of a patient.
    d. result in the provision of inappropriate care at the receiving facility.
    e. result in incomplete collection of the data needed for quality improvement.

21. Which of the following should be documented in cases involving patient refusal of care or transport? (Circle all that apply.)
    a. assessment findings, including history and physical examination findings
    b. that an explanation was given to the patient of the potential outcome of failure to obtain medical care
    c. a description of the patient's mental status
    d. that the patient was obviously intoxicated
    e. the patient's signature on the patient refusal statement

22. List five factors in the prehospital setting that are associated with an increased likelihood of inquiry or litigation.

   (a)

   (b)

   (c)

   (d)

   (e)

23. It is important to record "serial assessments" on the PCR, particularly **(a)** _____ and **(b)** _____. Discuss why.

Answers to questions from chapter 14 can be found on page 429.

Section 3A

SCENE AND PATIENT ASSESSMENT

CHAPTERS

15. Scene Assessment, Safety, and Control
16. Mechanism of Injury

Chapter 15

Scene Assessment, Safety, and Control

OBJECTIVES

1. Identify the types of potentially hostile or dangerous scenes.
2. Discuss scene safety in terms of priorities, potential hazards, and methods to minimize risks.
3. Describe precautions that should be taken when approaching a scene of potential gang violence.
4. Describe special considerations when entering the following potentially dangerous environments:
   a. Hazardous materials
   b. Radiation
   c. Farm emergencies
5. Identify clues to the nature of illness that should be pursued at the scene of medical calls.
6. Discuss appropriate methods of scene control.
7. Describe appropriate methods for managing family and bystanders at the scene of an emergency.
8. Describe precautions that should be taken to minimize the likelihood of disease transmission at the scene.

CASE PRESENTATION #1 (QUESTIONS 1–6)

At 1:30 a.m. on a busy Saturday morning, you are dispatched to the scene of a possible aggravated assault. The location of the call is out of your normal response area; it is in an area that is known to have a high rate of violent crime. Dispatch indicates that the caller simply said that a man had been seriously hurt in a fight and that there was a lot of bleeding.

1. As you quickly get en route to the scene, your first question to the dispatcher should be:
   a. Are there other potential patients?
   b. Have law enforcement personnel been dispatched?
   c. Is the patient conscious?
   d. Is this a residential or a business area?

When you arrive at the scene, you note that you are in a poorly lighted area in an old, run-down, older business section of town. A young man approaches your vehicle and says he can take you to the patient. Police officers have not arrived yet.

2. Your first priority should be to determine:
    a. if the patient is breathing.
    b. if the scene is safe.
    c. the mechanism of injury.
    d. whether additional help is needed.

3. Would it be important to take time to get personal protective equipment in place before you enter the scene? Briefly explain your answer.

Police units have arrived now to secure the scene. Allegedly, the victim's assailant is still in the area. The victim's friends have moved him from the street to a place inside a dilapidated building. You approach the building with the police officers.

4. While the police officers are crossing the doorway, where should you and your partner be positioned? Why?

Once you are safely inside of the building, you begin your assessment of the patient. He is conscious, and his ABCs are intact. He has been beaten with a crowbar, mostly in the head and neck area. He has contusions and lacerations and is bleeding heavily from the face. There is a strong smell of alcohol on his breath. No other injuries to the chest or abdominal region are obvious. Vital signs are: BP 140/70; pulse 110; and respirations 26. You gain control of the bleeding, and you prepare to apply cervical spine precautions. While you are doing these things, the patient becomes violent; he tells you that he does not want to go to the hospital.

5. How should you respond to patient? Briefly explain your answer.

You are able to convince the patient to go to the hospital, and you leave the scene with no further problem. The patient is delivered to the emergency department in stable condition. On your next shift of duty, the medical director calls to let you know that the patient was admitted to the hospital with a closed head injury. He reinforces the importance and appropriateness of the actions you took with this patient.

6. How does the medical director's information relate to medical accountability of the system and to legal considerations for you as a practicing paramedic?

CASE PRESENTATION #2 (QUESTIONS 7-10)

You are dispatched to the scene of a possible shooting at 10 p.m. on a Friday night. The location of the emergency is a neighborhood that is known to have frequent gang-related calls. Because of the potential dangers involved, the police have been dispatched also. Allegedly, the victim is located inside a residence.

7. While you are en route to the scene, you recall some basic personal safety considerations regarding entering a hostile or dangerous gang area. Briefly discuss them.

When you arrive at the scene, police officers are present. They tell you where the patient is and how the approach has been planned. They inform you that they have concerns about both weapons and the potential for violence at the scene. They also express concern about the confined area in which the patient is located.

8. Besides working with police assistance, what could you and your partner quickly do in the event of a problem? Briefly explain your response.

The police officers lead you to the patient. He is a 14-year-old boy who has been shot in the chest. He is unconscious. There are many bystanders in the crowded room, which makes it difficult for you to access the patient and evaluate his condition. One of the bystanders begins to shout at you angrily.

9. What immediate step(s) should you take to control the scene? (Circle all that apply.)
    a. Ask for police assistance in removing the hostile bystander.
    b. Consider moving the patient to another area.
    c. Eliminate any obvious noise distractions that can be removed easily.
    d. Request that people step out of the way so that you can evaluate the patient.
    e. Restrain the hostile bystander yourself to get him out of the way.

10. Once the scene is controlled and you are evaluating and taking care of the patient, what other appropriate methods can be used to help relieve family and/or bystander anxiety?

CASE PRESENTATION #3 (QUESTIONS 11–13)

You are dispatched to an apartment complex near a college campus for treatment of a possible overdose victim. Upon arrival at the scene, you find a young woman lying on a couch in the living room. She appears to be unconscious. No bystanders are present.

11. After securing her ABCs, what are some clues at the scene that you should look for?

You find an empty syringe near the patient. There is no evidence of pills. The patient has needle tracks, and her pupils are pinpoint. Vital signs are: BP 120/76; pulse 82; and respirations 6 and shallow.

12. You should anticipate administering which of the following medications?
    a. activated charcoal
    b. epinephrine
    c. Narcan®
    d. nebulized albuterol

Meanwhile, the patient's roommate arrives on the scene. She tells you that the patient has been depressed and is a heavy drug user. She also tells you that her roommate is primarily a heroin user, but that she often takes several different drugs. She does not have any idea what drugs the patient might have taken today. While you are preparing the patient for transport, her roommate becomes upset and starts to cry.

13. What could you do to reassure her, and perhaps lessen her anxiety?

General Review Questions

14. Why is knowledge of the response area an important factor in scene management?

15. Name three scenes that can produce potentially hostile situations.

  (a)

  (b)

  (c)

16. Briefly describe special scene safety considerations for entering the following potentially dangerous environments:

  (a) Hazardous materials

  (b) Radiation

  (c) Farm emergencies

17. When you are responding to motor vehicle collisions, where should the ambulance be parked to ensure your safety?

  a. as close as possible to the accident scene
  b. between oncoming traffic and the emergency scene
  c. in the middle of the highway to block traffic
  d. wherever the police tell you to position the vehicle

18. Briefly discuss distractions at the scene that you can eliminate to gain scene control.

Answers to questions from chapter 15 can be found on page 431.

Chapter 16

Mechanism of Injury

OBJECTIVES

1. Describe the relationship between a high index of suspicion and mechanism of injury.
2. List the three time "phases" of a traumatic incident and the historical information included in each one.
3. Explain the significance of minimizing on-scene time in prehospital trauma care.
4. Explain how the three basic physics laws of force and energy relate to trauma and injury potential.
5. Name three types of collisions that can occur during change of speed impact.
6. Describe shear and compression forces and the types of injuries each can cause.
7. List important historical information to consider when evaluating mechanism of injury in motor vehicle collisions.
8. Describe the injury patterns produced by the following types of collisions:
   a. Head-on   c. Rear-end
   b. Side/lateral   d. Rollover
9. Explain the advantages and potential disadvantages of seatbelts and air bags.
10. Describe the forces, mechanisms, and injury patterns most often involved in vehicle-pedestrian accidents, falls, hangings, and explosions.
11. List important items of historical information to gather in penetrating trauma incidents and explain their relationship to potential injuries.

CASE PRESENTATION #1 (QUESTIONS 1–6)

You are dispatched to a motor vehicle collision that has occurred on a busy, two-lane state highway. Upon arrival, you find two vehicles involved in a head-on collision; each appears to have sustained significant damage on impact. The posted speed limit at the accident site is 55 miles per hour (mph).

1. As you survey the scene, what is important to recall about the impact of a head-on collision?

Further evaluation reveals the following information:

Car #1: The driver, who was alone in the vehicle, has been declared dead at the scene by a police officer. You confirm this and, according to local protocol, you do not resuscitate.

Car #2: Two people are inside—the driver and one passenger; the front end of the car is demolished.
Driver: A middle-aged man who was found down and under the steering wheel; he is unconscious, but is breathing and has a pulse.
Passenger: A school-aged child who was ejected from the vehicle and found 15 feet away. The patient is face down on the ground, and is bleeding from the head and crying.

2. Although multiple injuries are possible, based on the driver's position, you immediately suspect trauma to what region of the body? Briefly explain your response.

3. Considering the energy, impact, and change of speed, briefly describe the "three collisions" that were experienced by the passenger in Car #2.

For each of the following statements (4–6), circle the correct response, True or False. Briefly explain your answer.

4. Fatal injuries are probable for the passenger in Car #2.

    TRUE   **FALSE**

Briefly explain your answer: _____

5. Shear injuries occur infrequently in head-on collisions with rapid deceleration.

    TRUE   **FALSE**

Briefly explain your answer: _____

6. The speed at which these vehicles were traveling is a significant factor in terms of injury potential.

    TRUE   **FALSE**

Briefly explain your answer: _____

CASE PRESENTATION #2 (QUESTIONS 7 AND 8)

You have responded to a motor vehicle incident. On arrival, you find a small Toyota that is seriously damaged and positioned upside-down. The driver, who is the only occupant, is out of the car and is walking around. He has two minor head lacerations; he states that he feels fine and doesn't need to go to the hospital. He is alert and oriented, and vital signs are: BP 100/60; pulse 110; and respirations 20.

7. Based on this information, briefly explain why it would be important for you to encourage him to go to the hospital.

8. If the patient does not consent to treatment or transport, what information should be documented in the prehospital care report?

GENERAL REVIEW QUESTIONS

Each traumatic incident has three distinct phases that can affect patient outcome. Match the factor in Column 1 with its corresponding phase in Column 2.

Column 1

9. _____ Type and level of prehospital care given
10. _____ Age and physical condition of the victim in the car collision
11. _____ Position of the victim in the car before the collision
12. _____ Time from the incident until delivery of definitive care
13. _____ Energy transfer (to patient or elsewhere)
14. _____ Whether the victim was wearing a seatbelt
15. _____ Alcohol or substance abuse
16. _____ Current medications

Column 2

a. Pre-occurrence
b. Occurrence
c. Post-occurrence

17. The most important factor for increasing patient survivability in prehospital trauma care is:
   a. having an enhanced 9-1-1 system in your area.
   b. minimizing the time from occurrence of the incident to definitive care at the hospital.
   c. replacing blood loss using IV fluids and a PASG.
   d. recognizing the signs and symptoms of common injuries.

18. A Lincoln Continental that was traveling at 80 miles an hour skidded off the highway and struck a tree. The driver, who weighs 250 pounds, is alone in the vehicle. In terms of the law of kinetic energy, which factor is most important?
   a. the effect of hitting a stationary object
   b. the patient's weight
   c. the car's speed (80 mph)
   d. the size and type of automobile

19. Define the following terms; discuss associated organ injuries that are likely to occur with rapid change of speed:

   (a) Shear

   (b) Compression

20. You are dispatched to the scene of a motor vehicle collision. Two cars are involved in a rear-end collision. List at least three questions that you should ask yourself at the scene that could assist in your determination of the mechanism of injury.

21. Briefly describe the injury patterns that may be produced by the following types of collisions:

   (a) Rear-end collisions

   (b) Side impact/rotational collisions

   (c) Rollovers

   (d) All-terrain vehicle (ATV) collisions

   (e) Tractor rollovers

22. A distinct advantage of the lap belt/shoulder harness seatbelt is that:
   a. backward forces are greatly reduced.
   b. ejection possibility is reduced.
   c. head injuries are unlikely to occur.
   d. organ collision rarely occurs.

23. List two disadvantages of air bags.

   (a)

   (b)

24. Which of the following is *not* true about motorcycle accidents?
   a. Bigger bikes are associated with increased injury potential.
   b. Ejection and resultant severe injuries are highly likely.
   c. Head or spinal injuries rarely occur if a helmet is worn.
   d. Leather and vinyl clothing help to reduce abrasion injuries.

25. Describe the response reaction and injury potential for both adults and children who are involved in vehicle-pedestrian accidents?

   (a) Adults

   (b) Children

26. A 50-year-old man jumped 20 feet from a ladder and landed on his feet. He is conscious and is complaining of tingling and numbness in his legs. You immediately suspect:
   a. compression injury of the spine.
   b. flail chest.
   c. head injury.
   d. pericardial tamponade.

27. A 48-year-old man was trapped inside a building in which a major explosion occurred. You find him unconscious, with obvious head injuries. Briefly discuss three factors associated with an explosion that could have contributed to his injuries.

   (a)

   (b)

   (c)

28. Cavitation that occurs with penetrating trauma typically produces:
   a. a "through and through" type of injury.
   b. bloodless injuries of no immediate concern.
   c. pressure waves that push surrounding organs out of place.
   d. shear injuries of the aorta or kidneys.

29. Briefly list historical factors that are important for the paramedic to consider when treating patients with penetrating trauma resulting from either stab wounds or gunshot wounds.

   (a)   Stab wounds

   (b)   Gunshot wounds

Answers to questions from chapter 16 can be found on page 433.

Section 3B
Assessment of the Critical Patient

CHAPTERS

17. Initial Assessment
18. The Patient With Airway and Breathing Compromise
19. The Patient Without a Pulse
20. The Patient With Compromised Circulation
21. The Critical Trauma Patient
22. The Critical Pediatric Patient

Chapter 17

Initial Assessment

OBJECTIVES

1. Describe the purpose of the initial patient assessment.
2. List the steps of the initial assessment in sequential order and describe how each is performed.
3. Describe how to use one's senses to help recognize immediately life-threatening conditions.
4. Explain the acronym AVPU.
5. Describe how the initial assessment of a patient's airway differs between trauma and medical patients.
6. Describe the signs and symptoms and management of the following life-threatening conditions:
   a. Unconsciousness
   b. Airway obstruction
   c. Absent breathing
   d. Absent pulse
   e. Severe bleeding

CASE PRESENTATION #1 (QUESTIONS 1-10)

You are dispatched to a call for treatment of an unconscious patient. When you arrive, an engine crew is on the scene. An engine crew member meets you and states that the patient collapsed shortly before their arrival, and that he is now in a "semiconscious" state. He also tells you that the patient has long-standing heart problems, and that he complained of chest pain just before he passed out.

1. You arrive at the patient's side. Your first priority is to evaluate the patient's:
   a. airway.
   b. breathing.
   c. level of consciousness.
   d. pulse.

The patient is somewhat combative as you first approach him, and he responds to loud verbal commands. You note that his skin is sweaty and pale in appearance.

2. What is your next assessment priority?

His vital signs are as follows: BP 100/60; pulse 42 and weak; respirations 10 and shallow. His wife tells you that he was getting ready to play tennis when he suddenly felt weak and had chest pain. She is extremely anxious because his symptoms are very similar to those that occurred 5 years ago when he had his heart attack.

3. What should you do to manage his respiratory status? Explain why.

4. Given the urgency of the situation, what should you do or say to reassure the patient's wife?

You manage his respirations and prepare to perform a 12-lead ECG. The patient's wife tells you that the only medications he is taking are nitroglycerin and Inderal®. He took some nitroglycerin before the engine crew arrived, but experienced no relief of symptoms.

5. What are some possible reasons for the ineffectiveness of the nitroglycerin?

6. What additional assessment procedures should you perform to evaluate the patient's circulatory status?

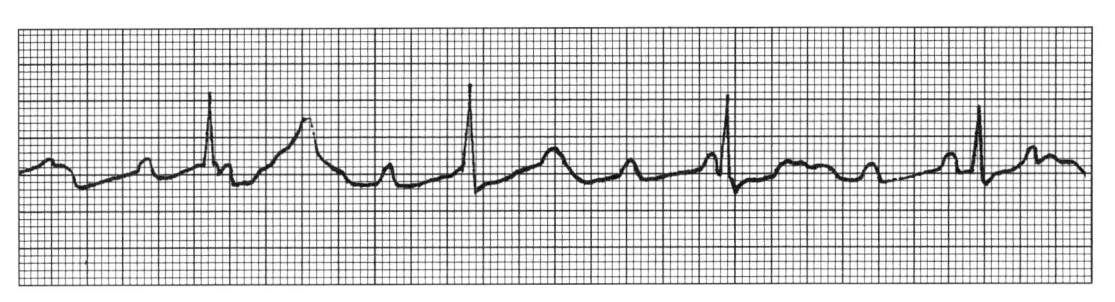

The patient's ECG results are shown in Figure 17-1.

Figure 17-1

7. This rhythm is best described as:
   a. sinus rhythm.
   b. sinus rhythm with first-degree heart block.
   c. second-degree heart block.
   d. third-degree heart block.
   e. a wandering atrial pacemaker.

Analysis of the 12-lead ECG shows the possibility of an acute myocardial infarction. You prepare for transport. The patient is awake now, but he is very confused and very pale.

8. You could anticipate orders from medical direction to include:
   a. atropine administration.
   b. adenosine administration.
   c. noninvasive pacing.
   d. lidocaine administration.
   e. a and c

9. Given the patient's history and physical findings, you would conclude that he is likely to be which of these—acidotic or alkalotic? Explain your response.

10. During transport to the emergency department, you should closely monitor his airway, breathing, and circulatory status by: _____

Case Presentation #2 (Questions 11-14)

On a hot Sunday afternoon, you are dispatched to a stadium for treatment of a medical emergency. The temperature is 102° F. A concert is taking place at the stadium, and more than 30,000 people are in attendance. On arrival, you are directed immediately to a first-aid station. You find the patient lying on a cot. She appears to be in her mid-twenties and is lying very still.

11. To evaluate her level of consciousness, what should you do first?
    a. Pinch both arms to elicit a response.
    b. Perform a sternal rub.
    c. Shake her gently, while talking to her.
    d. Immediately help her to sit up.

The patient easily responds to you. She is belligerent and verbally abusive toward you and your partner.

12. Given her responses, you know that which of the following is intact?
    a. airway
    b. breathing
    c. pulse
    d. a, b, and c

As you continue your assessment, you discover that the patient has been drinking and has been in the hot sun all afternoon. She ate a full lunch about an hour ago. When she passed out, her friends brought her to the first-aid station.

13. Your next assessment priority should be to:
    a. check the ECG.
    b. look for needle tracks.
    c. obtain further history from bystanders.
    d. obtain vital signs.

You find out that the patient is allegedly a drug user, but it is believed that she has taken no drugs today. Her pulse is 100, and is strong and regular; respirations are 16. She has no known medical problems and apparently was feeling fine until today.

14. Based on the information that you have accumulated thus far, and without a more detailed history and physical, you most likely suspect:
    a. drug overdose.
    b. heart attack.
    c. heat exhaustion.
    d. hypoglycemia.

General Review Questions

15. The primary objective of the initial assessment is to:
    a. correlate the relevance of the medical history with the current situation.
    b. determine if there are life-threatening problems that require immediate intervention.
    c. obtain an adequate history so that you can provide appropriate treatment.
    d. perform a physical examination that is consistent with the chief complaint.

16. An initial assessment procedure that differs for trauma patients versus medical patients is:
    a. the approach used for counting the respiratory rate and evaluating the respiratory status.
    b. the method that is used to determine the level of consciousness.
    c. that for the trauma patient steps of the assessment are performed en route to the hospital.
    d. the technique for opening the airway in unconscious patients.

17. Provide the meaning for each letter of the following acronym:

    A —

    V —

    P —

    U —

18. What is the first step that should be taken in an unconscious patient to relieve a suspected airway obstruction?

19. Your patient has been in a motor vehicle collision. He does not respond to any stimuli. His airway is clear, and he is breathing 6 times per minute. Lung sounds are clear. Your next step is to:
    a. assess for a tension pneumothorax.
    b. check circulation.
    c. prepare to intubate.
    d. ventilate with a BVM device or demand valve.

20. It is best to perform initial assessment of circulatory status by evaluating the patient's:
    a. blood pressure.
    b. capillary refill.
    c. pulse.
    d. pulse oximetry reading.
    e. skin color and temperature.

21. At which assessment location should the pulse be checked in the following patients?

    (a) Unconscious adult:

    (b) Conscious infant:

    (c) Conscious adult:

22. If the patient does not have a pulse, the first procedure that you should perform is:
   a. administration of intracardiac epinephrine.
   b. application of quick-look paddles to assess rhythm.
   c. a precordial thump.
   d. intubation.

23. A rapid, weak pulse could indicate: (Circle all that apply.)
   a. cardiac arrest.
   b. heart failure.
   c. inadequate circulating blood volume.
   d. life-threatening dysrhythmias.
   e. shock.

24. In the initial approach to assessment, the paramedic can use all four senses to form a first impression of the patient. Briefly discuss some examples of the use of the four senses in the initial assessment procedure.

Answers to questions from chapter 17 can be found on page 435.

Chapter 18

The Patient With Airway and Breathing Compromise

OBJECTIVES

1. Describe the normal anatomy of the respiratory system.
2. Describe the normal physiology of breathing.
3. List various causes of respiratory distress.
4. Describe the history and assessment of the patient experiencing respiratory distress.
5. Describe various abnormal breath sounds and their significance.
6. List signs and symptoms of respiratory distress.
7. Describe the management of various patient conditions that present with respiratory distress.
8. Identify normal and abnormal values for tidal volume, respiratory rate, blood gases, and pulse oximetry.

CASE PRESENTATION #1 (QUESTIONS 1–6)

You are dispatched to a cafe that is 2 minutes from your location for a "patient choking." On arrival, you find a 60-year-old woman who is lying on the floor and is surrounded by cafe employees. They tell you that, while the woman was eating, she suddenly became anxious, began clutching her throat, and was unable to talk. An employee who believed that the woman was choking quickly attempted to clear the patient's airway by using back blows and abdominal thrusts, until the patient lost consciousness just minutes before you arrived.

1. Was the initial treatment that was provided by the cafe employee an appropriate action? Explain your response.

Your initial assessment reveals that the patient is unconscious and is unresponsive to pain. She has a carotid pulse but is not breathing. Her skin is cyanotic and moist. Your partner immediately opens the patient's airway using the head tilt/chin lift method. Even after the patient's head has been repositioned and you have performed abdominal thrusts, you are unsuccessful in ventilating this patient using a BVM and 100% oxygen.

2. At this point, should you consider performing a cricothyrotomy? If not, describe the next appropriate intervention.

You successfully remove what appears to be a large food bolus from the patient's pharynx. She remains unconscious. Her pulse is weaker and slower. She is moving air, but her breathing rate is 6 per minute. Your partner, who is eager to assist and is a new EMT, performs rescue breathing for the patient. You observe that he appears somewhat nervous while ventilating the patient at a rate of 24 per minute. You instruct the EMT to ventilate the patient more slowly.

3. Explain the problem that can occur if the patient is ventilated too quickly. How can this be prevented from happening?

4. List the assessment findings that would indicate that this patient is being oxygenated adequately.

The EMT continues to provide respiratory assistance as you begin transport. You contact medical direction while en route. Your ETA at the hospital is 7 minutes.

5. Is there any indication that additional treatment should be provided en route? Explain your response.

The patient's condition has improved on arrival to the emergency department. She is breathing spontaneously and moans when you call her name loudly. Her vital signs are: BP 134/88; pulse 86 and regular; respirations 18 and normal. A cardiac monitor shows normal sinus rhythm. The physician orders a chest radiograph and arterial blood gas assessment to be performed while the patient is being monitored closely. Her pulse oximetry reads 94% on room air. The emergency physician praises you for a job well done and states that this patient's respiratory status is back to normal.

6. What would most likely be her pCO_2 reading, if her condition has returned to normal?

CASE PRESENTATION # 2 (QUESTIONS 7–14)

Around midnight, you are dispatched to a bar in a rough neighborhood. Your patient is a 26-year-old man who was stabbed in the chest during a fight with another patron. They were both reported to be intoxicated. Police are on the scene; when you arrive, they lead you to the patient. The patient is leaning against the wall screaming obscenities at his assailant and telling the police to arrest the man who tried to kill him. You attempt to calm the patient so that you can examine his chest, and your partner prepares to measure his vital signs.

7. At this point, what can you conclude about this patient's respiratory status from your observations?

8. Describe how you should assess this patient's chest injuries.

When the patient finally stops screaming, you note an audible hissing sound coming from his chest. On examination, the patient has an approximately 1-inch wound to the right anterior chest below the nipple. Bleeding is minimal. His breath sounds are slightly diminished on the same side. You administer high-concentration oxygen and prepare to dress his wound quickly while your partner measures his vital signs. His vital signs are: BP 100/60; pulse 112 and regular; respirations 24 and slightly labored.

9. Based on your assessment findings, what is this patient experiencing?
    a. flail chest
    b. pulmonary edema
    c. simple pneumothorax
    d. sucking chest wound

10. Describe how you would dress this patient's chest wound. Explain why you would use this technique.

You quickly load the patient and begin transport to a Level I trauma center. Your ETA is 12 minutes. While en route, you initiate an IV of Ringer's lactate and connect him to the cardiac monitor. The monitor reading indicates sinus tachycardia. When you are approximately 5 minutes from the hospital, the patient begins to develop increased respiratory distress. The right chest is now hyperresonant, with diminishing breath sounds. You also note subcutaneous emphysema in the tissue surrounding the chest wound.

11. Was your transport priority appropriate? Explain your response.

12. What is most likely causing this patient's worsening respiratory distress, and what should be the initial treatment?

13. List an additional assessment finding that would confirm your suspicions.

The patient responds favorably to your additional treatment. He is in stable condition when he is delivered to the emergency department. His vital signs are unchanged. After chest tube placement, he is taken to the operating room.

14. Describe the procedure that would have been indicated if your initial treatment had not relieved this patient's increasing respiratory difficulty.

CASE PRESENTATION #3 (QUESTIONS 15–19)

You are dispatched to a private residence in the middle of the night for a "breathing difficulty." The patient is a 2-year-old girl who has been ill for the past 3 days with a barking cough and low-grade fever that seems to be worse at night.

15. Based on the information provided by dispatch, you suspect that this patient is experiencing:
 a. asthma.
 b. croup.
 c. epiglottitis.
 d. pneumonia.

When you arrive, the father meets you at the door and leads you to a steamy bathroom where you find the mother and child. The patient is sitting upright on the mother's lap; she appears to be in mild respiratory distress. You note nasal flaring and a barking cough. Her apical pulse is 160, and her respirations are 40. Her skin is warm to the touch, and it is moist from the shower. No cyanosis is present. The mother feels that the child's condition has improved somewhat since she has been running the shower.

16. Is it possible that running the shower did improve the patient's condition? Explain your response.

17. Why should you limit your physical examination of this patient to the essentials? Why is it especially important to avoid examination of the oropharynx?

You bundle the child in a blanket and take her to the ambulance. You administer nebulized humidified oxygen while she is sitting on her mother's lap. Your ETA at the children's hospital is 7 minutes. You contact medical direction while en route. The physician orders no additional treatment.

18. What assessment findings related to the respiratory system would indicate progression of the obstruction?

19. If this patient's condition worsens en route, what medication may be indicated?

The patient is delivered to the emergency department in an improved condition. She is treated and dismissed the same night.

GENERAL REVIEW QUESTIONS

20. Label (Figure 18-1) the upper and lower airways.

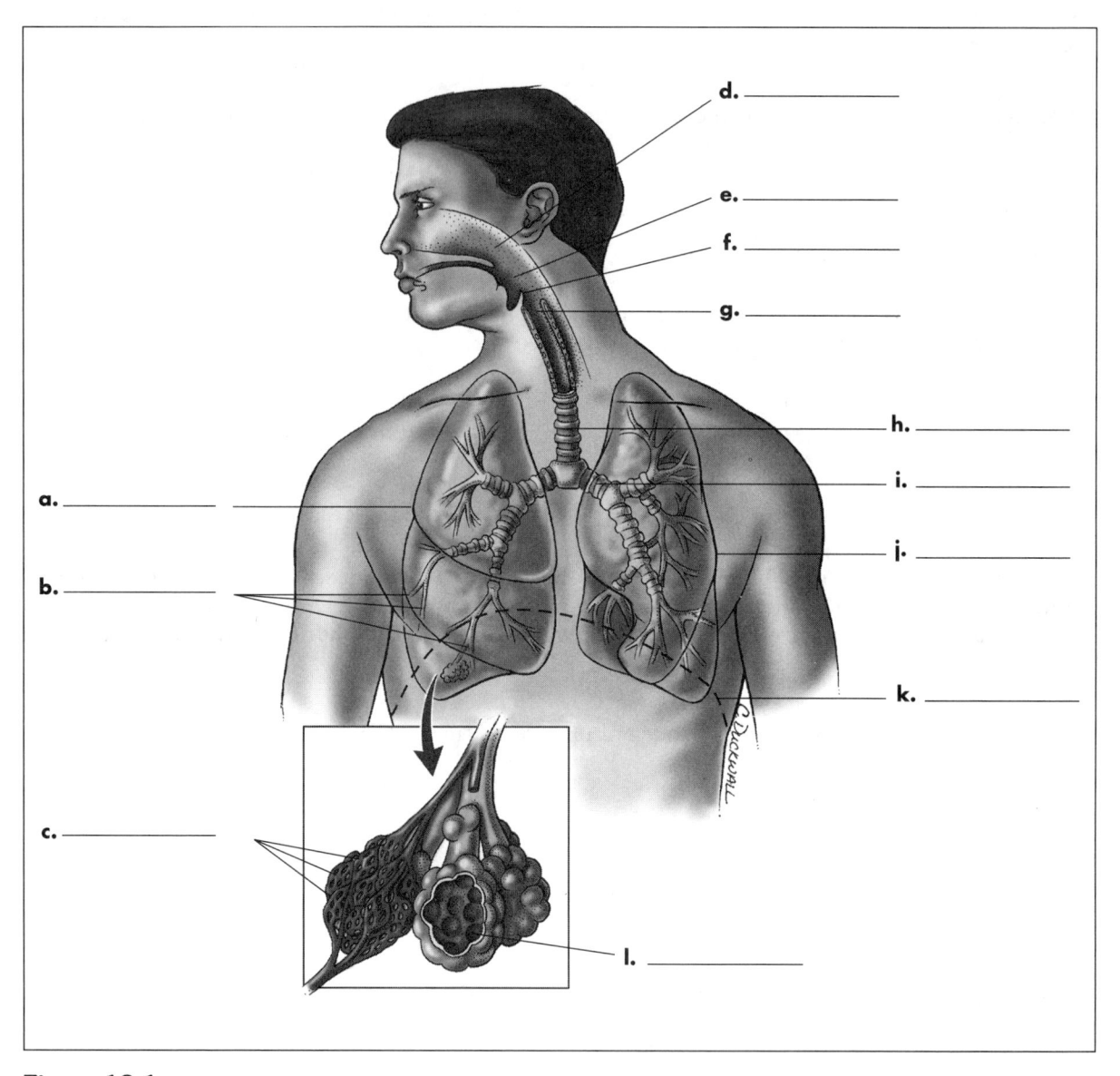

a. _____
b. _____
c. _____
d. _____
e. _____
f. _____
g. _____
h. _____
i. _____
j. _____
k. _____
l. _____

Figure 18-1

Match the term in Column 2 with its correct description in Column 1.

Column 1

21. _____ Membrane enclosing the lungs

22. _____ A dome-shaped muscle used in breathing

23. _____ Membrane lining the thoracic cavity

24. _____ Area between the membranes of the lungs and the thoracic cavity

Column 2

a. Pleural space
b. Visceral pleura
c. Diaphragm
d. Parietal pleura
e. Retroperitoneum

In the space provided, write the term for each description of abnormal lung sounds.

25. _____ Rattling sounds caused by excessive mucus in the larger airways

26. _____ Harsh sounds (like pieces of dried leather being rubbed together) that are created by inflammation of the pleura

27. _____ Fine, crackling sounds created by fluid in the smaller airways

28. _____ Often indicates upper airway obstruction, usually occurring when the tongue obstructs the airway of an unconscious, supine patient

29. _____ High-pitched sound, described as a seal bark, that results from an upper airway obstruction

30. _____ Whistling sounds that result from bronchoconstriction or from edema that narrows the airways

31. In the healthy adult at rest, what is the normal value for each of the following?

  (a) Tidal volume

  (b) Respiratory rate

  (c) Oxygen saturation

32. Identify the two situations in which chest thrusts are performed instead of abdominal thrusts to treat a conscious adult with an airway obstruction.

  (a)

  (b)

33. List four common causes of upper airway obstruction.

  (a)

  (b)

  (c)

  (d)

34. List the three lung diseases that are classified as chronic obstructive pulmonary disease (COPD).

  (a)

  (b)

  (c)

Briefly describe the appropriate treatment and rationale for each of the following patient conditions:

35. A conscious 56-year-old man is in *severe* respiratory distress after crashing his vehicle into a light pole at high speed. He has tenderness and bruising to his anterior chest and asymmetrical movement with respirations. Breath sounds are equal; neck veins and heart sounds are normal. Vital signs are: BP 122/80; pulse 96; and respirations 20.

36. A 32-year-old woman has been stabbed in the right chest with a screwdriver. She is awake but appears to be in *severe* respiratory distress (she is breathing 28 times per minute). Her pulse is weak and rapid, her skin is pale and diaphoretic, and her neck veins are flat. Breath sounds are decreased on the right and dull to percussion. She has postural vital signs.

37. A 19-year-old man is experiencing an acute onset of dyspnea. The patient is sitting upright and is clutching an empty metered dose inhaler. He is unable to answer your questions because of his labored breathing. He has audible wheezing bilaterally and retraction of the neck muscles on inhalation. The skin is moist, and nail beds are cyanotic. His vital signs are: BP 128/84; pulse 124 and regular; respirations 28 and labored.

38. A 64-year-old woman awakened in the middle of the night with severe shortness of breath. The patient experienced some relief when sitting upright. She is obviously struggling to breathe, and gurgling breath sounds are heard even without a stethoscope. She has pitting edema around both ankles and is cyanotic around the lips. She has been out of her two medications, Lanoxin® and Diazide®, for three days. Her vital signs are: BP 160/90; pulse 98 and irregular; respirations 26 and labored.

39. Which of the following is true regarding normal respiration?
   a. Changes in pO_2 play the most important role in the control of respiration.
   b. Muscle movement reduces lung volume during inspiration.
   c. Chemoreceptors in the lungs monitor the pO_2 level.
   d. The medulla is the center that primarily regulates breathing.

40. Signs and symptoms of complete airway obstruction include:
   a. a seal bark cough during inhalation.
   b. expiratory wheezing.
   c. fever with a productive cough.
   d. inability to cough or speak.

41. Which of the following may be elicited by palpation of the chest?
   a. diminished or absent breath sounds
   b. symmetry of chest wall movement
   c. presence of abnormal breath sounds
   d. distended neck veins

42. The purpose of the Sellick maneuver is to:
   a. prevent vomiting.
   b. obtain better visualization of the cords.
   c. improve oxygenation before intubation.
   d. clear an airway obstruction.

43. Pulse oximetry is most accurate when it is used to evaluate the adequacy of oxygenation in which of the following groups of patients?
   a. patients with carbon monoxide poisoning
   b. patients who are suffering from smoke inhalation
   c. infants and children
   d. patients who are being intubated

Answers to questions from chapter 18 can be found on page 436.

Chapter 19

The Patient Without a Pulse

1. Describe the anatomy and physiology of the cardiovascular system.
2. Define the following terms:
   a. Systole
   b. Diastole
   c. Cardiac output
   d. Stroke volume
   e. Preload
   f. Afterload
   g. Depolarization
   h. Repolarization
   i. Automaticity
   j. Contractility
3. Describe the normal sequence of electrical conduction in the heart.
4. Identify the assessment steps in determining that a patient is in cardiac arrest.
5. Describe the purpose and significance of early CPR and defibrillation.
6. Identify the critical findings, including cardiac rhythms, in pulseless patients from various causes.
7. Describe the different management approaches to various patient conditions that present with pulselessness.
8. Identify medications commonly used to correct ventricular fibrillation or pulseless ventricular tachycardia, pulseless electrical activity, and asystole.
9. Describe how the general management approach may vary in a patient who is pulseless as a result of associated trauma, electric shock, near-drowning, or hypothermia.

CASE PRESENTATION #1 (QUESTIONS 1–6)

On a cloudy day, you are dispatched to a high school football field for "players down" after being struck by lightning. The panicked caller reports that one victim appears to be dead and the other two are awake, but their conditions are unknown.

1. It would have been helpful if dispatch had discussed with the caller what two factors that have a significant impact on the pulseless patient's outcome?

   (a)

   (b)

As you approach the scene, you notice that one of the victims is sitting up and talking; another is lying on the ground but is moving his head and extremities. The third victim is receiving CPR from his coach.

2. Which patient has the highest priority? Explain your response.

You and your partner perform a rapid assessment of these patients. You evaluate the patient who is receiving CPR, while your partner evaluates the other two victims.

3. What are the initial steps in assessment of the patient who is receiving CPR?

Your partner reports that the other two victims are shaken but awake, and their vital signs are stable. An additional paramedic unit arrives on the scene just as you have completed your rapid assessment. You have worked with this crew before. You report that your patient is in full cardiopulmonary arrest. Responding according to standing orders, everyone springs into action. Quick-look ECG paddles reveal that the patient is in asystole. He is intubated and ventilated with 100% oxygen; an IV life line with normal saline is established at a TKO rate.

4. How should you confirm that this patient is in asystole?

5. Identify the procedure that is indicated for this patient's cardiac rhythm. Explain why it should be initiated in conjunction with drug therapy.

6. List the drugs indicated for use in this patient if he remains in asystole. List the drugs in the order in which they should be administered to the patient.

In spite of 10 minutes of aggressive resuscitation efforts, your patient remains in asystole. You begin transport to the nearest hospital and contact medical direction en route. Your ETA is 8 minutes. The patient's condition is unchanged on arrival at the emergency department. The patient never regains a pulse and is pronounced dead before you leave the ED for your next call.

CASE PRESENTATION #2 (QUESTIONS 7-11)

You are dispatched to a convention center where a national political rally is being held. The patient is a 58-year-old man who slumped over and stopped breathing after delivering a speech to a zealous crowd. A bystander determined that the patient was pulseless and immediately initiated CPR. The fire department first responders arrived on the scene within the first two minutes, attached an automatic external defibrillator (AED), and delivered three shocks to the patient.

7. Explain the advantages of the initial treatment that was rendered before your arrival.

After your arrival on the scene, your quick assessment reveals that this patient is still pulseless. CPR is resumed. The patient is connected to an ECG monitor, which indicates ventricular fibrillation. He is intubated with ease, but your partner has been unsuccessful at establishing an IV.

8. What initial drug is indicated, and how should it be administered?

In spite of initial drug therapy and a repeated shock, your patient remains in ventricular fibrillation. Your partner suggests that it is time to give an antidysrhythmic drug. He pulls lidocaine and Bretylium® from the drug box. He mutters that a higher dose of epinephrine might work on this patient.

9. Which antidysrhythmic drug should you choose, and why?

10. Would a high dose of epinephrine benefit this patient? Explain.

The next shock finally converts the patient to an organized junctional escape rhythm at a rate of 40 beats per minute. His blood pressure is 88/50. The patient's condition is unchanged on arrival at the emergency department. The physician establishes a central line.

11. What additional drug therapy might you expect this patient to receive, and why?

The patient is admitted to the intensive care unit (ICU) in stable condition, but he dies two days later from cardiogenic shock.

CASE PRESENTATION #3 (QUESTIONS 12–16)

You are dispatched to an outdoor concert because of a shooting. The gunman has been apprehended, and police are performing CPR on a 22-year-old man who has been shot in the chest. On arrival three minutes later, you confirm that the patient is in cardiopulmonary arrest with a wound to the anterior left side of the chest. There is minimal bleeding and equal rise and fall of the chest with artificial ventilation. Quick-look ECG paddles reveal the rhythm found in Figure 19-1.

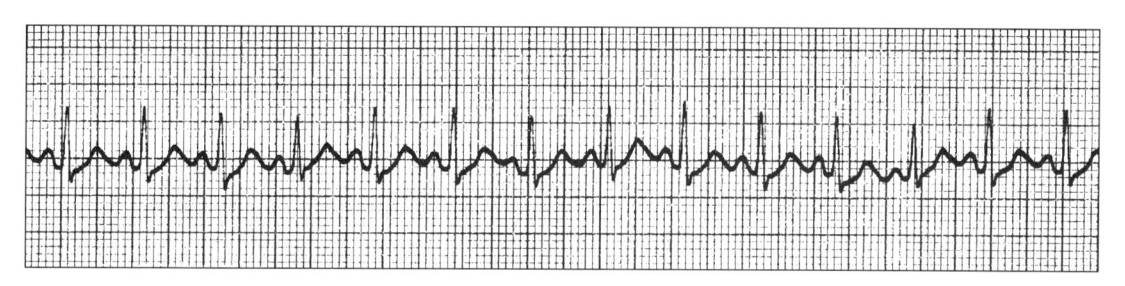

Figure 19-1

12. Which of the following statements provides the best description of this patient's cardiac rhythm?
    a. There is complete block between the atria and the ventricles.
    b. The injury has caused a temporary interruption of the normal electrical activity.
    c. The heart is experiencing an electrical disturbance that is resulting in an uncoordinated rhythm.
    d. An organized cardiac rhythm is present when a pulse cannot be detected.

13. Explain why your approach to this patient in traumatic cardiac arrest differs from that used with medical arrest.

The patient is intubated quickly and is hyperventilated with 100% oxygen. You have standing orders to administer the first dose of epinephrine; you do so through the endotracheal tube. The fire department first responders arrive, and you prepare to transport this patient to the hospital.

14. What should you keep in mind when you are instructing the first responders?

Patient transfer to the ambulance is difficult because of the lack of crowd control. Once in the ambulance, you notice that the tape around the endotracheal tube has pulled loose and the patient's chest is expanding less on the left side. Your partner reports that the patient's breath sounds also are decreased on the left side. The trachea is midline, and neck veins are flat.

15. What is the most likely cause of these findings, and how should the problem be treated?

Your ETA at the local trauma center is 4 minutes. Two large-bore IVs with Ringer's lactate are established en route and are run wide open. You contact medical direction to request a repeat dose of epinephrine. As you are pulling into the ED ambulance bay, your patient's rhythm changes to asystole. He has received a total of 800 ml of fluid and 2 mg of epinephrine. A thoracotomy is performed in the trauma room, which reveals that the bullet pierced the aorta. In spite of aggressive resuscitation efforts, this patient never regains a pulse.

16. Ethically speaking, was your decision to resuscitate this patient in the field an appropriate one? Explain your response.

GENERAL REVIEW QUESTIONS

17. In the space provided, number the following structures in the order in which blood flows through them. Start with the right atrium.

  a. _____ Right atrium
  b. _____ Left atrium
  c. _____ Pulmonary artery
  d. _____ Pulmonary vein
  e. _____ Aortic valve
  f. _____ Pulmonic valve
  g. _____ Lungs
  h. _____ Aorta
  i. _____ Left ventricle
  j. _____ Mitral valve
  k. _____ Right ventricle
  l. _____ Tricuspid valve

18. In the space provided, place an O beside those structures that carry oxygenated blood and a D beside those structures that carry deoxygenated blood.

    a. _____ Coronary arteries

    b. _____ Vena cava

    c. _____ Left atrium

    d. _____ Right atria

    e. _____ Aorta

    f. _____ Coronary veins

    g. _____ Left ventricle

    h. _____ Right ventricle

    i. _____ Pulmonary artery

    j. _____ Pulmonary vein

19. Match the term in Column 1 with its definition in Column 2.

    Column 1
    a. Stroke volume
    b. Cardiac output
    c. Depolarization
    d. Repolarization
    e. Automaticity
    f. Contractility
    g. Systole
    h. Diastole
    i. Preload
    j. Afterload
    k. Pericardium
    l. Asystole

    Column 2
    1. _____ The pressure in the ventricles after diastole
    2. _____ Period when the ventricles are at rest and are filling
    3. _____ Contraction-ejection phase
    4. _____ Amount of blood ejected from the ventricles
    5. _____ Amount of blood pumped in one minute
    6. _____ The ability to self-depolarize
    7. _____ Process resulting in muscle contraction
    8. _____ Process of returning cells to their resting state
    9. _____ The pressure against which the ventricles must pump
    10. _____ The force of ventricular contraction

20. List four situations in which sodium bicarbonate may be helpful in the treatment of cardiac arrest patients.

    (a)

    (b)

    (c)

    (d)

21. Calculate the cardiac output of a patient who has a stroke volume of 50 ml and a heart rate of 100.

Figures 19-2 to 19-4 are cardiac rhythms that may be seen in pulseless patients. Identify the advanced cardiac life support (ACLS) algorithm that you would use for each.

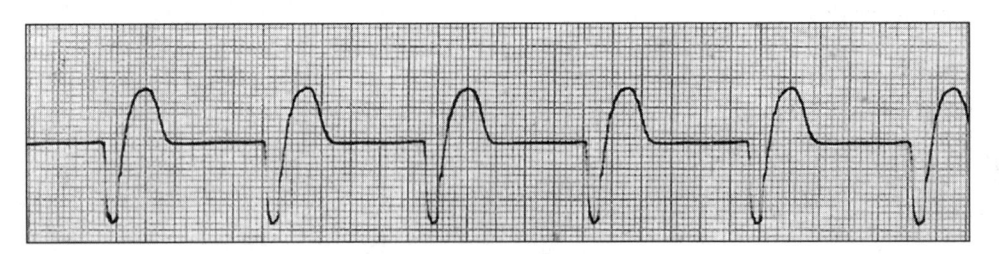

Figure 19-2 _____

22. _____

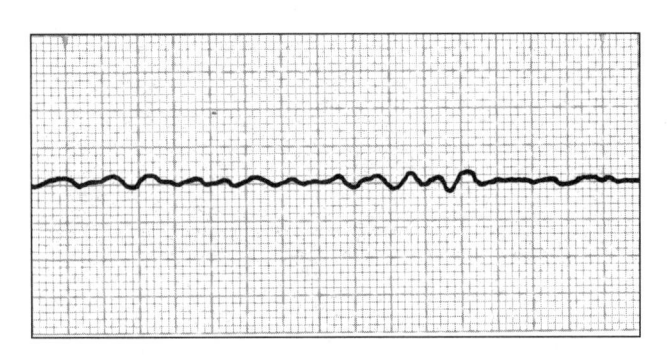

Figure 19-3 _____

23. _____

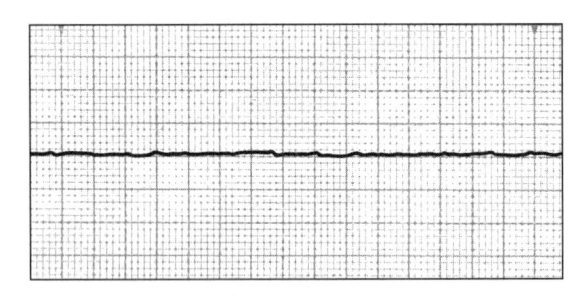

Figure 19-4 _____

24. _____

25. In what order does the electrical impulse normally travel through the following structures in the heart?
    1. Left and right bundle branches
    2. Sinoatrial (SA) node
    3. Atrioventricular (AV) node or junction
    4. Bundle of His
    5. Purkinje fibers
        a. 3, 2, 4, 1, 5
        b. 1, 2, 4, 5, 3
        c. 2, 3, 4, 1, 5
        d. 2, 3, 4, 5, 1

26. The primary pacemaker in the heart is the:
   a. AV node.
   b. Purkinje system.
   c. SA node.
   d. coronary node.

27. During the course of cardioversion, your patient suddenly develops ventricular fibrillation. You should:
   a. synchronize cardiovert quickly.
   b. begin CPR immediately.
   c. proceed with defibrillation.
   d. administer lidocaine bolus.

28. If myocardial infarction is extensive, it can lead to sudden death from:
   a. cardiogenic shock.
   b. lethal dysrhythmias.
   c. congestive heart failure.
   d. ventricular rupture.

29. The majority of adult patients who suffer medical cardiac arrest have an underlying rhythm of:
   a. asystole or ventricular fibrillation.
   b. pulseless electrical activity (PEA) or ventricular tachycardia.
   c. ventricular fibrillation or ventricular tachycardia.
   d. ventricular tachycardia or asystole.

30. Which of the following statements is accurate regarding near-drowning victims? (Circle all that apply.)
   a. They are often found in a ventricular fibrillation rhythm.
   b. They should not be intubated if there is water in the mouth.
   c. They have a better chance of survival if they are young.
   d. They usually have a dismal outcome if they were submerged in cold water.

31. Management of a patient in cardiopulmonary arrest who is hypothermic includes: (Circle all that apply.)
   a. ventilating with warm, humidified oxygen.
   b. withholding additional shocks if body temperature is lower than 86° F.
   c. administering additional medications if body temperature is lower than 86° F.
   d. withholding CPR until body temperature is higher than 86° F.

Answers to questions from chapter 19 can be found on page 439.

Chapter 20

The Patient With Compromised Circulation

OBJECTIVES

1. Explain the pathophysiology of compromised circulation.
2. Given a patient with assessment findings of compromised circulation, explain the importance of rapid recognition and treatment.
3. Identify signs and symptoms of compromised circulation from various causes.
4. Describe the history and assessment of the patient with compromised circulation.
5. Explain the relationship of vital signs to circulation and perfusion.
6. Describe and differentiate among the various causes of compromised circulation in the prehospital setting.
7. Describe the management approaches to various patient conditions that present with compromised circulation.
8. List the therapeutic effects, indications, contraindications, potential side effects, and correct dosages of various medications used to treat specific causes of compromised circulation.

CASE PRESENTATION #1 (QUESTIONS 1–8)

You are dispatched to a church for treatment of a patient with possible stroke. On arrival, you find a 68-year-old woman who is experiencing "lightheadedness." The symptom began suddenly, approximately 30 minutes ago, while she was singing in the choir. She is alert and appropriately answers questions. No motor or sensory deficits are noted during initial assessment. Although she appears to be in no significant distress, her skin is pale and cool.

1. What can you conclude about this patient's condition, based on her ability to provide appropriate responses to questions?

2. Is this patient's circulation adequate? Explain.

3. Once your initial assessment is complete, what three components of the history and physical examination should be your focus?

   (a)

   (b)

   (c)

Before further examination, the patient is placed on high-concentration oxygen via a nonrebreather mask. Breath sounds are clear bilaterally. She has no significant medical history and takes no medications. Your partner reports that the patient's vital signs are: BP 96/60; pulse 54 and regular; respirations 20 and unlabored. She is also connected to the cardiac monitor, which shows third-degree heart block. An IV life line is established.

4. Was your initial treatment appropriate? Why, or why not?

At the same time that the third-degree heart block is revealed, the cardiac monitor indicates a slight decrease in the patient's heart rate. She tells you that she feels extremely tired; she also appears drowsy. You quickly reassess her vital signs. Her blood pressure is now 88/50; pulse is 50; and respirations are unchanged. You contact medical direction and are ordered to administer atropine IV push and to prepare for transcutaneous pacing.

5. What is the current life threat for this patient?

6. Briefly explain the rationale for medical direction's orders.

7. As you are pacing this patient, capture of the heart is indicated by:
   a. twitching of the body as the current passes through the chest.
   b. the presence of pacing spikes on the ECG monitor.
   c. the apparent level of pain experienced by the patient.
   d. palpation of a pulse rate that is the same as the pacer rate.

The patient's condition improves while en route to the hospital. She is more alert, and her pulse rate and blood pressure have increased. She is delivered to the emergency department, where her condition is evaluated. She is then admitted for implantation of a permanent pacemaker.

8. What drugs would have been indicated if this patient had not responded to your interventions, or if a pacemaker had not been available?

CASE PRESENTATION #2 (QUESTIONS 9–17)

You are dispatched to a private residence for treatment of an unconscious person. No additional information is available at this time. The caller was disconnected, and attempts by dispatch to reestablish communication have been unsuccessful.

9. What should you and your partner be thinking and discussing while en route, to ensure that care at the scene proceeds smoothly?

On arrival, you find a 44-year-old man who is leaning forward and complaining of stomach pain. As you approach him, you immediately note that he is anxious and his skin is pale and diaphoretic.

10. List three specific questions that you should ask about this patient's medical history and current condition to determine whether he has a gastrointestinal problem.

(a)

(b)

(c)

11. What two additional life threats must you rule out with this line of questioning?

(a)

(b)

The patient describes the pain as a "burning" sensation that began several hours ago. He noticed that his bowel movement yesterday was black, and just minutes earlier he vomited what looked like "coffee grounds." The only medication he takes is Maalox® for frequent indigestion. His radial pulse is so weak and fast that it is difficult to palpate. You are unable to obtain a blood pressure reading by either auscultation or palpation. As you attempt to measure his blood pressure, the patient tells you that he is becoming very dizzy and needs to lie down.

12. This patient's findings are most consistent with:
   a. acute myocardial infarction.
   b. abdominal aortic aneurysm.
   c. gastrointestinal bleeding.
   d. diverticulitis.

13. What can you conclude about this patient's blood pressure, based on his pulse rate?

14. Should you perform a tilt test on this patient? Explain.

The patient is prepared for immediate transport. You quickly administer high-concentration oxygen with a nonrebreather mask at 15 liters per minute and connect the patient to the cardiac monitor. His cardiac rhythm reveals sinus tachycardia with an occasional unifocal PVC. Your partner places the PASG on the stretcher before loading the patient and contacts medical direction. Your ETA at the closest appropriate hospital is 7 minutes.

15. Should you establish an IV before departure? Explain.

16. Additional treatment for this patient to be provided en route may include: (Circle all that apply.)
   a. inflating the PASG.
   b. running IV fluids wide open.
   c. administerinng lidocaine bolus.
   d. placing the patient in the Trendelenburg position.

The patient is conscious on arrival at the emergency department. When giving report to the receiving physician, you inform her that you were able finally to palpate a systolic blood pressure of 90 after the patient had received two liters of lactated Ringer's solution. The physician, anticipating a course of transfusions and possible surgery for this patient, orders stat laboratory tests and radiographs.

17. Would you expect this patient's hematocrit to be low, normal, or high? Explain.

CASE PRESENTATION # 3 (QUESTIONS 18–23)

You are dispatched to a home for treatment of a child who is having breathing difficulty. Your patient is a 6-year-old girl who appears unconscious but responds by opening her eyes when you call her name loudly. The history from the patient's mother reveals that the patient was seen earlier today by a physician for treatment of an ear ache. The physician gave her a prescription for amoxicillin. After taking her second tablet minutes ago, the patient quickly developed abdominal cramping, hives, and tightness in her throat. Now, she is having stridorous respirations, and cyanosis is evident at the mouth and lips. It is readily apparent to both you and your partner that this patient is having an anaphylactic reaction.

18. Is this patient in shock? Explain.

19. Explain why it is important to cover this patient.

20. Explain the significance of the patient's cyanotic mouth and lips.

You immediately secure her airway and administer high-concentration oxygen. Her vital signs are: BP 88 by palpation; pulse 112 and weak; respirations 40 and labored. While your partner is establishing an IV, you contact medical direction and are ordered to administer an epinephrine IV push.

21. Explain why medical direction ordered epinephrine to be administered via IV push rather than subcutaneously.

22. Explain why this patient is hypotensive.

You administer Benadryl® after epinephrine. The patient's condition improves remarkably during the 10-minute transport to the hospital. She is sitting upright and is breathing easier. Her blood pressure has increased to 94/60 after administration of IV fluid boluses. Her respirations are 24, and breath sounds are clear. Her pulse still is elevated at a rate of 100. She is admitted to the emergency department for observation.

23. Most likely, this patient's pulse remains elevated as a result of:
   a. uncompensated shock.
   b. an adverse reaction to epinephrine.
   c. fear and anxiety.
   d. volume loss.

GENERAL REVIEW QUESTIONS

24. Compromised circulation results when the integrity of any of which three body systems is lost?

   (a)

   (b)

   (c)

25. Identify three areas of the body in which pallor, or loss of normal skin color, is most noticeable.

   (a)

   (b)

   (c)

26. In what situation would fluid challenge be inappropriate for a patient in cardiogenic shock?

27. Briefly explain why demand transcutaneous pacing is used more frequently than non-demand transcutaneous pacing.

By placing **a, b, c, d,** or **e** in the space provided, indicate the type of shock that each hypotensive patient most likely is experiencing.

   a. Cardiogenic
   b. Hypovolemic
   c. Anaphylactic
   d. Septic
   e. Neurogenic

28. _____ A 77-year-old with a fever of 104° F, bilateral rales, and productive cough of green sputum for 4 days.

29. _____ A 32-year-old with a large-caliber gunshot wound to the abdomen.

30. _____ A 24-year-old paramedic student who passes out after seeing his first severely traumatized patient.

31. _____ A 29-year-old with bilateral wheezing, systemic rash, and itching that began after he ate at a Chinese restaurant.

32. _____ A 12-year-old who has no feeling in his legs after falling from a horse.

33. _____ A 57-year-old who is complaining of the acute onset of severe chest pain that is radiating to the neck, and shortness of breath.

34. _____ A 1-year-old with vomiting and diarrhea for 3 days, sunken fontanelle, and tenting skin.

35. _____ An 80-year-old with shortness of breath (SOB), bilateral rales, frothy sputum, and peripheral edema to both ankles.

For each of the following patients, give the most appropriate initial drug therapy from the list of drugs provided below. Assume that the airway has been managed and that an IV has been initiated.

   a. Adenosine
   b. Atropine
   c. Dopamine
   d. Epinephrine
   e. Levophed
   f. Lidocaine
   g. Morphine

36. ____ A 67-year-old who is complaining of weakness and mild SOB. ECG: sinus bradycardia at a rate of 40; BP 80/56; respirations 20.

37. ____ A 36-year-old with an acute onset of chest palpitations. ECG: PSVT; BP 120/60; pulse 180, regular; respirations 18.

38. ____ A 20-year-old in sustained ventricular tachycardia after smoking crack. BP 140/90; pulse 160; respirations 22.

39. ____ A 60-year-old with severe SOB. History of congestive heart failure; he is out of medications. ECG: atrial fibrillation with PACs, rate 110; BP 134/88; respirations 28, labored.

40. ____ A 72-year-old unconscious person, cause unknown. No pulse or respirations; ECG: ventricular tachycardia.

41. Tissue perfusion distal to a musculoskeletal injury of the elbow is best assessed by:
   a. asking the patient to move fingers.
   b. assessing capillary refill of the nail beds.
   c. checking blood pressure.
   d. palpating a radial pulse.

42. Which of the following fractures poses the greatest potential for hypovolemic shock?
   a. femur
   b. humerus
   c. shoulder
   d. tibia

43. Which of the following is the *least* important finding for a patient with a history of alcoholism who is complaining of abdominal pain and has obvious signs of compromised circulation?
   a. a rigid abdomen
   b. melena for 3 days
   c. an appendectomy surgery scar
   d. negative orthostatic vital signs

44. Which of the following drugs is used for post resuscitation persistent hypotension?
   a. epinephrine
   b. dopamine
   c. procainamide
   d. norepinephrine

Answers to questions from chapter 20 can be found on page 441.

Chapter 21

The Critical Trauma Patient

OBJECTIVES

1. Describe the relationship of time (the Golden Hour) to the care of the critical trauma patient.
2. Discuss the goals of trauma assessment in the prehospital setting.
3. Discuss the relevance of trauma scoring systems in the prehospital setting.
4. Given a scenario involving a trauma patient, calculate the Glasgow Coma Score and the Revised Trauma Score.
5. Describe the systematic process used to rapidly assess and manage trauma during:
   a. Initial assessment
   b. Focused history and physical examination
   c. Continued assessment
6. Explain why it is important to re-evaluate the critical patient.
7. Identify "load and go" trauma emergencies, and describe patient management in these situations.
8. Discuss assessment factors to consider for the critically injured pediatric patient.
9. Discuss assessment factors to consider for the critically injured pregnant patient.
10. Identify two specific traumatic conditions that can occur in the last trimester of pregnancy and the appropriate field management of them.

CASE PRESENTATION #1 (QUESTIONS 1–9)

You are dispatched to a motor vehicle collision that has occurred during rush hour. The collision occurred at a busy intersection, and it appears that the two cars involved hit each other head-on. A first responder unit is on the scene. Damage to both vehicles is extensive.

1. You ask dispatch to send a second ambulance. Your next priority is to:
   a. ascertain the number of victims.
   b. determine if the scene is safe.
   c. evaluate damage to the vehicles.
   d. set up emergency flares.

2. Briefly discuss scene safety factors that should be considered at the scene of a motor vehicle collision.

The driver of one car (Victim #1) was ejected through the windshield and is lying about 15 yards from her car. The other driver (Victim #2) is unconscious and is slumped over the steering wheel. There are no passengers in either car. The second ambulance has not arrived yet.

3. With two potentially critical patients who need treatment, what should you and your partner do?

Your initial assessment reveals the following:

<u>Victim #1</u> — An unconscious 38-year-old woman who responds to painful stimuli. Airway and breath sounds are clear, and carotid and radial pulses are present (rate 100). Other findings include an obvious distended abdomen and an open right femoral fracture that is bleeding heavily.

<u>Victim #2</u> — A 22-year-old man who responds to verbal stimuli but is confused. Skin is pale and diaphoretic; airway is intact, and respirations are 28 and shallow. Radial pulse is not palpable; carotid pulse is present but weak, at a rate of 130. Obvious bruising to the chest is noted, and the steering wheel is bent. Further initial observations include a large gash on the forehead and a right forearm fracture.

4. While the first responders stabilize Victim #1's C-spine, you should:
    a. control hemorrhage from the femoral fracture.
    b. apply a PASG to the backboard.
    c. obtain a blood pressure reading.
    d. start an IV of Ringer's lactate.

5. Are either of these victims classified as "load and go" patients? Explain your answer.

After you have completed the initial assessment, the second ambulance arrives. After you give the team a brief report, they assume the care of Victim #1. You and your partner rapidly extricate Victim #2 while maintaining spinal immobilization.

6. Once you are in the ambulance with Victim #2, you perform a focused history and examination. Describe what it should include.

Assessment reveals that the patient's blood pressure is 60/40 and his level of consciousness is deteriorating. At this point, he opens his eyes only in response to painful stimuli. His speech is inappropriate, and he pushes your hands away as you attempt to apply a painful stimulus. Breath sounds are equal but diminished bilaterally. His neck veins are flat; there is no deviation of the trachea. His abdomen is distended slightly, and his pelvis is stable.

7. This patient's vital signs and assessment findings are most likely caused by:
    a. closed head injury.
    b. massive hemothorax.
    c. right forearm fracture.
    d. tension pneumothorax.

8. Calculate this patient's Glasgow Coma Scale and Revised Trauma Score.

You assist ventilations using high-concentration oxygen, apply the ECG monitor, and leave the scene. Your partner contacts medical direction to discuss the patient and requests permission to transport him to a Level I trauma center. Meanwhile, you attempt to start two IV lines of Ringer's lactate.

9. Is the decision to leave the scene and start IVs while en route an appropriate one? Why, or why not?

The patient's condition continues to deteriorate while you are en route. When you transfer him from the stretcher to the hospital cart, he has a cardiac arrest. The emergency physicians crack his chest, perform open cardiac massage, and rush him to the operating room. You leave the hospital shortly after this.

About two hours later, you return to this facility with another patient. You find out that your previous patient had a tear in the aortic arch and died on the operating table. The physician informs you that, given the patient's lethal injury, your early recognition of the life-threatening problem and quick transport to the appropriate facility afforded him the best possible chance for survival.

CASE PRESENTATION #2 (QUESTIONS 10–18)

Late one evening, you are dispatched to a possible shooting in an area known for gang activity. As you approach the location, you observe that there are no street lights. A stranger waves at you and yells, "Over here!" You do not see a police unit.

10. Before you exit the vehicle, you should: _____

While you call dispatch, the stranger approaches the ambulance and tells you that the victim is located in his backyard. He tells you that there is only one victim and that he is unconscious after having been shot in the chest. The police arrive and secure the scene. You and your partner are led to the patient by police.

11. Describe the focus of your initial patient assessment.

The patient responds to verbal stimuli and appropriately answers questions. His radial pulse is present and thready at a rate of 150. Respirations are 30 and labored. He has a small entrance wound located on the left side of his chest at about the fourth intercostal space. There is no obvious exit wound. His skin is very diaphoretic. The stranger saw the incident and informs you that the patient was shot with a .22 caliber gun, from a distance of about 30 feet.

12. Given this information, you next treatment priority is to:
    a. get the stretcher and move the patient to the ambulance.
    b. inflate the PASG.
    c. obtain an ECG reading.
    d. start an IV of Ringer's lactate.

Your focused assessment reveals no other bullet wounds. Blood pressure is 80/40; neck veins are distended; breath sounds are absent on the left side; also, there is a deviated trachea to the right. You quickly contact medical direction and report your findings.

13. Based on this patient's presentation, you most likely suspect:
    a. cardiac tamponade.
    b. flail chest.
    c. ruptured spleen.
    d. tension pneumothorax.

14. What lifesaving procedure might medical direction order you to perform at the scene?

Your partner administers oxygen, starts an IV, and hooks up the ECG, while you quickly prepare equipment for the procedure. The patient becomes unresponsive. His ECG rhythm is shown in Figure 21-1.

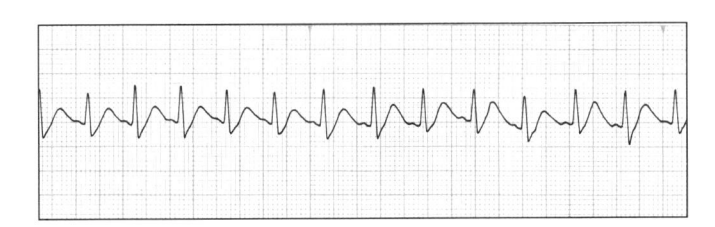

Figure 21-1

15. This ECG rhythm reveals _____. Is this rhythm expected given his condition? Briefly explain your response.

You insert the needle into his chest, and the patient immediately begins to moan and has less breathing difficulty. You leave the scene and start a second IV while en route.

16. At this point, should you apply a PASG? Explain your answer.

17. What reassessment of the patient is indicated to be performed en route to the trauma center?

You arrive at the trauma center 23 minutes after the call was dispatched. The patient's level of consciousness and vital signs continue to stabilize. Your on-scene time was 15 minutes.

18. Was the on-scene time acceptable in this case? Why, or why not?

A chest radiograph is ordered immediately, and physician evaluation confirms the diagnosis of an initial tension pneumothorax, now open.

Case Presentation #3 (Questions 19–21)

You respond to a call involving a motor vehicle collision. The driver of the car is nine months pregnant. The patient is conscious, alert, and oriented, and is complaining of severe abdominal pain. Her skin is very diaphoretic, and her abdomen is rigid. Her vital signs are as follows: BP 70/40; pulse 150; and respirations 28 and shallow.

19. Considering her presentation, what specific conditions related to her pregnancy should you consider?

20. What could be the effects of her clinical condition on the fetus?

21. Your treatment while en route should include: _____

General Review Questions

22. Define the "golden hour" for the trauma patient.

23. Describe the relationship of the golden hour to the appropriate care of the critical trauma patient.

24. There are four major goals in the care of the trauma victim. Briefly list these.

   (a)

   (b)

   (c)

   (d)

25. The most important aspect of the history in care of the trauma patient is:
   a. identification of the mechanism of injury.
   b. a list of medications that are being taken currently.
   c. information about previous medical problems.
   d. the time when the last meal was eaten.

26. Discuss the importance of re-evaluation of the critical trauma patient en route to the hospital.

27. Which of the following patient findings would be considered a "load and go" situation(s)? (Circle all that apply.)
   a. airway compromise
   b. bilateral femoral fractures
   c. a fractured humerus
   d. a tender, rigid abdomen
   e. an unstable pelvis

28. The leading cause of trauma in pediatric patients is:
   a. burns.
   b. drownings.
   c. gunshot wounds.
   d. motor vehicle collisions and falls.
   e. stab wounds.

29. Immobilizing the spine of a pediatric patient poses two potential problems. List and briefly discuss each one.

(a)

(b)

For each of the following statements (30–32), circle the correct response, True or False. Briefly explain your answer.

30. Abdominal organs have a greater potential for injury in children than in adults.

TRUE   **FALSE**

Briefly explain your answer: _____
_____

31. In the pediatric patient, shock is defined by a specific blood pressure value.

TRUE   **FALSE**

Briefly explain your answer: _____
_____

32. Pediatric long bone fractures should be splinted as found (when possible).

TRUE   **FALSE**

Briefly explain your answer: _____
_____

Answers to questions from chapter 21 can be found on page 444.

Chapter 22

The Critical Pediatric Patient

OBJECTIVES

1. Identify the epidemiology of critical illness and trauma in pediatric patients.
2. Describe how the anatomy of the pediatric airway differs from that of an adult and how this may affect the management of children with airway compromise.
3. Discuss how to recognize and manage conditions associated with airway obstruction.
4. Discuss how to recognize and manage conditions associated with circulatory compromise.
5. Discuss the limitations of fluid replacement in a pediatric patient.
6. List the potential causes of diminished consciousness in a pediatric patient.
7. Describe how to manage diminished consciousness in a pediatric patient.
8. Describe how to evaluate the need for neonatal resuscitation.
9. Discuss the management techniques used for neonatal resuscitation.

CASE PRESENTATION # 1 (QUESTIONS 1–7)

A hysterical mother calls 9-1-1 because her 18-month-old child is seizing. Dispatch is unable to obtain any additional information because of the mother's emotional state. While en route to the scene, you and your partner review the possible causes of seizure in this age group. You then ask the paramedic intern to tell you what history questions she may need to ask the patient's mother on arrival that will help in determining the possible cause of this child's seizure.

1. List six important historical points that the paramedic intern should repeat to you.

    (a)

    (b)

    (c)

    (d)

    (e)

    (f)

On arrival, you learn that the patient was seen a few days ago at the neighborhood pediatric clinic because he was running a high fever. The young mother tells you that she has been unable to get her son to take the medicine that the clinic prescribed for an ear infection because he did not like the taste. On examination, the patient appears postictal. His airway is intact, chest is clear, pupils are equal and reactive, and his neck is supple. His vital signs are: pulse 134 and regular; respirations 26 and unlabored.

2. Identify other procedures that should be included in this patient's examination.

The paramedic intern reports that the child has a rectal temperature of 105° F. You contact medical direction as you begin transport to the nearest hospital. The physician orders you to initiate cooling measures with tepid water and to stop when the child's temperature has dropped to 102° F. The intern appears puzzled by the order.

3. How should you explain the rationale for the physician's orders?

The patient remains postictal. Just as the intern begins the cooling procedure, the patient starts to seize again. As the intern manages the patient's airway and protects him from injury, you again contact medical direction. The physician orders you to administer diazepam .5 mg per kilogram rectally and to continue cooling measures after the seizure activity has stopped.

4. Explain the significance of the patient's second seizure.

5. List two possible side effects for which you should be alert after administering diazepam to this patient.

(a)

(b)

The patient's seizure lasts less than one minute. His respiratory rate is 22 with adequate air movement. His temperature is now 101.8° F. You check a fingerstick glucose level, which reads 40 mg/dl. Your ETA at the hospital is 3 minutes.

6. Are any additional advanced life support treatment measures required at this time? Explain your response.

By the time you deliver the patient to the hospital, he is beginning to awaken. His overall condition is stable. Based on your report, the physician confirms your suspicions that this patient was most likely having febrile seizures and praises you for transporting him quickly. As you are preparing the ambulance for your next dispatch, you and your partner critique this call with the intern.

7. Explain to the intern why it was especially important to transport this patient quickly.

CASE PRESENTATION #2 (QUESTIONS 8–14)

You are dispatched to the home of a 25-year-old who is in active labor. This is her first pregnancy and, until today, she has had regular prenatal care with no problems. She is at 37 weeks gestation.

8. Identify problems for which this infant will be at special risk, if delivery occurs prematurely.

On arrival, you are greeted by a neighbor who screams, "The baby just popped out and doesn't look very good." As you enter the room, you find the newborn lying between the mother's legs.

9. What essentials of care will you begin providing immediately to the infant, regardless of the need for resuscitation?

10. To determine if this newborn needs resuscitation, you should assess:
    a. skin color, respiratory status, and heart rate.
    b. respiratory rate and depth, and heart rate.
    c. muscle tone, reflex irritability, and heart rate.
    d. respiratory rate, skin color, and muscle tone.

On initial assessment, the infant is limp and blue. Her vital signs are: respirations 24 and shallow; pulse regular at 86 per minute. The mother is stable and is being comforted by her neighbor.

11. What should be your first treatment priority for the infant at this time? Explain your response.

12. Explain the significance of the fact that pulmonary compliance is lower in the premature newborn than in the full-term newborn.

After a few minutes, the infant responds favorably to the initial treatment. Her body is pink, but her extremities are still blue. Her pulse rate is now 120. Additional EMS help has arrived to assist you with transport preparation. You contact medical direction while en route and are directed to the nearest hospital with a neonatal intensive care unit. Your ETA is 5 minutes.

13. Based on your reassessment findings, how might you alter the airway management of your infant patient while en route?

Both mother and infant remain stable while en route. On arrival at the hospital, the infant is moving her upper extremities and is crying. Her respiratory rate is 36 and heart rate is 140. She still has mild peripheral cyanosis. Even though it is past the 1- and 5-minute time intervals after delivery (within which you normally calculate an Apgar score), your partner wants to practice and have you check his calculations.

14. The Apgar score for this infant, based on your assessment findings on arrival at the hospital, is:
    a. 5.
    b. 7.
    c. 9.
    d. 10.

CASE PRESENTATION #3 (QUESTIONS 15–20)

You are dispatched to an apartment for treatment of a "sick child" and arrive to find an ill-appearing 18-month-old. The mother tells you that her baby has been vomiting and has had diarrhea for 3 days. The child lies very still while you examine him. He has cracked lips, sunken eyes, and tenting skin. His pulse is rapid and weak, and respirations are 44 and shallow. You manage his airway and prepare to initiate an IV before transport.

15. Identify the child's ECG rhythm, which is shown in Figure 22-1.

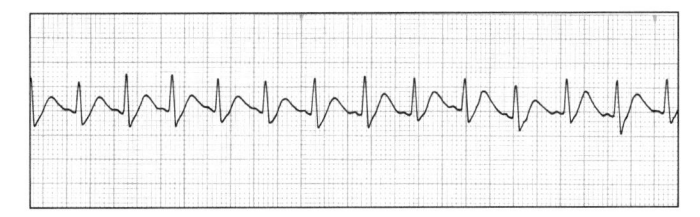

Figure 22-1

16. Most likely, what is wrong with this child? List clinical findings to support your answer.

17. Priority sites for IV access in this child include:
    a. brachial and scalp veins.
    b. dorsal hands and saphenous veins.
    c. external jugular and brachial veins.
    d. brachial and saphenous veins.

18. Describe appropriate initial fluid therapy for this child.

19. List clinical findings that would indicate successful fluid resuscitation in this patient.

20. Early signs of IV fluid overload for which you should be alert in this patient include:
    a. rales and cardiac wheezing.
    b. peripheral edema and jugular vein distention.
    c. tachypnea and tachycardia.
    d. pink, frothy sputum and rales.

Your ETA at the hospital is 6 minutes. Medical direction orders no additional treatment at this time. The patient becomes more active and aware of his surroundings while en route. On arrival at the hospital, his pulse rate is 124 and respiratory rate is 30.

CASE PRESENTATION #4 (QUESTIONS 21–27)

You are dispatched to a private residence at 5:00 a.m. for an "unresponsive infant" call. You are met by anxious parents who lead you to the crib of their 4-month-old infant. The mother is crying as she tells you, "I think my baby is dead and I just don't understand. She was fine when I put her back to bed after her midnight feeding." You find the infant lying supine in her crib. Her skin is mottled, and you note bloody froth around her mouth. You cannot detect a pulse, and she is not breathing. You and your partner suspect that you are dealing with a case of Sudden Infant Death Syndrome (SIDS).

21. List history and physical findings in this patient that are characteristic of SIDS.

You immediately contact medical direction for orders on how to proceed. The physician orders you to provide limited resuscitation and transport quickly to the nearest hospital. Your partner begins CPR. You are unable to establish an IV, but you manage to intubate the child with ease. Standing orders allow you to administer the initial dose of epinephrine. The patient weighs approximately 22 pounds.

22. The appropriate endotracheal tube size to select for this patient is:
    a. 2.5 mm.
    b. 3.5 mm.
    c. 4.5 mm.
    d. 5.0 mm.

23. The appropriate route and milliliter dose of epinephrine for this patient is:
    a. endotracheal, 0.1mg/kg (1:1000).
    b. subcutaneous, 0.1 mg/kg (1:1000).
    c. endotracheal, 0.1 mg/kg (1:10,000).
    d. endotracheal, 0.5 mg/kg (1:10,000).

24. Describe the proper CPR technique for this child.

25. Explain why the physician ordered you to resuscitate and transport this child.

26. Describe appropriate behavior that you and your partner should demonstrate toward this child's parents.

You continue resuscitation efforts during the 3-minute transport to the hospital. Shortly after your delivery of this patient to the emergency department, the physician stops resuscitation efforts. As you attempt to discuss the case with your partner while preparing the ambulance for your next call, he angrily says, "I don't want to talk about it."

27. Explain the possible reason for your partner's behavior. Provide suggestions that may be helpful in this situation.

GENERAL REVIEW QUESTIONS

For each of the following patient presentations (28–32), identify the respiratory condition that each patient most likely is experiencing. Describe the appropriate prehospital management approach for each.

Choices: croup, epiglottitis, asthma, bronchiolitis, foreign body obstruction

28. A 2-year-old who awakened his parents at 2 a.m. with a barking cough. The patient has a 2-day history of mild fever and cough. He is breathing 44 times per minute and has inspiratory stridor.

   (a) Condition:

   (b) Management:

29. A 5-year-old who is sitting quietly with his head extended and tongue protruding while drooling. In a muffled voice, he tells you that he has pain on swallowing, which began this morning.

   (a) Condition:

   (b) Management:

30. An 8-year-old who is in acute respiratory distress after playing with a friend's cat. He has audible wheezing and accessory muscle use. His Atrovent® inhaler, which he tells you usually corrects this condition, is at home.

   (a) Condition:

   (b) Management:

31. A 2-year-old with the acute onset of choking and gagging, which began while he was playing unsupervised, minutes earlier. He now has stridor and a weak cough.

   (a) Condition:

   (b) Management:

32. A 9-month-old with tachypnea, wheezing, prolonged expiration, and a 2-day history of mild fever and runny nose.

   (a) Condition:

   (b) Management:

For each of the following statements (33–38) related to airway management in a pediatric patient, circle the correct response, True or False. Briefly explain your answer.

33. Use of the Sellick maneuver in the very young to reduce the risks of vomiting and aspiration requires caution.

TRUE   **FALSE**

Briefly explain your answer: _____

_____

34. Placement of an orogastric or nasogastric tube increases the effectiveness of ventilation.

TRUE   **FALSE**

Briefly explain your answer: _____

_____

_____

_____

35. Blind nasotracheal intubation is best reserved for children who are younger than eight years of age.

TRUE   **FALSE**

Briefly explain your answer: _____

_____

_____

36. Cuffed endotracheal tubes are not used in children older than eight years of age.

TRUE   **FALSE**

Briefly explain your answer: _____

_____

_____

37. Surgical cricothyrotomy is contraindicated in children younger than 12 years of age.

TRUE   **FALSE**

Briefly explain your answer: _____

_____

38. The best method for verifying proper endotracheal tube placement is pulse oximetry.

TRUE   **FALSE**

Briefly explain your answer: _____

_____

39. Describe three situations in which intubation and assisted ventilation should be considered in an infant or child with a depressed level of consciousness.

(a)

(b)

(c)

40. The leading cause of death after the first year of life is:
  a. birth defects.
  b. cardiac arrest.
  c. SIDS.
  d. trauma.

41. The initial steps in treatment of the conscious pediatric patient should be aimed at gaining the child's confidence and cooperation:
  a. when life-threatening problems are absent.
  b. only when the parents are present.
  c. in all situations.
  d. only in life-threatening situations.

42. Which of the following does *not* lead to stridor in a pediatric patient with upper airway obstruction?
  a. edema
  b. fatigue
  c. foreign body
  d. infection

43. Which of the following characteristics is *not* commonly associated with status asthmaticus?
  a. absence of wheezing
  b. distended chest
  c. exhaustion
  d. carpopedal spasms

Answers to questions from chapter 22 can be found on page 446.

Section 3C

Continued Patient Assessment

CHAPTERS

23. Clinical Significance of Vital Signs
24. Focused and Continued Assessment
25. Pediatric Assessment
26. Geriatric Assessment

Chapter 23

Clinical Significance of Vital Signs

OBJECTIVES

1. Identify normal and abnormal vital signs in patients of varying ages.
2. Describe how age, physical conditioning, the use of medications, and the patient's medical condition can affect vital sign measurements.
3. State ways in which pulse, respiration, and blood pressure measurements can aid in determining the probable cause of a patient's problem.
4. Describe how vital signs can help identify a patient in shock.
5. Explain how the size of a blood pressure cuff can produce false blood pressure readings.

CASE PRESENTATION #1 (QUESTIONS 1–6)

You are dispatched to a residential area for treatment of a child with a history of asthma who is having "trouble breathing." The patient's mother provides you with the following history as she leads you to her daughter's bedroom: The patient's asthma attack began approximately one hour ago while she and her sister were pillow fighting. The patient used her Atrovent inhaler once, but when she showed no improvement, her mother decided she needed to call 9-1-1. Your patient is a frail 8-year-old girl who is working very hard to breathe; her respiratory wheezing is audible across the room. You immediately administer high-concentration oxygen while your partner measures her vital signs.

1. In performance of your assessment, which of the following principles may *not* apply?
    a. Be honest when providing information to the patient.
    b. Obtain all additional history from the patient.
    c. Protect the patient's modesty when examining her.
    d. Provide simple explanations of what you are doing.

2. Is it important to count this patient's respirations for one full minute before initiating any treatment? Explain your response.

3. Would you expect her pulse rate to be low, normal, or high? Explain your response.

4. Describe what size cuff your partner should use to measure this patient's blood pressure. Explain why this is so.

The patient's blood pressure is 90 systolic; pulse rate is 140 and irregular; respirations are labored at a rate of 36 per minute. You administer nebulized albuterol while your partner prepares to establish an IV of normal saline. The cardiac monitor reveals sinus dysrhythmia. You contact medical direction and begin transport. Your ETA is 7 minutes.

5. Should you be concerned about this patient's irregular pulse? Explain your response.

6. Describe vital sign changes that may occur while you are en route to the hospital that would alert you that your patient is:

  (a) approaching impending respiratory arrest

  (b) responding effectively to your treatment

The patient arrives to the emergency department in markedly improved condition and later is discharged.

CASE PRESENTATION #2 (QUESTIONS 7-11)

You are dispatched to a laundromat to treat a patient who called because of chest pain. Your patient is a 65-year-old man who is complaining of severe, "tearing-like" pain to his anterior chest that is radiating to his back between the shoulder blades. The pain began suddenly about an hour ago while he was taking his clothes from the dryer. He has a history of hypertension for which he takes propranolol. On examination, he is in obvious distress. His skin is very diaphoretic. His pulse is 72 and regular; respirations are 24 and shallow; blood pressure is 112/70. Because you are suspicious that this patient may be experiencing a dissecting aortic aneurysm, you measure his blood pressure in the opposite arm; it reads 120/82.

7. Explain the effect that each of the following factors could have on this patient's pulse rate and blood pressure.

    (a) Age

    (b) Medications

8. Explain your rationale for measuring this patient's blood pressure in both arms.

9. After noting the discrepancy in this patient's blood pressure in both arms, would you assess him as being critically ill? Explain your response.

Recognizing the need for rapid transport, you quickly administer high-concentration oxygen and contact medical direction. An IV life-line with Ringer's lactate is established using a large-bore catheter, and an ECG monitor, which reads sinus tachycardia, is connected while en route. Minutes after departure from the scene, your patient becomes very restless. You immediately note that his skin color has become very pale and that there is neck vein distention. You quickly reassess his vital signs. His pulse is now 88 and weak; blood pressure is 92/80 and palpable; and respirations are unchanged.

10. Explain the significance of the change in this patient's blood pressure.

As you are reporting to medical direction about the change in this patient's condition, your partner informs you that he can no longer palpate a carotid pulse and the patient has stopped breathing. The cardiac monitor has not changed. You establish an airway and begin chest compressions.

11. Your initial drug therapy should be:
    a. atropine.
    b. dopamine.
    c. epinephrine.
    d. lidocaine.

Your patient's condition is unchanged on arrival to the emergency department two minutes later. Immediately on arrival, the emergency physician performs a pericardiocentesis and aspirates 100 mL of blood. Despite continued efforts at resuscitation, the cardiac rhythm changes to asystole, and this patient never regains a pulse.

CASE PRESENTATION #3 (QUESTIONS 12-15)

You are called to the scene of a motor vehicle collision on a busy expressway. The fire department arrives just minutes before you do and secures the scene. Your patient is a 30-year-old man who was the driver of a truck that plowed into a utility pole. He is outside of the vehicle walking around when you arrive. He was not wearing a seatbelt, and you note a spidered windshield and significant damage to the front of the vehicle. The patient is conscious but restless. He is sweating profusely. His only obvious injury is a contusion to the forehead. His vital signs are: BP 146/90; pulse 124 and regular; respirations 22 and unlabored.

12. The patient is ambulatory at the scene and has no obvious sensory motor deficits; is it necessary to provide spinal immobilization? Explain your response.

13. What is the significance of this patient's elevated vital signs?

14. This patient's skin condition, which is associated with the mechanism of injury and tachycardia, is suggestive of what type of shock?
    a. cardiogenic
    b. hypovolemic
    c. neurogenic
    d. septic

15. What is the priority of transport for this patient?

The patient is quickly packaged for transport. The PASG is placed on the stretcher, and high-concentration oxygen is administered via nonrebreather mask. The cardiac monitor and an IV of Ringer's lactate are established en route. Your ETA at the hospital is 3 minutes. The only significant finding that was revealed during your focused examination was bruising to the patient's chest and abdomen. His breath sounds were clear bilaterally, and his abdomen was mildly distended but nontender. The patient's condition was unchanged on arrival to the emergency department.

GENERAL REVIEW QUESTIONS

Fill in the blank with the correct vital sign.

    a. Pulse   **b.** Respirations   **c.** Blood pressure

16. _____ Which is the vital sign that is assessed most inaccurately?

17. _____ Which is the first to change when sufficient fluid volume has been lost to affect vital signs?

18. _____ Which is determined by cardiac output and total peripheral resistance?

Listed below are skin and vital sign assessment findings in patients who have sustained trauma. Indicate whether the clinical findings are more consistent with:

    a. Hypovolemic shock   **b.** Neurogenic shock

19. _____ skin warm and dry; pulse 50 and regular; blood pressure 80 and palpable; respirations 12 and shallow

20. _____ skin cool and diaphoretic; blood pressure 60 and palpable; respirations 22; pulse 120 and weak

21. _____ skin hot and dry; pulse 68 and full; respirations 20 and normal; blood pressure reading 84/50

In each of the following patient scenarios, indicate whether the blood pressure would measure a:

    a. False high reading   **b.** False low reading   **c.** Normal reading

22. _____ using an adult blood pressure cuff on a child

23. _____ using an obese cuff on a 120-pound adult

24. _____ using a neonate cuff on a toddler

In each of the following patient scenarios, indicate whether you would expect the heart rate to be:

    a. Tachycardia   **b.** Bradycardia   **c.** Normal

25. _____ a 20-year-old who was stabbed in the abdomen. Skin is pale and sweaty. BP is 76/50; respirations 24.

26. _____ a 35-year-old who is unable to move his legs after falling 20 feet from a roof. Skin is warm and dry. BP is 88/60; respirations 20.

27. _____ a 55-year-old with acute onset of chest pain and nausea. Skin is diaphoretic. BP is 112/80; ECG reveals normal sinus rhythm.

28. _____ a 45-year-old who became unconscious after exposure to organophosphate insecticides. BP is 80 and palpable.

29. _____ a 12-year-old who became unconscious after experiencing a blow to the head. Pupils are unequal. BP is 144/90; respirations 10 and shallow.

30. _____ a 22-year-old who has overdosed on amitriptyline. BP is 100/60; respirations 16.

31. _____ a 4-year-old who is postictal after a febrile seizure. Rectal temperature is 104° F.

32. _____ a 50-year-old homeless person who was found unconscious in a park after sleeping outside in the snow. BP is 84 and palpable.

33. When fewer beats are palpable during pulse taking than can be visualized on cardiac monitor or auscultated with a stethoscope, this is known as _____; it occurs with _____ cardiac rhythm.
   a. mean arterial pressure; sinus bradycardia
   b. pulse deficit; atrial fibrillation
   c. pulse pressure; atrial fibrillation
   d. pulsus paradoxus; paroxysmal sinus tachycardia

34. Common respiratory causes of tachypnea include: (Circle all that apply.)
   a. pneumonia.
   b. pulmonary embolism.
   c. pulmonary edema.
   d. hypothermia.

35. Which of the following sets of adult vital signs indicates a positive tilt test? (Circle all that apply.)
   a. BP: supine 140/90; sitting 128/80; Pulse: supine 100; sitting 122
   b. BP: supine 120/70; sitting 124/70; Pulse: supine 60; sitting 78
   c. BP: supine 130/82; sitting 108/70; Pulse: supine 80; sitting 88
   d. BP: supine 150/90; sitting 130/70; Pulse: supine 100; sitting 124

36. Your patient has experienced the loss of approximately two liters of blood from a lacerated artery. What effect would you expect this amount of blood loss to have on this patient's cardiac output?
   a. decreased output
   b. increased output
   c. no relationship
   d. unchanged output

37. Disease states that commonly result in tachycardia include: (Circle all that apply.)
   a. heat stroke.
   b. hyperthyroidism.
   c. increased intracranial pressure.
   d. third-degree heart block.

Answers to questions from chapter 23 can be found on page 448.

Chapter 24

Focused and Continued Assessment

OBJECTIVES

1. Discuss the reason for performing a focused history and physical examination.
2. Describe the four main steps in conducting a focused history and physical examination.
3. Compare and contrast the two types of questions used in history taking.
4. List appropriate questions to use in obtaining the history of present illness or event.
5. Define *OPQRST* and explain its use in evaluating the history of the present illness or event.
6. Discuss components of and questions used to obtain the SAMPLE history.
7. Differentiate between the focused assessment performed for a responsive medical patient and one who is unresponsive or has an altered mental status.
8. Discuss the reasons for reconsidering the mechanism of injury.
9. State the reasons for performing a rapid trauma assessment.
10. Define *DCAP-BTLS* and its purpose in patient assessment.
11. Describe the areas included in the rapid trauma assessment and discuss what should be evaluated.
12. Discuss the purpose of the continued assessment.
13. Describe when and why a detailed physical examination is necessary.
14. Differentiate patients requiring a detailed physical examination from those who do not.
15. Discuss the value of vital signs in the focused physical examination and continued assessment.

CASE PRESENTATION #1 (QUESTIONS 1–7)

You are dispatched to a call for a person who is experiencing breathing difficulty at an apartment complex. On arrival, a young girl meets you outside and says she will take you to her roommate who is having the problem. You find a 32-year-old woman sitting on the couch leaning forward; it is apparent that she is breathing rapidly and is struggling to catch her breath.

1. Your initial priority is to:
   a. check her radial and carotid pulses.
   b. evaluate her airway.
   c. listen to her breath sounds.
   d. obtain a quick SAMPLE history.

The patient is alert and oriented. She tells you that the breathing difficulty began about 45 minutes ago while she and her roommate were watching a movie. She has never experienced a problem like this before. Her respiratory rate is 32, and radial pulse is 110. You administer oxygen and begin the focused history and physical examination.

2. At this point, what questions related to this current episode would be important to ask the patient?

The SAMPLE history reveals that she has no previous medical history of asthma or other medical problems. There is no history of trauma and no obvious cause for an airway obstruction. She had been to see the physician earlier that morning for a bladder infection. He prescribed antibiotics, fluids, and rest.

3. At this point in the assessment, what would you suspect is the cause of her medical condition?

As you continue the physical examination, your partner leaves to get the stretcher to prepare to take the patient to the hospital.

4. (a) What vital signs should you obtain now?

   (b) What steps in the physical examination are important to perform on this patient?

Further information reveals the following: blood pressure 94/60; pulse still 110 and slightly thready. Skin color is normal, although you note that the patient has a rash around her neck and in the upper chest area. She is also complaining of itching. In continuing to evaluate her respiratory status, you find that she has mild wheezing on both sides of her lungs. The ECG reveals sinus tachycardia.

5. You make the patient as comfortable as possible and establish an IV of Ringer's lactate. What drug order do you anticipate receiving from medical direction?
   a. atropine
   b. Benadryl®
   c. epinephrine
   d. lidocaine
   e. b and c

6. Briefly describe the continued assessment of this patient while en route to the hospital.

Shortly before reaching the hospital, the patient's condition improves. She has minimal itching and tells you that she feels "very sleepy."

7. Explain why the patient may be experiencing these symptoms.

The patient is treated in the emergency department for the allergic reaction and is released later that same day.

CASE PRESENTATION #2 (QUESTIONS 8–14)

You are dispatched to treat an injured person. A man has fallen from the roof of a two-story house while doing some repair work. He is lying on his back next to the house. It appears that he fell about 20 feet. You perform a rapid trauma assessment and stabilize his C-spine. Your initial assessment shows that he is awake and alert, is breathing at a rate of 22 breaths per minute, and has a strong pulse rate of 100.

8. What else should be evaluated in the initial assessment?

9. What questions should be asked regarding the fall itself?

The initial survey reveals no evidence of life-threatening conditions or of a load-and-go situation. The patient is complaining of severe pain in the left ankle and lower back area. He tells you that he turned to get a hammer, slipped on some loose shingles, lost his balance, and fell. He landed just as you found him and had not been moved before your arrival.

10. What is your next priority?

11. Describe aspects of the focused history and physical examination that would be important for this patient:

   (a) Vital signs

   (b) Head

   (c) Neck

   (d) Chest/Back

   (e) Abdomen

   (f) Pelvis

   (g) Extremities

The patient tells you that he ate lunch about an hour ago and now feels nauseated. He has a history of high blood pressure and takes Catapres®. There are no known allergies. On your focused examination, you find that he has clear breath sounds, a soft abdomen, and no signs of a possible pelvic fracture. However, examination of the extremities reveals decreased sensation and movement in both lower extremities, in addition to the obvious ankle fracture. He has normal sensation and movement in the upper extremities. His blood pressure is 94/60.

12. Using the SAMPLE history, document the information you have obtained while evaluating this patient's condition.

   S — _____
   A — _____
   M — _____
   P — _____
   L — _____
   E — _____

13. Having completed the focused history and physical examination, you prepare to transport the patient. Your next priority should be to:
   a. obtain an ECG reading.
   b. package his neck and back.
   c. stabilize the ankle fracture.
   d. start an IV of Ringer's lactate.

During transport to the hospital, you reevaluate the patient and find that he is becoming somewhat confused, agitated, and restless. You increase the oxygen percentage, but the symptoms remain the same. You also note that his left pupil is larger than the right and is less reactive to light.

14. These signs and symptoms could indicate:
    a. a closed head injury
    b. hypoxia
    c. internal bleeding
    d. shock
    e. all of the above

You inform medical direction of the changes in the patient's status and change your travel mode to lights and sirens. The patient is delivered in serious but stable condition to the emergency department.

Admission diagnosis: Fractured T-12 associated with quadriplegia, closed head injury, and a fractured left ankle.

GENERAL REVIEW QUESTIONS

15. The four main steps in the focused history and physical examination are:

    (a)

    (b)

    (c)

    (d)

16. Describe the information that can be obtained by using the mnemonic "OPQRST" for a chief complaint of pain.

    O — _____
    P — _____
    Q — _____
    R — _____
    S — _____
    T — _____

17. Which of the following may affect a blood pressure reading? (Circle all that apply.)
    a. anxiety
    b. heart failure
    c. inappropriate cuff size
    d. stress
    e. trauma

18. Which of the following conditions typically is *not* accompanied by jugular venous distention?
    a. cardiac tamponade
    b. congestive heart failure
    c. flail chest
    d. tension pneumothorax

19. The mnemonic DCAP/BTLS can be useful in the physical examination. Define the mnemonic, and describe how it is used.

20. Which of the following statements best describes the purpose of the continued assessment?
    a. Focus on the chief complaint for a SAMPLE history and physical examination.
    b. Identify immediately life-threatening conditions involving the airway, breathing, or circulation.
    c. Using a more detailed method, reevaluate the areas identified in the focused examination.
    d. Evaluate changes in vital signs and the ECG reading only.

21. Briefly describe aspects of the physical examination that are important for a medical patient with a cardiovascular or respiratory complaint.

22. Briefly describe the difference between open-ended and direct questions, and explain how they are used to obtain a thorough patient history.

Answers to questions from chapter 24 can be found on page 451.

Chapter 25

Pediatric Assessment

1. Describe the unique physiological, anatomical, and psychological characteristics of the pediatric patient.
2. Describe appropriate interaction with the pediatric patient's parents or guardian.
3. Identify ways to become better prepared to deal with pediatric patients.
4. Describe how the assessment process and management of the pediatric patient should be altered based on the child's developmental level.
5. Describe the essential components of the history and physical examination of a pediatric patient.
6. Identify priorities of care for a pediatric patient based on assessment findings.

CASE PRESENTATION #1 (QUESTIONS 1–6)

You are dispatched to the scene of a motor vehicle collision in a parking lot. Your patients are a mother and her 3-year-old son, who were rear-ended by a hit-and-run driver. The toddler was thrown from his car seat to the floor when the restraint failed. Concerned bystanders have removed both patients from the vehicle. When you arrive, the mother is sitting on the curb crying; she is holding her child. She insists that she is unhurt and demands that you hurry and check her son because he is "not acting right." The patient appears somewhat dizzy and begins to cry as your partner manually stabilizes his head and neck.

1. List additional behavioral signs that you should observe directly in your pediatric patient while asking the mother to describe what behaviors are different from normal.

2. Which of the following principles is important for you to remember while you are examining this toddler?
   a. Separate the child from his mother.
   b. Provide detailed explanations to the mother.
   c. Limit your examination to pertinent essentials.
   d. Perform a thorough head-to-toe examination.

His mother seems relieved when her son begins crying; she explains that it is not normal for him to be sleepy at this time of the day. His skin feels cool. His respirations are 40, pulse is 160 and difficult to palpate, and capillary refill is 3 seconds. The patient's crying and pulling away make it difficult for you to listen to breath sounds and obtaining a blood pressure reading. The only obvious sign of trauma is a bruise to the abdomen, which possibly was caused by the seatbelt. Evaluation of the mother reveals no significant findings at this time. Based on your findings, you and your partner prepare for immediate transport.

3. Explain why you feel a sense of urgency in transporting this patient to the hospital.

After airway management interventions and complete spinal immobilization, you contact medical direction. Your ETA at the nearest trauma center is 5 minutes. As you prepare to establish an IV line on your pediatric patient while en route, he begins to cry again. Attempting to reassure the child, your partner tells him, "It will only hurt a little."

4. Was this an appropriate response from your partner? Explain your response.

5. Explain why it is important to perform multiple serial examinations on this pediatric patient during transport.

The patients are delivered to the emergency department in stable condition. While you are restocking the ambulance for the next call, your partner confides in you that he is very uncomfortable when dealing with pediatric patients because he has no children of his own.

6. What suggestions can you make to your partner that may help him address this problem?

CASE PRESENTATION #2 (QUESTIONS 7-11)

You are dispatched to a 5-year-old who is having difficulty breathing. On arrival, you are met at the door by an anxious mother. She leads you to her daughter, who is in obvious respiratory distress.

7. Most likely, from whom will you obtain most of the history—the mother or the child? Explain your response.

8. List the five components of respiratory status that should be included in your physical examination of this patient.

(a)

(b)

(c)

(d)

(e)

The patient has a history of asthma. An hour ago, she used her inhaler once at the onset of this episode, with only minimal relief. She is alert but restless. Her vital signs are: BP 110 palpable; pulse 140; respirations 36 and labored. She has expiratory wheezing bilaterally and intercostal muscle retractions on inspiration. She has mild cyanosis of the lips, and her oxygen saturation level is 94%. You contact medical direction; you are ordered to administer nebulized albuterol. The patient literally grabs the nebulizer from you and self-administers. Within minutes of completion of the treatment, the patient's respiratory rate slows. You prepare to transport.

9. Explain why it is important to reassess more than just the respiratory rate in this patient.

10. Was it appropriate to allow this patient to self-administer the albuterol? Explain your response.

Once the patient's condition has improved, the mother says, "I should have called sooner when her inhaler didn't help."

11. What should you remember about parental dignity when responding to the mother?

The patient is observed in the emergency department and later is discharged.

GENERAL REVIEW QUESTIONS

Match the behavior below with the developmental age in which it is most likely observed. Choices a through e may be used more than once.

      a. Infant
      b. Toddler
      c. Preschooler
      d. School-aged child
      e. Adolescent

12. _____ Becomes upset and begins to scream for his mother as you attempt to restrain a possible fractured leg

13. _____ Begins to cry when you and your partner enter the room and when her mother suddenly begins to cry

14. _____ Becomes extremely upset over a superficial abrasion to the face

15. _____ Becomes very anxious when you expose her chest for auscultation

Based on developmental age, describe the general principles that you should follow to effectively approach or interact with each of the following patients.

16. An 8-year-old with mild respiratory distress resulting from an asthma attack. She is in the school gym for a physical education class.

17. A 2-year-old who has sustained a first-degree burn on his index finger after dipping it in his mother's hot coffee.

18. A 16-year-old who has moderate vaginal bleeding and low abdominal cramping. She is at the movie theater with her parents.

Describe how each of these anatomic differences can make endotracheal intubation in children more challenging than in the adult.

19. Larger tongue

20. Smaller cricoid ring

21. Smaller airway and shorter distances between structures

22. To obtain the most accurate respiratory rate assessment in small children, you should count:
    a. 10 seconds and multiply by 6.
    b. 15 seconds and multiply by 4.
    c. 30 seconds and multiply by 2.
    d. for a full minute.

23. What is an important clinical indicator of early shock in a pediatric patient?
    a. bradycardia
    b. hypotension
    c. mottling and pallor
    d. tachycardia

24. Which of the following is true about measuring capillary refill using the nail beds?
    a. It is an absolute sign of poor perfusion.
    b. It is less reliable if the extremity is cold.
    c. The extremity that is used should be below the heart.
    d. The normal response time is 4 to 5 seconds.

25. A bulging fontanelle in an 18-month-old who is in a sitting position may be an indication of:
    a. hypoxia.
    b. hypothermia.
    c. hypovolemia.
    d. meningitis.

26. Of the following patients with mild respiratory distress, who will require more ventilatory effort because of high lung compliance?
    a. a 2-year old with a cold
    b. a 5-year-old with asthma
    c. an infant with meningitis
    d. a neonate after delivery

27. The best way to determine if the central blood supply is well oxygenated is to check the:
    a. mucous membranes inside the eyelids and lips.
    b. nail beds of the lower extremities.
    c. respiratory rate and quality.
    d. skin temperature of the hands and feet.

28. Mentation and level of consciousness in children: (Circle all that apply.)
    a. can be evaluated by noting responses to noise and touch.
    b. cannot be documented objectively using the AVPU scale.
    c. are important indicators of general perfusion status.
    d. require parental input for confirmation of variations in infants.

29. The respiratory rate in children: (Circle all that are true.)
    a. is often variable or cyclic.
    b. is normally faster than in adults.
    c. may be elevated in the presence of fever.
    d. may slow with advancing hypoxia.

Answers to questions from chapter 25 can be found on page 453.

Chapter 26

Geriatric Assessment

1. Identify changes in anatomy and physiology that occur with aging.
2. Describe the special problems associated with assessment of the elderly and techniques to overcome them.
3. Describe the incidence and unique features of selected medical and trauma-related problems in the elderly patient.
4. Describe the special problems that exist regarding management of various illnesses and injuries in the elderly patient.
5. Identify the special problems associated with medication use by the elderly.
6. Identify factors associated with elder abuse and neglect.

CASE PRESENTATION #1 (QUESTIONS 1–7)

You are dispatched to a retirement community for treatment of a resident who has fallen. On arrival, you find a 72-year-old woman complaining of right hip pain. She slipped and fell several hours ago but refused to allow anyone to call 9-1-1 until now. You note that she is grimacing as she walks.

1. What correctable environmental problems may have led to this patient's fall?

2. Why do you think this patient may have been reluctant to call 9-1-1?

3. What significant questions related to the fall should you immediately ask the patient? Why?

On initial assessment, the patient is alert and oriented. Her pulse is 62 and thready, blood pressure is 124/88, respirations are 20, and breath sounds are clear. When measuring her vital signs, you note that her skin is clammy.

4. What is the significance of the findings in your initial assessment?

You quickly administer high-concentration oxygen via nonrebreather mask and attach the ECG monitor, which shows normal sinus rhythm. Your partner performs a rapid assessment of the patient's hip. The right leg appears shorter than the left and is externally rotated. The patient claims that the only medication she takes is a stool softener. Based on the mechanism of injury and this patient's clinical findings, you suspect that she has a fractured hip with underlying blood loss. She is immobilized on a padded backboard and is transported to the nearest hospital. You contact medical direction and, while en route, you establish an IV infusion of Ringer's lactate.

5. Is this patient at high risk for this type of injury? Explain your response.

6. Was spinal immobilization appropriate for this patient? Explain your response.

7. Would an IV fluid bolus be appropriate for this patient? Explain.

You arrive at the hospital 6 minutes later. The patient's condition is unchanged. You later learn that she is admitted to the orthopedic unit in stable condition after successful surgery has been performed to pin her fractured hip. Her blood loss passed into the surrounding tissue at the fracture site and was not significant.

CASE PRESENTATION #2 (QUESTIONS 8–10)

You are dispatched to a trailer park to care for an elderly patient. The daughter called 9-1-1 because her 80-year-old mother appears to be having difficulty breathing. On arrival, she tells you that she has been stopping by to check on her mother at least once a day ever since her father died a month ago. Before that time, the patient was physically active. As you enter a room where the patient is lying in bed, you immediately note a strong smell of urine and the patient's unkempt appearance; there are several empty beer cans on the floor. Using an agitated, slurred speech, she denies that she is having trouble breathing and states that she wants you to leave her alone. You note that her respirations are fast and shallow at approximately 34 per minute and that she is coughing up thick, brown sputum. She says that she just has a cold and informs you that she has been taking over-the-counter medications.

8. List possible reasons for this patient's mental status change, based on your assessment to this point.

The patient's pulse is 120 and regular, her blood pressure is 96/70, and her temperature is 101.2° F. Her skin is dry and pale, and she has slightly cyanotic axillary nail beds. Breath sounds are congested, with bilateral rhonchi and rales. You suspect that this patient has pneumonia. You administer high-concentration oxygen via nonrebreather mask, establish an IV at a TKO rate, connect her to the ECG monitor, and transport her to the nearest hospital, which is 5 minutes away. No additional orders are received from medical direction.

9. Describe changes in this patient's respiratory system that have resulted from aging that may have contributed to her contracting pneumonia.

10. Is this patient seriously ill? Explain your response.

The patient's condition is unchanged on arrival at the emergency department. She is admitted to the ICU. Three days later, she dies from respiratory failure caused by the worsening of her pneumonia.

CASE PRESENTATION #3 (QUESTIONS 11–17)

You are dispatched to the residence of a 69-year-old woman whose neighbor called because he had not seen her in several days and she was not answering her telephone. On arrival, you find the patient lying on the floor. She is conscious but mumbles incoherently when you ask her questions. The neighbor quickly blurts out, "She is hard of hearing."

11. What can you do to facilitate history taking from this hearing-impaired patient?

12. What significant question should you ask the neighbor regarding this patient's mental status?

13. Besides the neighbor, you should be alert for what other sources of information in the environment that may help in clarifying the cause of this patient's condition?

The patient's vital signs are: pulse 68 and regular; blood pressure 200/120; respirations 18 and unlabored. Her skin is warm and dry; there is no evidence of trauma on physical examination. It appears that she has right-sided facial drooping and decreased reflexes on the right with a depressed gag reflex. Her pupils are equal and reactive. The neighbor indicates that this behavior is drastically different for this patient, and that she is normally "sharp as a tack."

14. Is the information that was obtained from the neighbor significant? Explain your response.

15. Outline the steps that you should take in managing this patient's airway.

Before departure, you manage her airway, connect her to the cardiac monitor, and establish an IV at a TKO rate. A quick glucose determination measures 120. Your partner points out a bruise on the patient's arm that was apparently caused by the tourniquet that you used when starting her IV.

16. What is the significance of this finding?

17. Based on this patient's clinical findings, she is most likely experiencing:
    a. acute alcohol intoxication.
    b. Alzheimer's disease.
    c. cerebral vascular accident.
    d. psychiatric illness.

While en route to the hospital, you reassess the patient for changes in airway, breathing, circulation, level of consciousness, and vital signs, as well as for changes on the cardiac monitor. On arrival at the emergency department, her condition is unchanged.

GENERAL REVIEW QUESTIONS

For each of the body systems listed below, describe changes in anatomy and physiology that may occur as a normal consequence of aging, and discuss potential problems that these changes may create.

18. Gastrointestinal system

19. Skin

20. Respiratory system

21. Cardiovascular system

22. Renal system

23. Central nervous system

24. Musculoskeletal system

For each of the following statements (25–29), circle the correct response, True or False. Briefly explain your answer.

25. The elderly are less prone to serious head injury because there is shrinkage of brain tissue that is associated with aging.

TRUE   **FALSE**

Briefly explain your answer:_____

_____

_____

_____

26. Positive tenting of the skin is an obvious sign of dehydration in the elderly.

TRUE   **FALSE**

Briefly explain your answer:_____

_____

_____

_____

27. Depression is common in the elderly and may mimic senility or organic brain syndrome.

      TRUE   **FALSE**

Briefly explain your answer: _____

_____

28. Drug management of wheezing in the elderly is the same as that for other age groups.

      TRUE   **FALSE**

Briefly explain your answer: _____

_____

_____

_____

29. Elderly patients are at increased risk for adverse drug reactions, and the effects of drugs may be exaggerated in such patients.

      TRUE   **FALSE**

Briefly explain your answer: _____

_____

_____

30. Which of the following signs and symptoms are commonly associated with acute myocardial infarction (AMI) in an elderly person?
    a. decreased level of consciousness and radiating chest pain
    b. mild chest pain and severe shortness of breath
    c. severe chest pain and mild shortness of breath
    d. shortness of breath, fatigue, and epigastric discomfort

31. The leading causes of death among the elderly are:
    a. cancer, heart disease, and stroke.
    b. chronic obstructive lung disease, stroke, and falls.
    c. heart disease, stroke, and drug overdose.
    d. hypertension, cancer, and trauma.

32. A common psychiatric problem among the elderly is:
    a. Alzheimer's disease.
    b. delirium.
    c. depression.
    d. schizophrenia.

33. The primary finding in elder abuse is:
    a. dehydration.
    b. malnutrition.
    c. poor hygiene.
    d. unexplained trauma.

34. Which of the following is true about the aging process? (Circle all that apply.)
   a. The left ventricle thickens and becomes more rigid.
   b. There is decreased total body water and fat.
   c. There is a significant increase in oxygen uptake.
   d. There is a significant decline in metabolic rate.

35. Elements of aging that may make it difficult to assess the elderly include: (Circle all that apply.)
   a. decreased or absent pain perception.
   b. dementia.
   c. diminished sight and hearing.
   d. depressed temperature regulation mechanisms.

36. Contributing factors to medication errors in the elderly include: (Circle all that apply.)
   a. depression.
   b. limited income.
   c. poor vision.
   d. self-selection of drugs.

Answers to questions from chapter 26 can be found on page 455.

Section 4A

PATIENT PRESENTATIONS—MEDICAL

CHAPTERS

27. Dyspnea
28. Nontraumatic Bleeding
29. Syncope
30. Altered Mental Status
31. Chest Pain
32. Palpitations and Dysrhythmias
33. Headache
34. Weak, Dizzy, and Malaise
35. Diabetic Emergencies
36. Abdominal, Genitourinary, and Back Pain
37. Pregnancy and Childbirth
38. Fever
39. Eye, Ear, Nose, and Throat Complaints—Medical
40. Nontraumatic Extremity Complaints
41. Poisoning and Overdose
42. Drugs of Abuse
43. Environmental Emergencies
44. Aquatic Emergencies
45. Behavioral Emergencies

Chapter 27

Dyspnea

OBJECTIVES

1. Describe the normal physiology of breathing.
2. Define dyspnea.
3. Describe the history and assessment of the patient complaining of dyspnea.
4. Define and list signs and symptoms of respiratory failure.
5. Describe and differentiate among various causes of dyspnea in the prehospital setting.
6. In an examination of a patient with dyspnea, explain the significance of a silent chest, abnormal breath sounds, vital signs, and cardiac rhythm.
7. Describe general prehospital management of the patient with dyspnea.
8. Describe the different management approaches to various patient conditions that present with dyspnea.
9. List the indications, actions, potential side effects, and precautions for various medications used to treat specific causes of dyspnea.

CASE PRESENTATION # 1 (QUESTIONS 1–6)

You are dispatched to a "difficulty breathing" call at an elementary school. On arrival, you find a seven-year-old boy sitting in the playground, laboring to breathe. The teacher reports that the patient has a history of asthma and that the school nurse is attempting to locate his Proventil® inhaler.

1. What immediate interventions are appropriate for this patient?

2. What is the action of Proventil®?

Further physical assessment reveals cool and wet skin with mild circumoral cyanosis. You note retraction of the neck muscles on inhalation, and you find breath sounds difficult to auscultate. Your partner reports the following vital signs: BP 98/60; pulse 124 and regular; respirations 36 and shallow.

3. Explain why you may have difficulty auscultating the patient's breath sounds.

4. Are the patient's vital signs normal? Explain why, or why not.

As your partner prepares to initiate an IV of normal saline, you contact medical direction. The physician orders you to administer nebulized albuterol. After administering the medication as ordered, you reassess the patient.

5. What physical assessment findings indicate an improvement in this patient's condition?

Within minutes after treatment, the patient states, "I can breathe much better now." His breath sounds are audible with mild wheezing. His vital signs are: BP 92/60; pulse 98; and respirations 22 and less labored. As you are preparing to transport the patient to the emergency department, the school nurse knocks on the window of the mobile intensive care unit (MICU) screaming, "I found his Proventil® inhaler!"

6. Should you administer the Proventil® to this patient? Explain why, or why not.

The patient is admitted to the emergency department for observation and is later discharged.

CASE PRESENTATION #2 (QUESTIONS 7–14)

You are dispatched to a "respiratory emergency" at a private residence. On arrival, you find a thin, middle-aged woman sitting on the sofa in obvious respiratory distress. Her lips are pursed as she struggles to breathe, and you can hear wheezing without the use of a stethoscope.

7. List six additional signs of impending respiratory failure which you should be alert for when you are assessing this patient:

    (a)

    (b)

    (c)

    (d)

    (e)

    (f)

She is wearing a nasal cannula attached to a cylinder that is dispensing oxygen at a rate of 4 liters per minute. She is alert but extremely anxious. Her skin is diaphoretic, and she has peripheral cyanosis. She is so short of breath that she can answer your questions only by nodding her head yes or no. You determine that she has been ill for several days but that she has become progressively worse in the past few hours. When you ask about medications, she hands you a paper bag from which you remove two packs of cigarettes, partially empty medication bottles labeled "prednisone" and "Theo-Dur®," and an Alupent® inhaler.

8. Based on your assessment findings, you suspect that this patient is experiencing:
    a. anaphylaxis.
    b. decompensated COPD.
    c. pulmonary embolism.
    d. pneumothorax.

9. What additional history related to her medications would be helpful to know as you determine appropriate treatment for this patient?

Your partner replaces the patient's nasal cannula with a nonrebreather mask while you quickly measure her vital signs. Your findings are: BP 160/94; pulse 110 and irregular; respirations labored at a rate of 26 per minute.

10. Was your partner's action appropriate? Explain why, or why not.

11. Is cardiac monitoring indicated for this patient? Explain why, or why not.

The patient shows slight improvement after the concentration of oxygen is increased. You begin transport to the hospital; the patient has been admitted here multiple times in the past. This is also the closest hospital, giving you an ETA of 5 minutes. You start an IV TKO while en route and contact medical direction. You have albuterol and aminophylline on the MICU. The physician orders you to administer nebulized albuterol while en route.

12. In your opinion, why did the physician order albuterol instead of aminophylline for this patient?

On your arrival to the emergency department, blood tests and radiographs are ordered. You are still in the emergency department when the patient's arterial blood gas report comes back from the laboratory.

13. What would you expect this patient's pCO_2 and pO_2 to be? Explain why.

14. Explain why the use of pulse oximetry would have been helpful in monitoring this patient en route.

CASE PRESENTATION #3 (QUESTIONS 15-19)

You are called to a retirement center at around midnight. The attending nurse has told dispatch that the patient has a history of cardiac problems and she thinks that he is having another heart attack. On arrival, you find an alert, oriented 70-year-old man who is moderately short of breath. He denies any chest pain but admits it is getting more difficult for him to breathe. You immediately administer high-concentration oxygen with a nonrebreather mask; you initiate an IV of D5W TKO and connect him to the cardiac monitor, which shows atrial fibrillation at a rate of 90–100 with occasional unifocal PVCs. His BP is 150/90, pulse is strong and irregular, and respirations are 22 per minute and labored. Rales are audible to the level of the scapulae and his SaO_2 is 84%. The only medication he takes routinely is a diuretic.

15. Should you suspect myocardial infarction in this patient? Explain why, or why not.

16. What additional assessment findings would lead you to believe that this patient is also experiencing pulmonary edema?

Medical direction orders you to administer nitroglycerin sublingually and to begin transport. Your ETA at the hospital is 4 minutes.

17. After administering nitroglycerin, for what serious side effect should you monitor this patient closely? Explain why.

18. List two alternative medications that medical direction could have ordered for this patient instead of nitroglycerin. Explain why they would have been effective.

The patient's condition is unchanged on arrival to the emergency department. On your next shift, you learn that in spite of aggressive treatment in the hospital, this patient's condition worsened and he died a few hours after having been admitted to the ICU.

General Review Questions

Circle the correct answer within the parentheses ( ).

19. Breathing is usually (<u>a voluntary</u> or <u>an involuntary</u>) activity.

20. The most important stimulus for breathing is the blood level of (<u>carbon dioxide</u> or <u>oxygen</u>).

21. Dyspnea is noted when the resistance to air flow (<u>increases</u> or <u>decreases</u>).

22. An easily observable clinical sign of respiratory decompensation is (<u>the use of accessory muscles</u> or <u>peripheral cyanosis</u>).

23. Respiratory failure is imminent in a patient with dyspnea when (<u>tachycardia</u> or <u>bradycardia</u>) is also present.

Match the abnormal breath sound in Column 2 with the area in the respiratory tract or the common disorder with which it is associated in Column 1.

Column 1

24. ____ Upper airway
25. ____ Bronchi
26. ____ Alveoli
27. ____ Asthma
28. ____ Epiglottis
29. ____ Croup

Column 2

a. Wheezing
b. Stridor
c. Rales
d. Rhonchi

30. List at least five personal history questions that you should ask a patient who is experiencing dyspnea.

(a)

(b)

(c)

(d)

(e)

Describe the appropriate treatment for each of the following patients. Each is presenting with a chief complaint of dyspnea.

31. A 46-year-old fireman who was overcome by smoke. There are no burns present about his face, but he is coughing sooty sputum. Breath sounds are clear.

32. A 2-year-old boy with a fever of 103° F and a sore throat for 2 days. He is leaning forward and is drooling from the side of his mouth.

33. A 60-year-old man with a history of bronchitis. He is using accessory muscles to breathe and has moderate wheezing.

34. A 25-year-old man who broke out in hives minutes after eating shrimp. He is awake and alert with bilateral wheezing.

35. A 30-year-old patient with blunt trauma to the chest that was sustained in a motor vehicle collision. The patient has tracheal deviation to the left and absent breath sounds on the right.

36. A 16-year-old girl who became anxious about an examination at school. She is complaining of numbness around her lips and fingers. She is breathing at a rate of 36 per minute. Breath sounds are clear.

37. Dyspnea is defined as:
   a. cessation of breathing.
   b. underinflation of the lungs.
   c. an uncomfortable sensation while breathing.
   d. low blood levels of oxygen.

38. A patient with anemia may develop dyspnea because of:
   a. an increased metabolic acidosis.
   b. poor blood flow to the lungs.
   c. a decreased ventilation/perfusion ratio.
   d. a reduced oxygen-carrying capacity of the blood.

39. In an acute asthma attack, the most accurate available indicator of acuity is based on:
   a. the time of onset.
   b. a comparison of episodes.
   c. the presence of chest pain.
   d. the duration of the episode.

40. Dyspnea that is precipitated by exertion associated with an increased heart rate may be:
   a. cardiac in nature.
   b. a sign of pneumonia.
   c. an allergic reaction.
   d. of minimal concern.

41. Which of the following patients presenting with a chief complaint of dyspnea has a history suggestive of pulmonary embolism?
   a. a 4-year-old who has a skin rash and mild facial swelling
   b. a victim of a motor vehicle collision who has decreased breath sounds on one side
   c. a 62-year-old emphysema patient who is coughing up green sputum
   d. a 27-year-old who has hemoptysis two days after surgery for a fractured leg

Answers to questions from chapter 27 can be found on page 457.

Chapter 28

Nontraumatic Bleeding

OBJECTIVES

1. Define hemostasis, and discuss how it is accomplished by the body.
2. List diseases or conditions that may be associated with inadequate clotting ability.
3. Define the following terms:
   a. Epistaxis
   b. Hematemesis
   c. Hematuria
   d. Hemoptysis
   e. Melena
4. Discuss assessment procedures to perform on a patient who has nontraumatic bleeding and key assessment findings.
5. Identify causes, potential sites, signs and symptoms, and field treatment for patients who present with:
   a. Epistaxis
   b. Hematemesis
   c. Hematuria
   d. Hemoptysis
   e. Melena

CASE PRESENTATION #1 (QUESTIONS 1-9)

You are dispatched to a medical emergency. On arrival at the scene, you find a middle-aged man sitting at the kitchen table. He is conscious and alert. The patient apparently lives alone, and no bystanders are present. His chief complaint is that he has abdominal pain and is vomiting "coffee ground material."

1. While establishing ABCs and checking vital signs, you recall that his chief complaint could indicate:
   a. cerebral vascular accident.
   b. heart attack.
   c. internal bleeding.
   d. neurologic problems.

Vital signs are as follows: B/P 128/70; pulse 110; respirations 24 and shallow. His skin is slightly pale.

2. Which of these findings could indicate the presence of early shock?
   a. blood pressure alone
   b. blood pressure and pulse rate
   c. pulse rate alone
   d. respiratory rate alone
   e. respiratory and pulse rates

Further history reveals that the patient has been vomiting for the past 2 days. He says that he had been taking a lot of Maalox® for his stomach, and he has been unable to keep food down. He also tells you that he has a history of ulcers and has been taking Tagamet®.

3. Further patient questioning is needed; however, the most important question to ask now is:
   a. Have you been coughing at night?
   b. How long have you been taking Tagamet®?
   c. What does your stool look like?
   d. When were you diagnosed with ulcers?

You continue to question the patient and discover that he has a long history of alcohol abuse; he developed ulcers about a year ago. The medication that was prescribed for him seemed to be effective until recently, when he started having abdominal pain again. He says that he has noticed that it occurs when he has been drinking heavily. He denies melena.

4. Based on the information obtained to this point, his bleeding is most likely coming from the:
   a. gallbladder.
   b. lower colon.
   c. rectum.
   d. spleen.
   e. stomach.

5. Identify the steps of a physical examination that would be especially important for this patient.

6. Briefly discuss the relationship between alcohol abuse and the development of ulcer disease.

On physical examination, you find that the patient has moderate abdominal tenderness and a palpable enlarged liver, but he does not show any signs of peritonitis. You take his vital signs again, in a supine position and then in a sitting position. They are as follows: Lying: B/P 128/70; pulse 110. Sitting: B/P 96/50; pulse 138.

7. Do the changes in the patient's vital signs indicate a negative or a positive tilt test? Briefly explain your answer.

8. You prepare the patient for transport. Field treatment should include:
   a. dopamine drip.
   b. epinephrine drip.
   c. a high concentration of oxygen.
   d. an IV of Ringer's lactate or normal saline.
   e. c and d
   f. a and c

9. You contact medical direction and give your report. You are told to transport the patient using lights and sirens. Briefly discuss the rationale for this order from medical direction.

CASE PRESENTATION #2 (QUESTIONS 10–15)

You are dispatched for treatment of a patient with possible heart attack. On arrival at the scene, you find a 68-year-old woman lying on her bed. The patient is conscious and states that she has been coughing up blood. She says that she is very "weak" and has been sick about 3 days.

10. With a chief complaint of hemoptysis, what conditions should you consider as possible causes?

The patient provides the following information: Her illness began 3 days ago with a "chest cold," which was associated with a productive cough, chest discomfort, and fever. Earlier today, she noticed that her sputum contained "blood streaks," and she became very concerned. She has no history of respiratory disease; she has had no major medical problems. She has never smoked. Vital signs are as follows: B/P 152/86; pulse 120 and weak; respirations 28 and shallow. Oral temperature is 103° F. You note that she has crackles in the bases of both lungs.

11. Based on this information, you most likely suspect:
    a. chronic obstructive pulmonary disease.
    b. congestive heart failure.
    c. gastrointestinal bleeding.
    d. pneumonia.

12. Is this condition typically associated with hypovolemia? Briefly explain your response.

13. Your field management of this patient could include:
    a. oxygen administration.
    b. epinephrine IV push.
    c. IV of normal saline or Ringer's lactate and oxygen, administered TKO.
    d. nitroglycerin.
    e. a and c
    f. b and c

The patient remains stable en route to the hospital; however, on arrival at the emergency department, she begins to experience increased breathing difficulty.

14. Briefly describe why the patient began to experience breathing difficulty.

15. Now that you know the outcome of this call, is there anything that you would like to have done differently? Briefly explain your response.

GENERAL REVIEW QUESTIONS

16. A common cause of epistaxis is:
   a. bronchitis.
   b. gastrointestinal bleeding.
   c. hypertension.
   d. liver disease.
   e. pulmonary embolus.

17. In early pregnancy (first trimester), vaginal bleeding may be caused by:
   a. abruptio placentae.
   b. ectopic pregnancy.
   c. hyperemesis gravidarum.
   d. placenta previa.
   e. preeclampsia.

18. List two causes of hematuria, other than trauma:

   (a)

   (b)

19. Define hemostasis, and briefly describe three factors that affect it.

20. The earliest indication of hypoperfusion in a patient who is experiencing nontraumatic bleeding is:
   a. falling blood pressure.
   b. mentation changes.
   c. rapid respirations.
   d. tachycardia.

21. List at least three conditions or diseases that can alter the body's blood clotting ability.

22. Your patient is a 72-year-old man who is complaining of rectal bleeding. He states that he has had the problem for several days, and he is currently feeling light-headed. He describes that his stool is "streaked with bright red blood." You suspect that he is bleeding from the:
   a. colon.
   b. esophagus.
   c. liver.
   d. stomach.
   e. upper small intestine.

23. Discuss appropriate field treatment for a patient who is experiencing epistaxis.

24. The EMS provider should be alert to three potentially life-threatening complications of nontraumatic bleeding. These include:

   (a)

   (b)

   (c)

For each of the following statements (25–27), circle the correct response, True or False. Briefly explain your answer.

25. For treatment of patients with hemoptysis, a mask should be placed on the faces of both the patient and the EMS provider.

   TRUE   **FALSE**

Briefly explain your answer:_____
_____
_____
_____

26. All patients with nontraumatic bleeding should receive oxygen.

TRUE　　　　　　　　**FALSE**

Briefly explain your answer: _____

_____

_____

27. Foamy pink-tinged sputum indicates rapid bleeding from the lungs.

TRUE　　　　　　　　**FALSE**

Briefly explain your answer: _____

_____

_____

_____

Answers to questions from chapter 28 can be found on page 459.

Chapter 29

Syncope

OBJECTIVES

1. Define *syncope* and discuss its pathophysiology.
2. Identify the possible causes of syncope.
3. Discuss the following conditions in terms of pathophysiology, clinical significance, and prehospital management:
   a. Vasovagal response
   b. Orthostatic hypotension
4. Identify key historical questions to ask a patient who has experienced syncope.
5. Describe aspects of the physical examination that are indicated for a patient experiencing syncope.
6. Discuss the clinical significance of orthostatic vital signs (tilt test) as related to syncope.
7. Discuss the significance and probable cause of syncope in a patient who has no warning signs.
8. Describe the prehospital management of a patient with syncope.

CASE PRESENTATION #1 (QUESTIONS 1–8)

You are dispatched to a residence for treatment of a patient with a possible heart attack. The fire department crew was at the scene 2 minutes before your arrival. You find them with an elderly man who is sitting in a chair. He is conscious but appears to be confused. A member of the crew informs you that the patient said he "passed out" before their arrival.

1. Briefly discuss critical observations and findings that you should make in your initial assessment.

2. You establish ABCs, administer oxygen, and obtain vital signs. Your next priority is to:
   a. assess the patient's altered mental status.
   b. obtain the patient's medical history.
   c. obtain a 12-lead ECG reading.
   d. perform a blood glucose determination.

The patient is alert but disoriented to place and time. Vital signs are: BP 96/60; pulse 44 and weak; respirations 24 and shallow. His skin is slightly pale and moist.

3. List at least 5 questions about his syncopal event that you should ask the patient quickly.

   (a)

   (b)

   (c)

   (d)

   (e)

Further history reveals that the episode began about an hour ago. The symptoms started suddenly without any warning. The patient states that, while reading the paper, he began to feel "pressure in his chest." When he attempted to get up from his chair, he experienced dizziness and sat down again. When his wife arrived home 45 minutes later, she called 9-1-1. He has a history of hypertension and takes Catapres®. His medical history reveals no other pertinent information. You apply an ECG monitor.

ECG lead II reveals the following:

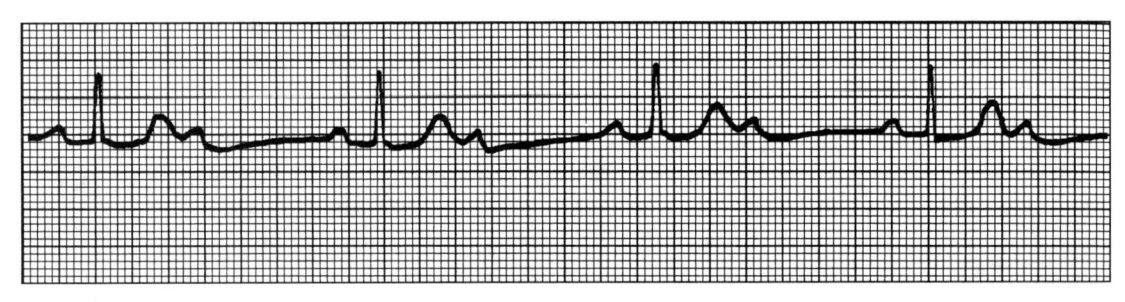

Figure 29-1

4. The best description for this ECG is:
   a. sinus bradycardia.
   b. first-degree heart block.
   c. second-degree heart block, type I.
   d. second-degree heart block, type II.
   e. third-degree heart block.

5. Based on the history and physical findings, what is the most likely cause of his syncopal episode? Explain why.

6. You quickly get the patient on the stretcher, establish an IV, and contact on-line medical direction (OLMD). You anticipate that _____ will be ordered initially.
   a. atropine 0.5 mg IV push.
   b. dopamine 200 mg IVPB.
   c. epinephrine 1.0 mg IVPB.
   d. transcutaneous pacing.

While en route to the hospital, the patient's overall condition and mental status improve. Vital signs are: BP 114/60; pulse 62; respirations 20, not labored. ECG: second-degree heart block, Type II. His blood sugar is 120.

7. OLMD now could direct you to administer:
   a. 50% dextrose IV push.
   b. Levophed drip.
   c. lidocaine IV push.
   d. nitroglycerin, sublingual or spray.

On arrival at the hospital, the patient's mental status and vital signs are stable. His chest pain is still present, although it is diminished somewhat.

8. What would you anticipate to be the next priority for emergency department personnel?

CASE PRESENTATION #2 (QUESTIONS 9–15)

You are dispatched to an office complex for a medical emergency. On arrival at the scene, you find a 28-year-old woman who is lying on a couch. She is conscious and alert. Her chief complaint is that she "passed out." You begin to obtain her vital signs. Her skin is pale and slightly cool to the touch.

9. List four key questions that you should ask this patient initially.

   (a)

   (b)

   (c)

   (d)

Her vital signs are: BP 100/50; pulse 120; respirations 26 and shallow. You discover that the syncopal episodes have been going on for about 30 to 45 minutes. She denies any history of diabetes, seizure, or heart problems. For the past 8 to 10 hours, she has had intermittent left lower quadrant abdominal pain that was associated with nausea. The pain now has subsided.

10. Based on the above information, it would be most important to ask her:
   a. Have you been taking any medication?
   b. Is there a history of heart problems in your family?
   c. When was your last meal?
   d. When was your last normal menstrual period?

On physical examination, you find that the patient has a tender abdomen and a positive tilt test. Her blood sugar reading is 130.

11. Explain the significance of a positive tilt test in this case.

You discover that her last menstrual period was about 8 weeks ago; there is no obvious external vaginal bleeding, discharge, or dysuria present.

12. Based on the patient's history and your physical findings, you *most likely* suspect a/an:
    a. acute appendicitis.
    b. hypoglycemic episode.
    c. kidney infection.
    d. ruptured ectopic pregnancy.

You prepare for transport and contact OLMD. The patient's BP is now 78/50, pulse is 130, and respirations are 26.

13. This patient is in what type of shock?
    a. anaphylactic
    b. cardiogenic
    c. hypovolemic
    d. neurogenic

14. Describe appropriate treatment for this patient.

15. Briefly describe the pathophysiology that led to her syncopal episode.

CASE PRESENTATION #3 (QUESTIONS 16–19)

You are dispatched for a medical emergency. On arrival, you find an elderly woman sitting at the kitchen table, where she was making homemade jam. She tells you that she ate breakfast, and that she had been sitting at the table working for about an hour. When she got up to get another ingredient, she felt her "head swim" and experienced blurry vision. She quickly sat down and felt better, but she called 9-1-1 because the episode frightened her. She has been in good health and takes no medications.

16. Based on the information provided in this case, this patient most likely is experiencing:
   a. cerebral vascular accident.
   b. hypoglycemia.
   c. hypovolemia.
   d. orthostatic hypotension.

Further questioning reveals that she has never experienced a similar episode. Also, you verify that there are no major medical problems.

17. Briefly explain why this patient may have experienced this syncopal episode.

18. Other pertinent questions to ask this patient include:

   (a)

   (b)

   (c)

   (d)

   (e)

19. The patient's condition most commonly is seen in what age group of patients?
   a. geriatric patients
   b. middle-aged people
   c. pediatric patients
   d. young adults

General Review Questions

20. Define syncope and discuss its pathophysiology.

    (a)

    (b)

21. Briefly define vasovagal episode. List two possible causes.

22. You obtain the vital signs of a patient, first in a supine position, then when sitting. Which of the following could indicate a positive tilt test? (Circle all that apply.)
    a. dizziness upon sitting up
    b. a pulse increase of 30 beats
    c. a systolic BP drop of 20 points
    d. a widened pulse pressure

23. List five possible causes of syncope; briefly explain the rationale for each.

    (a)

    (b)

    (c)

    (d)

    (e)

24. Any patient who develops syncope while supine without warning symptoms must be assumed to have a _____ cause and must be treated accordingly.

25. Briefly describe why pregnant patients sometimes experience syncope.

Answers to questions from chapter 29 can be found on page 461.

Chapter 30

Altered Mental Status

OBJECTIVES

1. Explain the pathophysiology related to altered mental status.
2. Describe the pathophysiology and identify subjective and objective findings of the following potentially life-threatening causes of altered mental status:
   a. Cerebrovascular accident
   b. Hypoglycemia
   c. Hypoperfusion
   d. Hypoxia
   e. Meningitis
   f. Seizures
   g. Toxins
   h. Tumors
3. Identify the key historical features in the assessment of a patient with altered mental status.
4. Outline the components of a rapid, directed physical examination in evaluating patients with altered mental status.
5. Given any of the following descriptive mental status terms, identify the corresponding patient behavior:
   a. Lethargic
   b. Awake
   c. Oriented
   d. Alert
   e. Confusion
   f. Agitation
   g. Aware
6. Describe the prehospital management of patients with altered mental status.

CASE PRESENTATION #1 (QUESTIONS 1–8)

At 10:00 a.m., you are dispatched for a medical emergency at a middle school. On arrival, you and your partner are led to the school nurse's office. The patient is a 13-year-old boy who appears to be unconscious. He is lying on his side on a cot. On quick observation, you note that he is breathing and that his skin is very pale. You also determine that he has a weak and rapid radial pulse.

1. While your partner is gathering information from the school nurse, you should:
   a. check the patient's blood pressure.
   b. further evaluate the patient's respiratory status.
   c. prepare to start an IV line.
   d. take an oral temperature.

The nurse tells you that about 15 minutes ago she received an urgent page to go to the patient's classroom. She found the patient on the floor beside his desk having what she describes as a generalized seizure. She stayed with the patient and protected his airway until the seizure activity ceased. He was taken on a stretcher to her office, where he had two more seizures. You administer oxygen and closely monitor the patient's respiratory status, watching for further seizure activity.

2. What historical information would be important to determine next?

The patient begins to have another generalized seizure. You and your partner continue providing patient care. The nurse provides further information: The patient does not have a history of seizure disorder, but recently he was diagnosed as a Type I diabetic, and he now takes insulin. The patient is now postictal and responds only to physical stimuli. Blood pressure is 92/60; pulse is 130.

3. Is it likely that the seizure activity is related to his medical history of diabetes? Briefly explain your response.

Your partner quickly prepares to check the patient's blood sugar and to establish an IV life line.

4. Would you expect his blood sugar to be low or high? Briefly explain your response.

Rapid glucose determination reveals a blood sugar of 25. The IV has been established successfully. According to local protocol, you can administer 25 grams of 50% dextrose for this blood sugar reading. Your partner administers the medication.

5. When administering this drug, you should be particularly careful to observe for:
   a. hypotension.
   b. respiratory depression.
   c. tachycardia.
   d. tissue infiltration.

Within two minutes, the patient begins to moan and appears to be waking up. Your questioning reveals that he is aware of who he is, but he is very confused about where he is and what happened. He last remembers sitting at his desk and listening to the teacher. The nurse now tells you that she has been unsuccessful in reaching the boy's parents.

6. Can you legally proceed to take the patient to the emergency department without parental permission? Explain your response.

7. If you should choose to transport the patient to the hospital, what would be important to monitor during your continued assessment?

The patient's mental status continues to improve, and he arrives at the emergency department in good condition. The admitting diagnosis is hypoglycemia.

8. Briefly explain how this condition causes altered mental status.

CASE PRESENTATION #2 (QUESTIONS 9–15)

You are dispatched to an outdoor concert for treatment of a possible drug overdose. As you arrive on the scene, there is a large crowd surrounding the patient. Police are also on the scene because violent activity has erupted from the crowd. The police escort you to the patient, who is an approximately 20-year-old woman. As you begin your assessment, she opens her eyes to your verbal command but quickly "passes out" again. Her airway is intact; respirations are 6 and shallow. Pulse is strong, at a rate of 70 beats per minute (bpm). She is not responding to your questions.

9. You assist her ventilations. As you continue your assessment, your next step should be to:
    a. obtain an ECG reading.
    b. obtain a blood pressure reading.
    c. look for drug paraphernalia.
    d. obtain information from bystanders.
    e. c and d

The patient's boyfriend tells you that she has been very upset lately because her parents are divorcing. While they were at the concert, a stranger approached and asked if they wanted to try something in a syringe for a "perfect high." He says that they had used some drugs in the past but had never taken intravenous drugs. When he told the stranger that he didn't want to try the drug, his girlfriend became very upset. He then went to the concession stand to get something to eat. When he returned, he found her this way. Another bystander tells you that he thought she shot up some type of "heroin."

10. You notice a place on her arm that looks like a puncture site; then you check her pupils. You would expect to find that her pupils are:
    a. dilated.
    b. of normal size.
    c. pinpoint.
    d. unequal.

11. If the patient did shoot up an intravenous heroin-type drug, how would this affect her mental status? Briefly explain your response.

Further examination reveals a blood pressure of 100/70, pale skin, and diminished breath sounds bilaterally. The blood sugar reading is 100. ECG shows normal sinus rhythm. Pupils are found to be pinpoint. You start an IV of Ringer's lactate and load the patient on a stretcher.

12. You would anticipate an order from medical direction for:
    a. activated charcoal.
    b. dextrose 50%.
    c. naloxone.
    d. syrup of Ipecac.

13. What changes in the patient's condition should you expect to notice after administering this medication?

During transport to the hospital, she becomes somewhat agitated, and you are forced to apply soft wrist restraints. You also notice that she has a very strong smell of alcohol on her breath. Her respiratory status improves; she now is breathing unassisted at a rate of 16. She tells you that she does not want to go to the hospital because she will get in a lot of trouble with her parents.

14. What advice should you give her? Explain your response.

15. What aspects of this call would be important to document on your patient care report?

She finally agrees to transport. She is in stable condition upon arrival at the emergency department. When you return to the hospital later in the evening, you are told that she was treated for her overdose and admitted to the psychiatric division for depression.

GENERAL REVIEW QUESTIONS

16. Discuss how altered mental status might be described by a patient or family member.

17. The sudden onset of localizing neurologic signs that are not associated necessarily with unresponsiveness is usually the result of:
   a. acute myocardial infarction.
   b. cerebral vascular accident.
   c. hypoglycemia.
   d. meningitis.
   e. status epilepticus.

18. When obtaining the history of a patient with altered mental status, what initial questions should you ask of others on the scene?

19. The occurrence of several generalized seizures without a period of consciousness between them is called:
   a. focal episodes.
   b. Jacksonian seizures.
   c. postictal state.
   d. status epilepticus.

20. Acute intracranial hemorrhage that produces an altered mental status may be caused by:
   a. blockage of blood vessels.
   b. embolism from the heart.
   c. rupture of blood vessels.
   d. thrombosis.
   e. all of the above

Match the descriptive term for mental status in Column 1 with its corresponding patient behavior description in Column 2.

Column 1

21. ____ Lethargic
22. ____ Awake
23. ____ Oriented
24. ____ Alert
25. ____ Confusion
26. ____ Agitated
27. ____ Aware

Column 2

a. Restless, unable to remain still; unable to control behavior
b. Understands present circumstances, such as who the current president is
c. Obviously alert, or a sleeping patient who can be easily awakened
d. Can be awakened, but returns to sleep when external stimulation ends
e. Awake and responds to surroundings; may be acting appropriately or inappropriately
f. A slowed thinking process; person is unable to think clearly
g. Able to identify from most to least difficult, the date, day of the week, month, year, place, and event

28. Describe how bradycardia and tachycardia can cause altered mental status.

29. During the physical examination of patients with altered mental status, describe what should be evaluated in the following areas:

   (a) State of mental functioning

   (b) Breathing/respiratory status

   (c) Skin

   (d) Pupils

   (e) Muscle strength

30. Which of the following conditions cause(s) altered mental status resulting from increased intracranial pressure? (Circle all that apply.)
   a. brain tumor
   b. cerebral vascular accident
   c. hypoperfusion
   d. meningitis
   e. subarachnoid hemorrhage

31. Discuss the general field management of a patient with altered mental status.

Answers to questions from chapter 30 can be found on page 463.

Chapter 31

Chest Pain

OBJECTIVES

1. Explain the pathophysiology of the various types of chest pain.
2. Identify the key historical features in the assessment of chest pain.
3. Describe a rapid, directed physical examination when evaluating patients with chest pain.
4. Identify the subjective and objective findings associated with potentially life-threatening processes in patients with chest pain.
5. Describe the prehospital management of patients with chest pain.

CASE PRESENTATION #1 (QUESTIONS 1–9)

You are dispatched to a call on the ninth floor of an office building. Upon arrival, you find a 62-year-old man sitting at a conference table. He is anxious and is complaining of chest pain. During your initial assessment, he remains conscious and alert. You note that he is pale and slightly sweaty, and his respirations are labored.

1. Given this initial information, could the patient be in shock? Explain your answer.

2. The initial treatment priority for this patient is to:
   a. administer oxygen.
   b. obtain a 12-lead ECG.
   c. request an order for morphine sulfate.
   d. start a TKO IV.

You obtain additional history and discover that his pain started about an hour ago after lunch. He describes the pain as very severe, radiating to his left arm, and associated with nausea. He denies any cardiac medical history and any major medical problems. His vital signs are: BP 86/60; pulse slow and weak; respirations 26 and shallow.

You apply monitoring leads and prepare to perform a 12-lead ECG. The rhythm is shown in Figure 31-1.

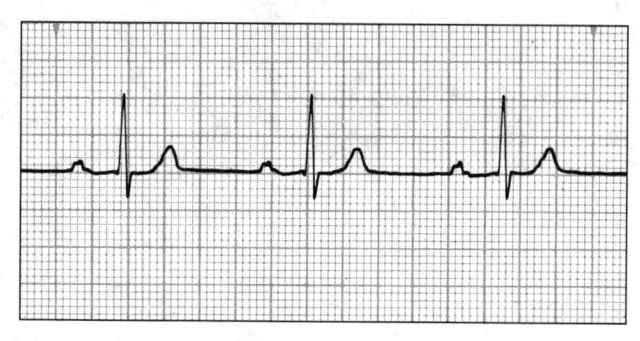

Figure 31-1

3. His ECG rhythm indicates which of the following?
   a. second-degree heart block, Mobitz I
   b. second-degree heart block, Mobitz II
   c. sinus bradycardia with first-degree heart block
   d. third-degree heart block
   e. none of the above

4. What could be the cause of the slow heart rate?

5. Should you prepare to treat his condition? Explain your response.

6. Which of the following drugs is indicated initially for treatment of this patient's rhythm?
   a. atropine
   b. dopamine
   c. epinephrine
   d. lidocaine

7. Briefly outline your field management of this patient at this point.

8. Could it be beneficial to perform a 12-lead ECG in the field on this patient? Why, or why not?

9. You anticipate that, in the emergency department, the immediate priority for this patient will be to obtain or receive:
    a. a chest radiograph.
    b. immediate admission to a coronary care unit.
    c. rapid administration of IV fluids.
    d. a repeat 12-lead ECG, along with thrombolytic therapy.

CASE PRESENTATION #2 (QUESTIONS 10-15)

You are dispatched to a "heart attack" call. On arrival, you find an 84-year-old woman who is lying on the couch in her living room. She is awake and alert and is complaining of severe chest pain. A female caretaker is present at the scene. She informs you that she takes care of both the patient and her husband, who previously has had a stroke.

10. While assessing the patient's vital signs, the most important historical information to obtain is:
    a. Are there any known allergies?
    b. Does the pain radiate?
    c. When did the pain start? Describe the pain.
    d. What is the patient's medical history?

Her vital signs are as follows: BP 180/70; pulse 90 irregular and weak; respirations 22. She states that she has had this pain for about 15 minutes, and she describes it as indigestion. She says she has never experienced pain like this before.

11. You administer oxygen to the patient. Your next priority should be to:
    a. ask about other associated symptoms.
    b. continue obtaining patient history.
    c. obtain an ECG reading.
    d. start an IV at a TKO rate.

The patient's ECG is shown in Figure 31-2.

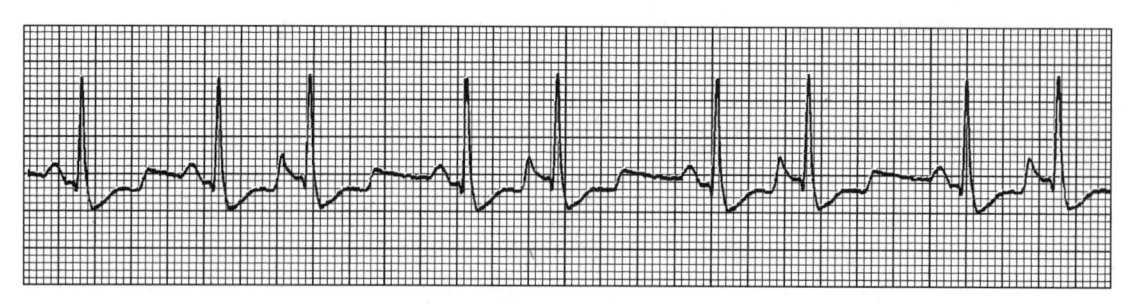

Figure 31-2

12. This rhythm is best described as:
    a. atrial fibrillation.
    b. sinus arrhythmia.
    c. sinus with PACs.
    d. sinus with PVCs.

As you continue assessment, the patient reveals that she broke her hip 3 weeks ago and has been receiving physical therapy at home. Up until then, she had been in good heath; there is no significant medical history. After she called 9-1-1, she took one of her husband's nitroglycerin tablets and is now feeling some relief. Her skin is warm and dry. There are no other associated symptoms except that she has had difficulty swallowing for the past few days.

13. Briefly list possible causes of her pain, and explain your rationale.

You administer oxygen and prepare to transport. The patient tells you that she really does feel fine and does not want to go to the hospital.

14. You suspect that her pain may be gastrointestinal in origin, and not cardiac. What should you advise, and why?

You are able to convince her to go to the hospital, and you start a precautionary IV. She remains stable while en route and on arrival at the emergency department. The medical director of your EMS systems provides regular feedback on the patients whom you bring to the hospital. In this case, you are informed that the patient was diagnosed with acute esophageal spasm and a hiatal hernia. She was treated and sent home a couple of days later.

15. Briefly discuss the relationship between her diagnosis and the presenting complaint of chest pain.

General Review Questions

16. Ischemia to the heart muscle may cause which of the following complications? (Circle all that apply.)
    a. hypoventilation
    b. hypoperfusion
    c. increased intracranial pressure
    d. life-threatening dysrhythmias
    e. pulmonary edema

17. Chest pain that is associated with ischemia may be described as:
    a. a "heavy sensation" in the chest.
    b. indigestion.
    c. pain that radiates to the arms.
    d. a "squeezing" sensation in the chest.
    e. all of the above

18. Life-threatening dysrhythmias that occur after a cardiac incident are the most common cause of sudden death caused by heart disease. Briefly discuss the significance of this in terms of prehospital monitoring and care.

19. Can chest pain occur at rest? Briefly describe the significance of this.

20. Pulse abnormalities in the presence of chest pain:
    a. are dangerous only when associated with hypotension.
    b. are normal findings and are usually not life-threatening.
    c. indicate the possibility of a dysrhythmia.
    d. should be evaluated using an ECG.
    e. c and d

21. In patients with chest pain, morphine sulfate usually is administered with:
   a. digoxin.
   b. epinephrine.
   c. Inderal®.
   d. nitroglycerin.

22. Your patient is a 64-year-old man who is in severe pain. He describes the pain as "tearing," and he says that it is located in his back and shoulder blades. What medical condition do you suspect first?
   a. acute aortic dissection
   b. cardiac ischemia
   c. pericarditis
   d. pulmonary embolus

23. Chest pain that is described as a sharp pain that worsens with deep inspiration or coughing typically is associated with:
   a. cardiac conditions.
   b. a gastrointestinal problem.
   c. pulmonary conditions.
   d. none of the above

24. Assessment of a patient who is experiencing chest pain is important. Briefly discuss key aspects of the historical assessment.

25. Why is pain relief important for a patient who is experiencing chest pain that you suspect is of cardiac origin? Briefly explain your response.

26. Briefly describe the differences in clinical presentation between angina pectoris and acute myocardial infarction.

Answers to questions from chapter 31 can be found on page 465.

Chapter 32

Palpitations and Dysrhythmias

OBJECTIVES

1. Describe the significance and common causes of palpitations.
2. Identify the key historical findings in the assessment of a patient with palpitations and dysrhythmias.
3. Identify four classifications of patient medications commonly used to treat palpitations and dysrhythmias.
4. Describe the rapid, directed physical examination of patients with palpitations and dysrhythmias.
5. Identify the subjective and objective assessment findings that indicate the need for prehospital intervention in patients with palpitations and dysrhythmias.
6. Describe the specific causes, signs and symptoms, potential problems, and prehospital treatment for the following:
    a. Bradycardias (sinus, junctional)
    b. AV heart block
    c. Narrow complex tachycardia
    d. Wide complex tachycardia
    e. Atrial fibrillation
    f. Premature ventricular contractions

CASE PRESENTATION #1 (QUESTIONS 1-9)

You are dispatched to a high-rise retirement complex for treatment of a possible heart attack victim. Your patient is a 66-year-old woman who lives alone. She answers the door when you arrive, quickly sits down in a chair, and tells you that she is having chest pain. You note that her skin color is good, but she is grimacing with the pain. She is alert and oriented.

1. What is your first priority with this patient?
    a. Apply the ECG monitor.
    b. Check for distended neck veins.
    c. Evaluate her pulse and breathing.
    d. Obtain a blood pressure reading.
    e. Perform a 12-lead ECG.

The patient tells you that her pain started about 45 minutes ago while she was washing the breakfast dishes. It is described as a "squeezing pain" in the center of her chest. She denies any dizziness but is slightly short of breath. Her vital signs are: BP 104/64; pulse 50; respirations 22 and shallow. Her breath sounds are clear and equal. The cardiac monitor shows a Mobitz II second-degree heart block, bradycardia.

2. What additional information would be appropriate to obtain during the focused history and physical examination?

She tells you that she has been experiencing intermittent chest discomfort for the past several weeks. However, the pain lasted only a few minutes and diminished when she sat down and rested. Otherwise, essentially she has been in good health; she takes no medications and walks 10 miles each week. She appears to be in good physical condition. There is no peripheral edema, and peripheral pulses are present and equal.

3. The patient's previous episodes of chest pain were likely to have been:
    a. angina pectoris.
    b. congestive heart failure.
    c. transient ischemic attacks.
    d. Wolff-Parkinson-White syndrome.

You establish an IV at a TKO rate and prepare the patient for transport. Noting that the patient is looking pale, you quickly recheck her blood pressure. It is now 84/50.

4. Briefly explain why the patient's blood pressure may have dropped.

5. Which of the following would you anticipate medical direction to order?
    a. adenosine rapid IV push
    b. atropine 0.5 mg IV push
    c. lidocaine 50 to 100 mg IV push
    d. transcutaneous pacing
    e. b and d

6. Bradycardias are treated only when the patient is symptomatic. Briefly explain why this patient's bradycardic dysrhythmia is treatable.

The patient's heart rate increases to 70 in response to your therapy. Her skin color is improved and she is breathing more easily, but she still is having chest pain.

7. Could this patient also receive nitroglycerin for her chest pain?

8. The use of atropine with Mobitz II and third-degree blocks may be associated with some increased risk. Briefly discuss this risk, including how you would monitor the patient for any complications.

You arrive at the hospital with the patient in stable condition. On follow-up, you learn that she was admitted to the coronary care unit for an acute inferior myocardial infarction.

CASE PRESENTATION #2 (QUESTIONS 9–15)

You are dispatched to a medical emergency. An elderly woman meets you at the door. She is upset and crying. The patient is her husband, who is lying in his bed, complaining of feeling "weak." He is awake and responds to verbal stimuli. Your initial assessment reveals that he is pale and sweaty and has a weak, rapid pulse. You quickly administer oxygen and apply the ECG monitor, which reveals the rhythm in Figure 32-1.

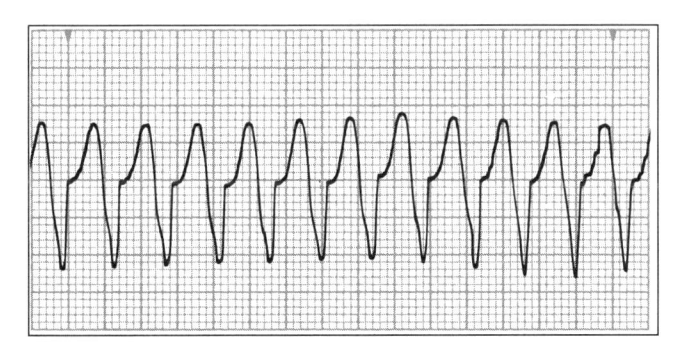

Figure 32-1

9. His ECG represents which of the following?
   a. atrial flutter
   b. paroxysmal supraventricular tachycardia
   c. sinus tachycardia
   d. torsades de pointes
   e. ventricular tachycardia

While you apply the cardiac monitor, your partner obtains the following vital signs and information: BP 70/40; pulse 150 and thready; respirations 30 and labored. The patient denies chest pain or palpitations. His wife says that while he was working in the garden, he started feeling weak and lightheaded, and he came inside to lie down. His medical history reveals "irregular heart rhythm" and hypertension; medications are Norpace® and Lopressor®.

10. Is this patient considered to be stable or unstable? Explain your response.

11. While your partner gets the stretcher, for what intervention should you prepare?
    a. adenosine rapid IV push
    b. defibrillation
    c. magnesium sulfate IV push
    d. synchronized cardioversion

12. The dysrhythmia that is seen in this patient is:
    a. often seen in elderly patients, but usually is not urgent.
    b. likely to progress to ventricular fibrillation.
    c. life-threatening and requires prompt intervention.
    d. controlled typically with medication only.
    e. b and c

While en route to the hospital, after three synchronized cardioversions, the patient's reading reveals the rhythm shown in Figure 32-2.

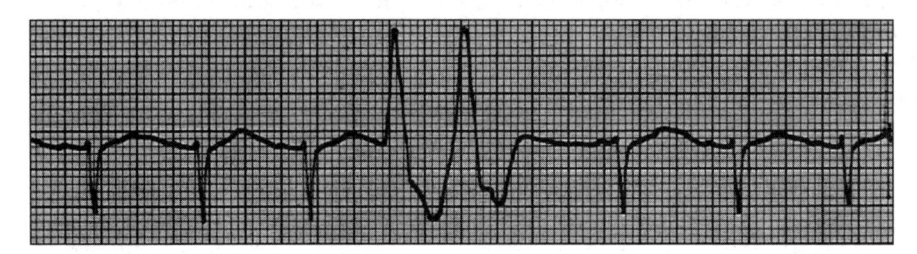

Figure 32-2

13. Identify the rhythm in Figure 32-2.

14. Medical direction orders you to administer a lidocaine bolus, followed by a lidocaine IV piggyback drip. What is the rationale for this order?

You have the lidocaine on board and are preparing to transport. The patient's blood pressure is now 92/60.

15. If his blood pressure had not increased, what medication would medical direction most likely have ordered? Explain your response.

The patient is stabilized in the emergency department and is admitted for observation. You later learn that he was discharged 3 days later in good condition, with changes in his medications.

GENERAL REVIEW QUESTIONS

16. Many dysrhythmias are perceived as, and described by, the patient as palpitations. Briefly discuss the significance of this, and identify some factors that contribute to the sensation.

17. Which of the following can cause bradycardia? (Circle all that apply.)
    a. closed head injury
    b. good physical conditioning
    c. ischemia to the heart
    d. stimulant drugs
    e. vagal stimulation

Match the patient medication used for palpitations and dysrhythmias in Column 1 with its description in Column 2. *Note:* **Answers may be used more than once.**

Column 1

18. ____ Cardizem®
19. ____ Lopressor®
20. ____ Lanoxin®
21. ____ Tocainide®
22. ____ Tenormin®

Column 2

a. Narrow range between therapeutic and toxic dosages
b. Slows conduction through the AV node
c. Indicated for ventricular dysrhythmias
d. Calcium channel blocker
e. Hypotension is a side effect
f. Beta blocker

23. List five key questions that should be asked to determine if prehospital field intervention for a dysrhythmia is indicated.

   (a)

   (b)

   (c)

   (d)

   (e)

Your patient is a 56-year-old man who was found unconscious. Witnesses tell you that the patient grabbed his chest and collapsed. He is responsive to verbal stimuli, his skin is diaphoretic, and he is having trouble breathing. He tells you that he has severe chest pain. His vital signs are: BP 74/50; pulse 46; and respirations 24. ECG reading shows sinus bradycardia with runs of ventricular tachycardia.

24. What is your first priority?
   a. atropine 0.5 mg IV push
   b. dopamine IV piggyback
   c. lidocaine 50 to 100 mg IV push
   d. magnesium sulfate
   e. transcutaneous pacing (TCP)

25. Sinus tachycardia is a normal response to the demand for an increased heart rate. Briefly discuss some common causes of tachycardia.

26. Which of the following dysrhythmias is usually chronic in nature and can lead to an embolic type of stroke?
   a. atrial fibrillation
   b. junctional tachycardia
   c. paroxysmal atrial tachycardia
   d. sinus tachycardia
   e. ventricular tachycardia

For each of the following statements (27–34), circle the correct response, True or False. Briefly explain your answer.

27. A common cause of premature ventricular contractions is hypoxia.

   TRUE   **FALSE**

   Briefly explain your answer:_____
   _____
   _____

28. Atrial fibrillation and atrial flutter are usually treated with cardioversion in the field.

TRUE   **FALSE**

Briefly explain your answer: _____
_____
_____
_____

29. The first drug of choice for treating narrow complex tachycardias (such as PSVT) is adenosine.

TRUE   **FALSE**

Briefly explain your answer: _____
_____
_____
_____

30. PVCs in the presence of chest pain are considered dangerous.

TRUE   **FALSE**

Briefly explain your answer: _____
_____
_____
_____

31. Palpitations are considered to be the most common symptom in patients with cardiac rhythm disturbances.

TRUE   **FALSE**

Briefly explain your answer: _____
_____
_____

32. Significant symptoms from cardiac rhythm disturbances generally result from either insufficient cerebral blood flow or inadequate myocardial perfusion.

TRUE   **FALSE**

Briefly explain your answer: _____
_____
_____

33. Drugs such as stimulants, tricyclic antidepressants, and cardiac medications may produce dysrhythmia in cases of overdose.

   TRUE   **FALSE**

Briefly explain your answer: _____
_____
_____

34. Narrow complex tachycardias usually are more life-threatening than are wide complex tachycardias.

   TRUE   **FALSE**

Briefly explain your answer: _____
_____
_____

Answers to questions from chapter 32 can be found on page 467.

Chapter 33

Headache

OBJECTIVES

1. Describe the pathophysiology of headache disorders.
2. Describe the general assessment of a patient with a headache and explain the significance of specific findings.
3. Describe the specific neurological patient evaluation and explain the significance of specific findings.
4. Given a description of several patients complaining of headache with different clinical findings, identify a patient who potentially has: subarachnoid or other intracranial hemorrhage; meningitis; hypertensive encephalopathy; preeclampsia; carbon monoxide poisoning; tension headache; sinusitis; migraine; glaucoma; and hemophilia.
5. List potential complications for patients who present with a headache disorder.
6. Describe the general management of patients with the following specific headache disorders:
    a. Subarachnoid (or other intracranial) hemorrhage
    b. Meningitis
    c. Hypertensive encephalopathy
    d. Preeclampsia (toxemia of pregnancy)
    e. Carbon monoxide poisoning and other toxins
    f. Tension headache
    g. Sinusitis and dental disease
    h. Migraine
    i. Glaucoma
    j. Hemophilia

CASE PRESENTATION #1 (QUESTIONS 1–6)

You are dispatched in the late afternoon to an office complex for a "sick call." On arrival, you are met at the door by a receptionist who leads you to the office of a stock broker. Your patient is a 35-year-old woman who is complaining of a severe headache. Because the patient is in no acute distress that requires immediate intervention, you continue your assessment. Your partner instructs the paramedic student intern to measure the patient's vital signs.

1. What general questions are important regarding the history of her headache?

2. Why is it important to determine whether this patient is pregnant or in the early post-partum stage?

The patient claims that her headache began about one hour ago and got progressively worse while she was dealing with a difficult client. When you ask her where the pain is located, she moves her hand across her forehead to the back of her head and neck. She has no associated symptoms or historical findings and has taken no medications. She also reports that she has had similar headaches previously when she was under a lot of stress. Her vital signs are: BP 140/88; pulse 102 and regular; respirations 20. You suspect that this patient is experiencing a tension headache. The paramedic student intern whispers to you that, because of her neck pain, his suspicion is that this patient has meningitis. Your partner confides in both of you that she is not sure whether this patient needs to be transported to the hospital.

3. What initial assessment findings would indicate that this is a life-threatening headache?

4. What specific assessment findings support your suspicion of tension headache?

This patient requests to be taken to the hospital where her private physician practices. You contact medical direction and receive instructions to comply with the patient's request. You manage the patient supportively by administering oxygen, applying a cardiac monitor, and transporting in a position of comfort. The patient is delivered to the emergency department in stable condition. She is treated with parenteral analgesics and is kept there for observation. While en route back to the station, you review the call with the paramedic student intern.

5. Explain to the paramedic student intern why you transported this patient to the hospital.

6. Explain to the paramedic student intern why you did not suspect that this patient had meningitis.

CASE PRESENTATION #2 (QUESTIONS 7-16)

You are called to a health club that is approximately 5 minutes away for treatment of a "man down." On arrival, you find a 22-year-old unconscious man on the racquetball court. According to his playing partner, the patient had complained of a sudden onset of "a horrible headache" just minutes before he collapsed. They had just started their first game. There are no obvious signs of injury. The patient has a strong, slow radial pulse, and respirations are fast and deep.

7. Is a neurologic examination an appropriate part of your initial assessment? If so, what should your neurologic examination include at this time?

8. Is the onset of his headache significant? Explain why, or why not.

While your partner is measuring vital signs, the patient begins to posture. His pupils are fixed and dilated. His vital signs are: BP 180/110; pulse 60; respirations 30 and deep. The patient is intubated. You quickly prepare to initiate an IV at a TKO rate and apply the cardiac monitor.

9. What should your treatment priorities be at this time? Explain your response.

10. What is the significance of posturing?

11. Is it appropriate to initiate an IV line on the scene?

As this patient is being prepared for transport, a first responder elicits additional history from the patient's racquetball partner, which reveals that the patient is taking the prescription drug Coumadin®.

12. Is the additional history that was solicited by the first responder significant? Explain why, or why not.

13. Does this additional history alter this patient's treatment? Why, or why not?

Upon contacting medical direction, you are instructed to transport this patient with lights and sirens to the Level I trauma center across town. This will add 4 minutes to your transport time, and you will bypass the closest hospital, which is smaller.

14. What is the most likely reason for your instructions from medical direction to bypass the smaller hospital?

15. Potential complications of this patient for which you should be especially alert while en route include:
    a. seizures.
    b. cardiac arrhythmias.
    c. vomiting.
    d. a and c
    e. all of the above

Approximately 2 minutes from the hospital, the cardiac monitor changes to the rhythm shown in Figure 33-1. You cannot palpate a pulse, and the patient has no spontaneous respirations.

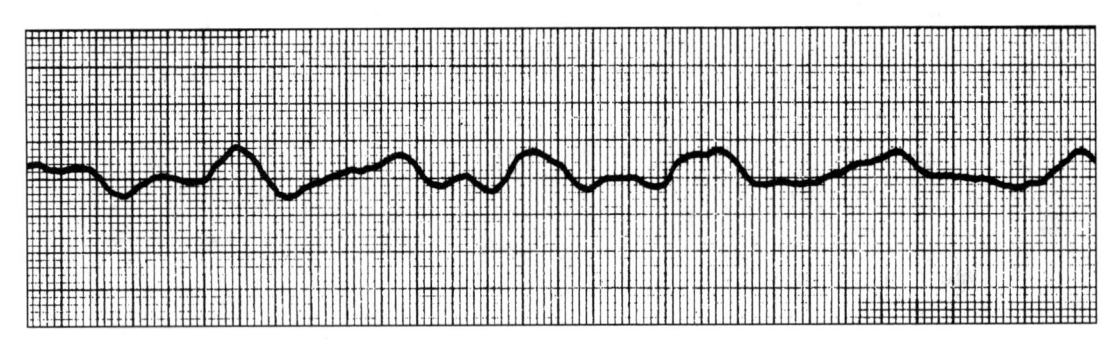

Figure 33-1

16. Your initial treatment is:
    a. synchronized cardioversion.
    b. to begin CPR.
    c. defibrillation.
    d. external pacing.
    e. administration of epinephrine.

The patient's condition is unchanged on arrival to the hospital. Despite the continuation of aggressive treatment by the emergency department staff, the patient dies.

CASE PRESENTATION #3 (QUESTIONS 17–21)

On a cold winter night, you are dispatched to an apartment complex in an impoverished neighborhood. The dispatcher informs you that three family members are complaining of headache, which began about an hour after they lighted their heater. Your ETA is 11 minutes.

17. Based on the information provided by dispatch, what is the most likely cause of the symptoms described by these patients?

While you are en route to the scene, dispatch informs you that the first responders have removed the patients from the apartment to the manager's office. On arrival, you find all three patients, including two teenaged boys and their mother, receiving high-concentration oxygen using nonrebreather masks. They are alert and appear to be in no acute distress. Fire department personnel have confirmed your suspicions of the underlying cause of these patients' headaches; they report that their vital signs are within normal limits.

18. Is the treatment administered by the first responders appropriate? Why, or why not?

19. On assessment, how might you expect the skin of these patients to appear?

20. Would the pulse oximeter be an appropriate device to use with these patients? Why, or why not?

21. Ideally, you would transport these patients to a hospital with what specific type of equipment?

Your transport time to the hospital is 15 minutes. While en route, the two teenaged patients tell you that their headache is almost completely gone. The mother also reports a significant decrease in her headache pain. When the patients are delivered to the emergency department, their condition has shown overall improvement.

General Review Questions

22. List two conditions with which nuchal rigidity may be present along with headache.

    (a)

    (b)

Match the patient presentation (all have a headache) in Column 1 with its probable condition in Column 2.

Column 1

23. ____ BP 220/130, blurred vision, altered mental status, confusion

24. ____ Severe, throbbing headache preceded by flashes of light

25. ____ Localized pain, redness, visual loss in one eye

26. ____ BP 194/110, facial and ankle edema, 7 months' pregnant

27. ____ Nasal congestion, tenderness over the cheeks and forehead

Column 2

a. Meningitis
b. Hemophilia
c. Sinusitis
d. Toxemia
e. Migraine
f. Glaucoma
g. Hypertensive encephalopathy

28. A patient with a history of hypertension and a BP of 220/110, who is complaining of severe headache and nausea, may be treated with _____ in the field.
    a. naloxone
    b. lidocaine
    c. nitroglycerin
    d. Lasix®

29. A potential complication for a patient with glaucoma who is complaining of severe headache is:
    a. seizure.
    b. blindness.
    c. neck stiffness.
    d. chills.

30. Which of the following is the clearest way to report an altered level of consciousness for a patient who presents with a severe headache?
    a. stuporous
    b. lethargic
    c. obtunded
    d. unresponsive to pain

31. Which of the following interview questions would most likely yield the best information from a patient who is complaining of a headache?
    a. Can you describe the pain?
    b. Does the pain radiate?
    c. Would you describe the pain as throbbing?
    d. Is the pain severe?

32. The most common cause of pain in patients with a headache is:
    a. dilation and distention of vessels.
    b. inflammatory processes.
    c. tension or traction on anatomic structures.
    d. constriction of vessels.

Answers to questions from chapter 33 can be found on page 470.

Chapter 34

Weak, Dizzy, and Malaise

OBJECTIVES

1. Describe the pathophysiology, common causes, and signs and symptoms for the following chief complaints:
   a. Weakness
   b. Dizziness/lightheadedness
   c. Malaise
2. Identify the structures that control the functions of equilibrium and spatial orientation.
3. Identify the historical and physical examination data to obtain for patients with these complaints.
4. Describe the significance and potential life-threatening conditions that can be associated with these complaints.
5. Discuss general field management for patients with these complaints and specific management of life-threatening conditions.

CASE PRESENTATION #1 (QUESTIONS 1-8)

You are dispatched to a medical emergency at a private residence. At the scene, you find the patient seated at his dining room table. He appears to be approximately 60 years old, and he is conscious and alert. His chief complaint is weakness.

1. You quickly recall that many conditions can cause this complaint. Briefly list these potential underlying conditions.

You take the patient's vital signs: BP 140/76; pulse 78 and regular; respirations 28 and slightly labored. The patient's skin color is normal, and he is not sweating.

2. Which question would be most relevant to ask first?
   a. Are there any associated symptoms?
   b. Do you feel dizzy or lightheaded?
   c. Is the weakness generalized or localized?
   d. What medical problems do you have?
   e. What medications are you taking currently?

3. As you continue to question the patient, your physical examination should include:

The patient states that he has felt a generalized weakness since yesterday. He denies any dizziness, nausea, vomiting, or specific area of pain. Breath sounds reveal rales in the lower bases, and the findings of the neurologic examination are normal. He tells you that he is a dialysis patient; he receives treatment three times each week. However, he has missed the last two treatments because he did not have a means of transportation to the dialysis facility. There is no other pertinent medical history.

4. Given the information gathered so far, what condition should you suspect?
   a. anemia
   b. cerebral vascular accident
   c. electrolyte imbalance
   d. inner ear disorder
   e. nerve compression

His ECG reveals the following rhythm shown in Figure 34-1:

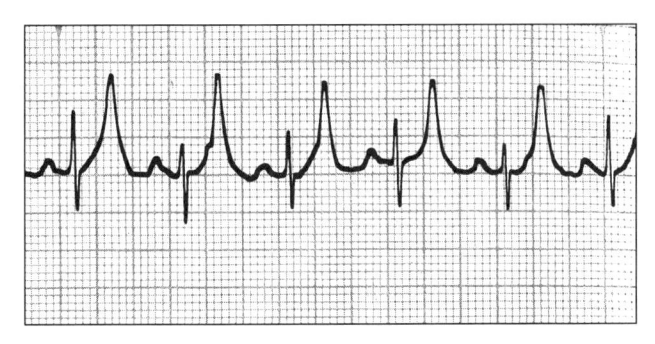

Figure 34-1

5. Name the rhythm and describe any abnormalities noted.

6. Given this rhythm and the information provided above about the patient's condition, you suspect that he has an electrolyte imbalance of:
   a. calcium.
   b. magnesium.
   c. potassium.
   d. sodium.

You send the ECG for evaluation to the on-line medical director (OLMD), administer oxygen, and establish a precautionary IV as you prepare to transport the patient.

7. You anticipate that the OLMD will order you to administer:
   a. bicarbonate.
   b. calcium.
   c. dopamine.
   d. epinephrine.
   e. a or b

8. While en route to the hospital, you should observe the patient closely for:

CASE PRESENTATION #2 (QUESTIONS 9–14)

You are dispatched to a call involving a possible unconscious patient. When you arrive at the scene, a member of the engine crew meets you at the front door and tells you that the patient is conscious, alert, and oriented. As you approach the patient, who is lying on her bed, you note that her skin is somewhat pale, but there is no indication of respiratory distress. She says that she just feels very dizzy. Her pulse is strong, and the rate is 80.

9. As you focus on her chief complaint, what questions would be important to ask her initially?

You check her lungs, and breath sounds are normal. She denies any vomiting, melena, or chest pain. She states that she has felt extremely nauseated because of her dizziness. She tells you that when she is lying down or sitting, she feels like "the room is spinning."

10. The description of this complaint indicates a condition known as:
   a. anemia.
   b. hypoperfusion.
   c. malaise.
   d. vertigo.

11. List potential causes of her chief complaint.

Further assessment reveals that her symptoms began rather suddenly (less than 3 hours ago) and have become progressively worse. She hasn't had any previous episodes, and there is nothing relevant in her medical history. Neurologic examination and ECG are normal; tilt test results are negative. You suspect that she is suffering from a condition that is affecting her balance. As you support her, you ask her to stand up and walk a few steps.

12. What is the relationship of this request to your assessment of her condition?

13. Should the patient be transported to an emergency department? Why, or why not?

Follow-up information obtained by your medical director reveals that the patient was diagnosed with an inner ear infection; she was treated and sent home.

14. Does this information have any bearing on your decision to transport? Briefly discuss your response.

General Review Questions

15. Generalized weakness implies a condition that affects:
    a. a specific nerve.
    b. only the brain.
    c. the entire body.
    d. none of the above

16. Briefly discuss how the following conditions may produce a symptom of weakness in a patient:

    (a) Anemia

    (b) Infection

    (c) Cardiac ischemia

17. "Lightheadedness" is a condition that is different from true vertigo; it causes two primary effects in a patient. These are:

    (a)

    (b)

18. What general conditions can lead to lightheadedness?

19. One of the more specific causes of malaise is:
    a. cerebral vascular accident.
    b. fever.
    c. hypoperfusion.
    d. inner ear infection.

20. Structures that control the functions of equilibrium and spatial orientation include:
   a. the brain stem.
   b. the cerebellum.
   c. the cerebral cortex.
   d. the middle ear and the inner ear.
   e. a and d
   f. all of the above

21. The most important step in the assessment of a patient with a complaint of weakness, dizziness, or malaise is to:
   a. determine the historical data that are related to the chief complaint.
   b. evaluate a 12-lead ECG.
   c. determine the patient's medical history.
   d. secure a rapid blood glucose determination.

22. For any patient who complains of weakness, dizziness, or malaise, two assessment procedures should be performed in the field. They are:

(a)

(b)

Answers to questions from chapter 34 can be found on page 472.

Chapter 35

Diabetic Emergencies

OBJECTIVES

1. Describe the function of insulin and glucagon.
2. Define *diabetes mellitus*.
3. Differentiate between Type I (insulin-dependent) and Type II (non–insulin dependent) diabetes in terms of pathophysiology, age of onset, required treatment, and tendency for ketoacidosis.
4. Describe the clinical characteristics of the common chronic complications associated with diabetes mellitus.
5. Identify the key historical features in the assessment of patients with medical problems caused by diabetes.
6. Given a patient with a diabetic problem, apply the principles of a rapid, directed physical examination.
7. Describe the principles of prehospital management of medical problems associated with diabetes.
8. Describe the pathophysiology and the associated clinical manifestations of potentially life-threatening diabetic emergencies.
9. Describe the indication and therapeutic action of common medications prescribed for diabetes.

CASE PRESENTATION #1 (QUESTIONS 1-7)

You are dispatched to a retirement home to care for a patient when the nurse reports that he may be having a stroke. On arrival, you are met by the same nurse, who informs you of the patient's history as she leads you to his room. The patient is a 65-year-old man who has had three episodes of vomiting over the past two days. He had complained of weakness that morning, and the nurse notes that he seems very lethargic. She believes that he is having a stroke because he awakened with right-sided facial paralysis as well. He has a history of diabetes mellitus, for which he takes Tolinase® once a day.

1. What chronic problem associated with diabetes might have led the nurse to suspect that this patient is having a stroke?

2. Based on what the nurse told you, does this patient have Type I or Type II diabetes? Explain your response.

You and your partner enter the patient's room to find an elderly man slumped over in bed. He answers most questions appropriately but is disoriented to his surroundings. He also has obvious facial drooping on one side. Additionally, he is unable to lift his right leg from the bed and says he feels dizzy every time he attempts to sit up. Peripheral pulses are strong and symmetrical. His skin is warm, dry, and inelastic. Pupils are equal and reactive to light. Vital signs are: BP 90/60; pulse 104 and regular; respirations 18 and normal. Blood glucose determination is greater than 350. You suspect that this patient, rather than having a stroke, is suffering from non-ketotic hyperosmolar coma.

3. List assessment findings that support your suspicion.

You place the patient on a cardiac monitor and administer high-concentration oxygen. Your partner initiates an IV of lactated Ringer's solution and administers a 500-mL bolus.

4. Was your partner's treatment approach for this patient an appropriate choice? Explain your response.

5. What baseline data should have been established before this patient was given a fluid bolus? Explain your response.

6. Improvement in which initial assessment findings would indicate a positive response to treatment?

When you call in your report to medical direction, the physician orders you to proceed immediately to the nearest hospital. Your ETA is approximately 6 minutes.

7. Explain the reasons for this physician's sense of urgency about getting this patient to the hospital.

You deliver the patient to the emergency department in a slightly improved condition. He is admitted to the hospital for continued treatment and observation.

CASE PRESENTATION #2 (QUESTION 8-16)

During the early afternoon, you are dispatched to an "unconscious person" call at a movie theater. On arrival, you are motioned to a 12-year-old girl who is lying on the floor in the lobby. As you approach the patient, you note that she is breathing and that there are no obvious signs of trauma. A crowd is gathered around her, and her friends are noticeably upset.

8. Because legally this patient is considered to be a minor, under what form of consent would you be operating while rendering care? Explain your response.

You and your partner initiate care while taking a history from her friends. The patient babbles incoherently and flails her arms as you attempt to manage her airway. You also note that her skin is pale and diaphoretic. Your partner obtains the following vital signs: BP 94/60; pulse 100 and regular; respirations 18 and normal. The patient's friends tell you that she seemed fine when they arrived an hour ago, but that she began acting "drunk" while waiting in line for popcorn. When you ask about her medical history, they tell you that she recently went on a special diet and began taking shots every day. You quickly perform a rapid glucose determination.

9. How would you expect her blood glucose measurement to read? Explain why.

10. Why should initial management of this patient precede a complete assessment?

This patient's rapid glucose measurement is 60 mg/dl. Your partner suggests that you administer glucose orally because it is quicker than establishing an IV.

11. Is this an appropriate action? Explain why, or why not.

12. Why should a red- or grey-topped tube be drawn before administration of D50?

13. What precautions should you take when administering D50 to this patient?

Almost immediately after you administer D50 to this patient, her level of consciousness improves.

14. As her level of consciousness improves, you should:
    a. provide reassurance and privacy.
    b. inform her of what happened.
    c. obtain a history of her last meal and medications taken.
    d. a and c
    e. a, b, and c

She is fully awake and oriented approximately 5 minutes later and refuses to be transported to the hospital. Her mother has arrived now and confirms that her daughter was diagnosed two months ago with Type I diabetes. Although you explain to both the patient and her mother that it is always safer to be evaluated thoroughly at the hospital, they adamantly refuse any further treatment. After consulting with medical direction, you comply with their wishes and discontinue the patient's IV.

15. Before you leave the scene, what information about her condition should you provide to this patient and her mother?

16. Before you leave the scene, what information is especially important to document on the patient care report?

CASE PRESENTATION #3 (QUESTIONS 17–21)

You are dispatched to a residential neighborhood for a "sick call." You are met at the door of the house by a man who called because his 55-year-old father is not feeling well. As you approach the patient, you note that he is awake and is breathing fast and deep. The patient tells you that he began feeling weak and nauseated several days ago and has been feeling progressively worse. He also has noticed an increase in his level of thirst and frequency of urination and, in spite of his nausea, he is always hungry. His vital signs are: BP 110/60; pulse 98; respirations 26 and nonlabored. His skin is warm and dry, and, as you are taking his history, you note a fruity odor to his breath. He was diagnosed 20 years ago with Type II diabetes, which he has controlled with dietary modifications.

17. Based on your assessment findings, most likely what is this patient experiencing? Explain your response.

A rapid glucose determination measures 400 via glucometer. Your partner applies high-concentration oxygen while you establish an IV of normal saline and begin fluid replacement.

18. Is it important to monitor this patient's cardiac rhythm? Explain your response.

19. Which of the following is indicated in the prehospital setting to assist in correction of this patient's acidosis?
    a. sodium bicarbonate
    b. sedation and intubation
    c. fluid and electrolyte replacement
    d. insulin

You contact medical direction. The physician agrees with your assessment and treatment. Your ETA at the emergency department is 12 minutes.

20. What is the total amount of fluid that may be administered to this patient while you are en route to the hospital?

While en route, you notice a draining, ulcerated area on his left foot. Further questioning reveals that the patient was aware of it but was unconcerned because it was not painful.

21. Could this patient's foot problem be related to his diabetes? Explain your response.

You apply a sterile dressing to his foot. The patient is delivered to the emergency department in stable condition. He is admitted for further definitive treatment, including continuation of fluid replacement, electrolyte monitoring, and insulin administration.

GENERAL REVIEW QUESTIONS

22. Differentiate between Type I and Type II diabetes by completing the following table:

	Type I (IDDM)	Type II (NIDDM)
Pathology		
Age of onset		
Required treatment		
Tendency for ketoacidosis		

23. Explain when insulin and glucagon are released into the bloodstream, and describe the function of each.

   (a) insulin

   (b) glucagon

24. List two chronic diseases that are major contributors to the decreased life expectancy of diabetics.

   (a)

   (b)

25. Describe the mechanism of action of oral hypoglycemic agents.

26. What special precaution should be taken before D50 is administered to infants and children?

27. Explain why rapid treatment of the hypoglycemic patient is essential.

All of the following patients have a history of diabetes; indicate each patient's probable glycemic status by writing **A** for hyperglycemic or **B** for hypoglycemic in the space provided.

28. ____ a 22-year-old who has taken her insulin but has not eaten
29. ____ a 26-year-old with a fruity odor to the breath and Kussmaul respirations
30. ____ a 17-year-old boy who has had the flu for three days
31. ____ a 20-year-old who passed out after drinking beer all day without eating
32. ____ a 34-year-old who has not taken her insulin for two days
33. ____ a 24-year-old obese person who has been fasting for two days

34. What group of signs and symptoms best indicates insufficient glucose to the brain?
    a. combativeness, tachycardia, warm and dry skin, and seizures
    b. sleepiness, bradycardia, and pale and diaphoretic skin
    c. combativeness, bradycardia, warm and dry skin, and seizures
    d. headache, confusion, tachycardia, and pale and diaphoretic skin

35. Chronic complications of diabetes occur because:
    a. these patients are in a constant state of acidosis.
    b. there is too much insulin circulating in the body.
    c. patients do not take their medication properly.
    d. the disease damages blood vessels to vital organs.

36. Which of the following situations would be least likely to precipitate hypoglycemia in a diabetic patient?
    a. decreased food intake
    b. a dose of insulin that is too small
    c. vigorous physical activity
    d. too much insulin

37. Diabetic ketoacidosis occurs because:
    a. there is too little glucose.
    b. there is too much insulin.
    c. dehydration is occurring.
    d. glucose cannot enter the cells.

38. Diabetes mellitus is a disorder of carbohydrate metabolism that is caused by:
    a. an excess of glucagon with increased blood sugar.
    b. an insulin deficit with increased blood sugar.
    c. a deficit of glucagon with decreased blood sugar.
    d. an excess of insulin with decreased blood sugar.

39. When you are giving D50 to a diabetic patient who is a known alcoholic, you also should administer:
    a. insulin.
    b. glucagon.
    c. thiamine.
    d. twice the usual dose.

40. Which of the following is *not* an oral hypoglycemic medication?

a. Diabinese®
b. Dymelor®
c. propranolol
d. Tolinase®

Answers to questions from chapter 35 can be found on page 473.

Chapter 36

Abdominal, Genitourinary, and Back Pain

OBJECTIVES

1. Describe the pathophysiology, characteristic features, and conditions associated with the following types of pain:
   a. Visceral
   b. Somatic
   c. Referred
2. Define the terms *guarding* and *rebound tenderness*.
3. Identify historical data that should be obtained from a patient with acute abdominal pain.
4. Discuss the significance of key findings from the history or physical examination that indicate a potential life-threat to patients with acute abdominal pain.
5. Identify specific signs and symptoms and conditions that indicate the presence of gastrointestinal or intra-abdominal bleeding.
6. Describe the physical examination of patients with acute abdominal pain.
7. Describe the pathophysiology, clinical characteristics, and potential complications associated with the following causes of abdominal pain:
   a. Acute pancreatitis
   b. Cholecystitis
   c. Appendicitis
   d. Intestinal (bowel) obstruction
   e. Abdominal aortic aneurysm
   f. Gastroenteritis
   g. Intestinal ischemia
   h. Ectopic pregnancy
   i. Diverticulitis
8. Discuss the appropriate field management of patients with acute abdominal pain.

CASE PRESENTATION #1 (QUESTIONS 1–10)

You are dispatched to a residence for a medical emergency. You arrive on the scene moments after the responding engine company gets there. You are met at the door by a crew member who tells you that the patient, a 60-year-old man, was found lying on the floor; he responds only to verbal stimuli. He has a weak and rapid pulse and is breathing on his own.

1. You arrive at the patient's side. Given this initial information, your immediate focus should be to:
   a. obtain a medical history.
   b. further evaluate the patient's pulse and breathing status.
   c. check the patient's blood pressure.
   d. obtain an ECG reading.

While you continue your initial assessment, the patient's wife tells you that, about two hours ago, her husband began having pain in the abdominal area. The pain was described as tearing and occurring intermittently; it was located in the center of his abdomen. He thought he was suffering from indigestion, so he took some Tagamet®.

2. Tagamet is classified as a medication that has which of the following properties?
   a. ACE inhibitor
   b. acid neutralizer
   c. antiinflammatory effect
   d. antisecretory capability

After taking the Tagamet, the patient laid down on the couch. Initially, he felt better; then he began to feel worse. According to his wife, the pain became constant and was focused in the middle back region. When he stood up, he became very dizzy.

3. Pain that is constant and that is located specifically at the site of the problem is called:
   a. atypical.
   b. referred.
   c. somatic.
   d. visceral.

You complete the initial assessment and obtain the patient's vital signs, which are: BP 94/60; pulse 130, thready and weak; respirations 28, shallow and labored. The patient is responsive to your questions but appears somewhat confused. His skin is pale and sweaty.

4. Could the patient be in shock? Explain your answer.

5. Is his immediate condition potentially life-threatening? Explain your answer.

You administer oxygen using a nonrebreather mask; you hook up the ECG monitor and establish an IV line. Additional information provided by his wife reveals that the patient had a heart attack 5 years ago and has been in good health since that time. He has no history of lung problems, diabetes, or other major illnesses. The only medications he takes are Catapres® and nitroglycerin PRN for chest pain.

6. Catapres is prescribed to:
   a. dilate the coronary arteries.
   b. improve conduction through the AV junction.
   c. lower the heart rate.
   d. lower the blood pressure.

You continue a quick focused assessment. The patient's abdominal area is mildly tender, but pain is focused in the back and flank areas, which are more tender than his frontal region. He denies any nausea, vomiting, or melena. Femoral and peripheral pulses are diminished bilaterally. You place him in a comfortable position and prepare to transport.

7. Based on your assessment up to this point, you suspect that he is most likely suffering from:
   a. acute appendicitis.
   b. cholecystitis.
   c. kidney stone.
   d. leaking or ruptured aortic aneurysm.

8. The IV that you established should be: (Circle the correct answer.)
   a. D5W.
   b. Ringer's lactate or normal saline.

   How should it be run?
   a. at a slow rate
   b. at a fast rate

9. During the course of treatment for this patient, should narcotics be used for pain control? Explain your answer.

You safely deliver the patient to the emergency department. He is evaluated and is prepared for the operating room. Surgical exploration reveals that the patient did have an abdominal aortic aneurysm; he recovers well postoperatively.

10. Why is immediate surgery indicated for his condition?

CASE PRESENTATION #2 (QUESTIONS 11–16)

You are dispatched to a residential area for a medical emergency. The patient greets you at the door. He appears to be about 30 years of age. His chief complaint is abdominal pain. Your initial assessment reveals that he is alert and oriented, has good skin color, and is not in acute distress. You help him to be seated comfortably, and you begin your assessment.

11. You focus your attention on his chief complaint. State four questions that you should ask the patient initially.

   (a)

   (b)

   (c)

   (d)

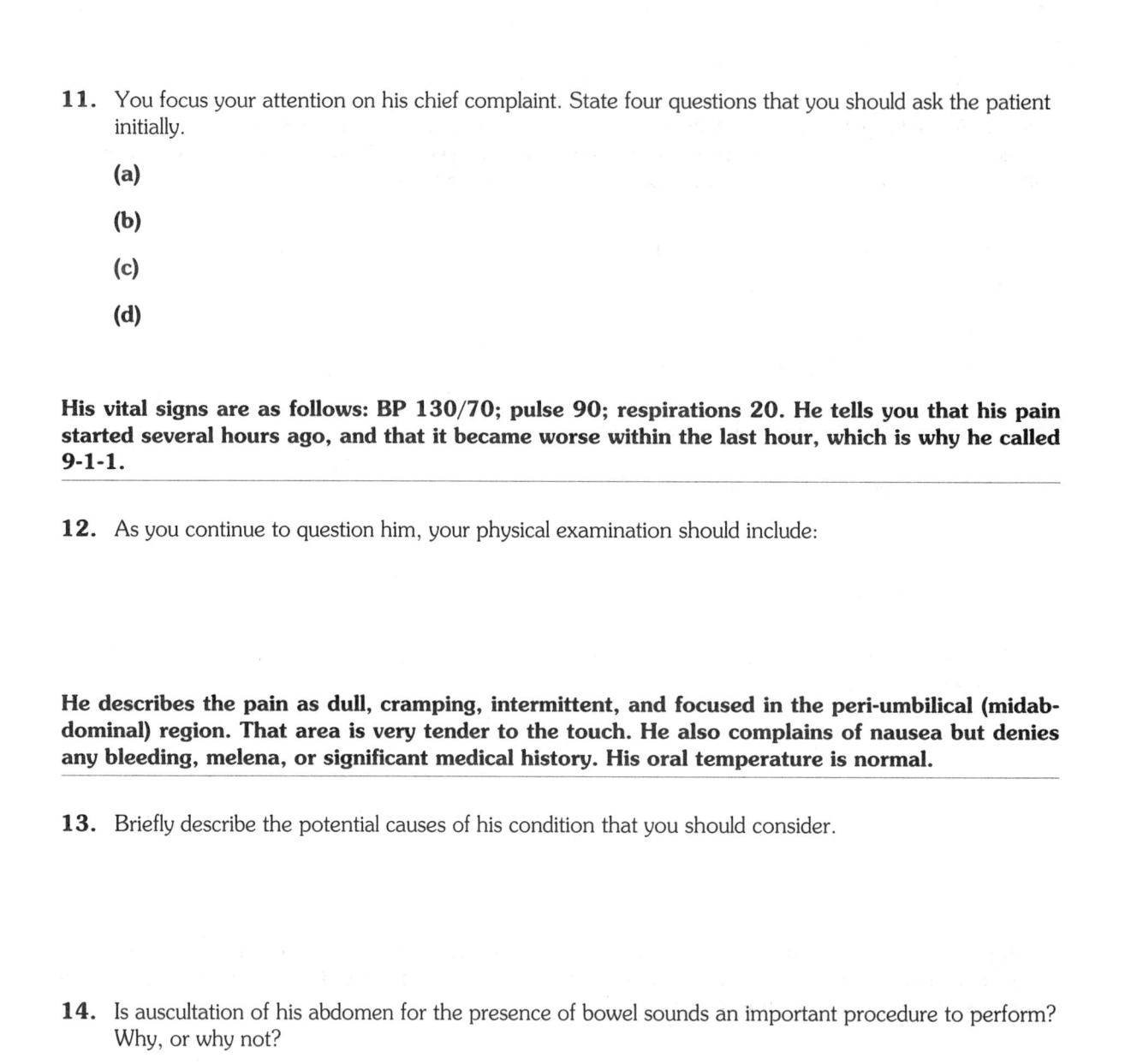

His vital signs are as follows: BP 130/70; pulse 90; respirations 20. He tells you that his pain started several hours ago, and that it became worse within the last hour, which is why he called 9-1-1.

12. As you continue to question him, your physical examination should include:

He describes the pain as dull, cramping, intermittent, and focused in the peri-umbilical (midabdominal) region. That area is very tender to the touch. He also complains of nausea but denies any bleeding, melena, or significant medical history. His oral temperature is normal.

13. Briefly describe the potential causes of his condition that you should consider.

14. Is auscultation of his abdomen for the presence of bowel sounds an important procedure to perform? Why, or why not?

Upon completion of your examination, the patient tells you that he feels better since taking some Tums®. After contacting medical direction, you administer oxygen, establish a TKO IV, and prepare for transport. The patient now states that he does not need to go to the hospital.

15. Describe how you should respond to the patient's refusal to be transported.

You are able to convince the patient to go to the hospital for further evaluation. You suspect that he has an acute appendicitis.

16. While en route to the hospital, for what potential problems should you be alert?

CASE PRESENTATION #3 (QUESTIONS 17–21)

You are dispatched to an office complex for a medical emergency. On arrival at the building, you are greeted by a nervous 22-year-old woman who leads you to the administrative office. The patient appears alert and oriented and is pacing the floor when you arrive. A bystander states that the patient is having severe pain in her side and back regions.

17. What is the initial treatment priority for this patient?

While questioning her, you obtain initial vital signs. They are: BP 150/90; pulse 116; respirations 20. Her skin is warm and dry. Results of the tilt test are negative. She tells you that the pain is on her right side, and it radiates to her back. Your partner asks her about her recent menstrual history.

18. Why is the patient's menstrual history relevant? Explain your answer.

You determine that her last menstrual period was normal, and that it ended last week. She denies vomiting, diarrhea, and fever. However, she has felt somewhat nauseated. The pain began about an hour ago. As you are attempting to examine and question the patient, she is unable to sit still or to get in a comfortable position.

19. What specific questions are important to ask next?

She denies vaginal bleeding, vomiting of blood, and melena. Medical history is also negative for these symptoms. She states that she has had some hematuria for the past 2 days.

20. Based on the information that you have gathered thus far, you suspect that most likely she is experiencing:
    a. acute myocardial infarction.
    b. ectopic pregnancy.
    c. kidney stone.
    d. perforated ulcer.

21. Does her condition warrant an evaluation in the emergency department? Why, or why not?

General Review Questions

22. Describe the characteristic features of the following types of pain in the abdominal and back areas:

    (a) Visceral

    (b) Referred

23. Pain that is sharp, knifelike, and constant and that often is aggravated by moving or coughing is typically of what origin?
    a. cardiac
    b. somatic
    c. referred
    d. visceral

24. Peritoneal inflammation most often is accompanied by visceral/somatic pain. (Circle the correct answer.)

25. Why is abdominal pain often referred to other areas? Briefly explain.

26. The primary purposes of asking about a patient's medical history are:

    (a)

    (b)

27. Explain why it is important to obtain careful historical data when you are evaluating the condition of a patient with abdominal pain that may represent a life threat.

28. Peritonitis can be caused by leakage of what into the intraabdominal cavity?
   a. blood
   b. gastric juices
   c. intestinal contents
   d. all of the above

29. Gastrointestinal bleeding may be caused by: (Circle all that are correct.)
   a. appendicitis.
   b. esophageal disease.
   c. rectal cancer.
   d. stomach ulcers.

30. What does melena indicate? Briefly describe.

31. Which of the following conditions is not usually life-threatening in the presence of abdominal pain?
   a. acute gastrointestinal bleeding
   b. gastroenteritis
   c. intestinal obstruction
   d. peritonitis
   e. ruptured ectopic pregnancy

32. During examination of the abdomen, the focus of the examiner should be:

For each of the following statements (33–39), circle the correct response, True or False. Briefly explain your answer.

33. Rebound tenderness should be assessed in the prehospital setting.

       TRUE   **FALSE**

Briefly explain your answer:_____

34. A high mortality rate is associated with ruptured abdominal aortic aneurysm.

TRUE   **FALSE**

Briefly explain your answer: _____
_____

35. Severe conditions that are associated with abdominal pain may produce hypoperfusion and dehydration.

TRUE   **FALSE**

Briefly explain your answer: _____
_____

36. Sepsis sometimes occurs with intra-abdominal disorders.

TRUE   **FALSE**

Briefly explain your answer: _____
_____
_____

37. "Guarding" on examination of the abdomen is a sign of peritonitis.

TRUE   **FALSE**

Briefly explain your answer: _____
_____
_____

38. Pain that is abrupt or explosive in nature and that reaches a peak within minutes usually constitutes a minor emergency.

TRUE   **FALSE**

Briefly explain your answer: _____
_____

39. A patient with acute myocardial infarction may present initially with a complaint of abdominal pain.

TRUE   **FALSE**

Briefly explain your answer: _____
_____
_____

Answers to questions from chapter 36 can be found on page 475.

Chapter 37

Pregnancy and Childbirth

OBJECTIVES

1. Define the following terms:
   a. Ovary
   b. Vagina
   c. Uterus
   d. Fallopian tubes
   e. Amniotic fluid
   f. Placenta
   g. Umbilical cord
   h. Supine hypotensive syndrome
2. Describe physiological changes that occur during pregnancy.
3. Describe the effects of decreased maternal circulation on the fetus.
4. Describe the pathophysiology, risk factors, signs and symptoms, complications, and management for:
   a. Spontaneous abortion
   b. Threatened abortion
   c. Ectopic pregnancy
   d. Hyperemesis gravidum
   e. Premature labor
   f. Toxemia of pregnancy (preeclampsia and eclampsia)
   g. Abruptio placenta
   h. Placenta previa
   i. Multiple pregnancies
5. Describe the pathophysiology and management for the following labor and delivery complications:
   a. Prolapsed cord
   b. Breech presentation
   c. Limb presentation
   d. Postpartum hemorrhage/infection
   e. Meconium-stained amniotic fluid
6. Identify the signs and symptoms and management of a patient in normal labor.
7. Describe the appropriate assessment of the pregnant patient.
8. Describe three phases of labor and delivery.
9. Describe the actions and uses of drugs used for labor and delivery complications.
10. Identify the signs and symptoms of imminent delivery.
11. Identify the appropriate equipment and steps that are necessary to manage an uncomplicated prehospital delivery.
12. Describe the appropriate steps involved in newborn care, including resuscitation.

CASE PRESENTATION #1 (QUESTIONS 1-10)

You are dispatched to an obstetric call. On arrival at the scene, you find the patient lying on a couch. Her friend tells you that the patient is in labor. The patient is moaning and appears to be in a great deal of pain. She is alert and oriented, and her overall skin color is normal. Her pulse is 100 and strong.

1. Your first priority is to:
    a. ask if this is her first pregnancy.
    b. listen to fetal heart tones.
    c. obtain a blood pressure reading and check her abdomen.
    d. time contractions while asking relevant history questions.

While your partner checks for crowning or bleeding, you obtain a medical history. This is the patient's first pregnancy, and she has received no prenatal care. She is 16 years old and moved in with her friend when she became pregnant. Her parents wanted her to have an abortion, but the patient said she "could not go through with it." Her labor started about 5 hours ago. Her blood pressure is 148/94.

2. What other pertinent questions should you ask at this time?

Contractions are at irregular intervals (about 8 to 15 minutes apart); each lasts about 45 seconds. The abdomen feels rigid during the contractions. There is no sign of crowning or vaginal bleeding. The bag of waters has not ruptured.

3. What steps in the focused history and physical examination should you perform next?

Based on the patient's responses, she is most likely at full term; however, the information is somewhat questionable. She has a history of headaches, her hands are extremely swollen, and you note that she has facial edema.

4. Based on the information that you have obtained thus far, you suspect that she has:
    a. abruptio placenta.
    b. placenta previa.
    c. preeclampsia.
    d. premature labor.

Your partner tells the patient that most likely she is in early labor, and because this is her first baby, it could be 10 to 20 hours before she is ready to deliver. He determines that her friend can stay with her and suggests that the patient go to the hospital in a few hours when her contractions become more regular.

5. What is your reaction and response to your partner's advice to the patient?

6. What complication that is associated with her suspected condition should you be concerned about?

7. Is this patient's risk for this condition higher than that of the average woman? Briefly explain your response.

You tactfully intervene in the conversation and suggest that the patient go to the hospital now. She agrees, and you prepare for transport.

8. Your field treatment should include: (Circle all that apply.)
   a. high-concentration oxygen.
   b. an IV line of Ringer's lactate TKO.
   c. monitoring of her contraction intervals.
   d. observation for any signs of seizure activity.
   e. placement of the patient on her right side onto the stretcher.

The patient remains stable while en route to the hospital. You later learn that she had a seizure about 15 minutes after hospital admission.

9. What emergency drugs most likely would have been administered for the seizure activity?

10. What should you discuss with your partner about this call?

CASE PRESENTATION #2 (QUESTIONS 11-15)

You are dispatched to an obstetric emergency. You arrive to find the patient sitting on a swing on the front porch. She is crying and is obviously pregnant near or at full term. You immediately note that her shorts are bloody. She appears pale and sweaty.

11. What is your initial response to this situation?

While your partner is taking her vital signs, you quickly obtain the history. The patient is so upset that it is difficult to get information. However, you are able to find out that she is at full term and began bleeding about an hour ago. She denies any pain and says she has gone through three feminine pads in the last hour. Each one has become rapidly soaked with blood.

12. Your initial suspicion is:
    a. abruptio placenta.
    b. ectopic pregnancy.
    c. hyperemesis gravidarum.
    d. placenta previa.
    e. toxemia of pregnancy.

Further evaluation reveals the following: BP 100/60; pulse 130; respirations are shallow. Her skin is clammy, and she says she feels weak.

13. What are the immediate priorities for this patient?

14. Is the patient's condition dangerous for the fetus? Briefly explain your response.

You have discovered that this is the patient's second pregnancy; the first one was uncomplicated. She is very scared and upset. While you quickly start an IV of Ringer's lactate and prepare for transport, the patient asks you if she or the baby is in any danger.

15. What is an appropriate response to her question?

You immediately transport her to the hospital. After a brief evaluation, she is taken to the labor and delivery suite for an emergency cesarean section.

CASE PRESENTATION #3 (QUESTIONS 16–18)

You are dispatched to an emergency obstetric patient. On arrival, you find the patient lying in bed. She appears to be in distress and is screaming, "The baby is coming!"

16. What is your first priority?

While quickly assessing the patient and taking vital signs, you obtain a history. This is her third pregnancy, and her other two children were born without complications. Your partner is examining the perineal area and notices that an arm is the presenting part.

17. What is your next step?
   a. Get the obstetric (OB) kit and prepare for immediate delivery.
   b. Gently pull on the arm, and prepare to deliver the baby.
   c. Insert your gloved hand into the vagina and open the baby's airway.
   d. Prepare for immediate transport to the hospital.

18. Why is this such a dangerous situation?

You start an IV of Ringer's lactate and administer 100% oxygen. While en route to the hospital, the patient tells you that she feels like pushing. You are immediately in touch with medical direction. On inspecting her, you find that the baby's shoulder is now protruding, and delivery appears to be imminent. You prepare to deliver while your partner continues to transport with red lights and siren. You arrive at the hospital, and the mother is rushed into labor and delivery for an immediate cesarean section.

GENERAL REVIEW QUESTIONS

Match the term in Column 1 with its description in Column 2.

Column 1

19. _____ Ovary
20. _____ Vagina
21. _____ Uterus
22. _____ Fallopian tubes
23. _____ Amniotic fluid
24. _____ Placenta
25. _____ Umbilical cord

Column 2

a. The organ that connects the fetus to the placenta and transports blood
b. Pear-shaped muscular organ of menstruation; it also houses the fetus during pregnancy
c. Fluid contained in the gestational sac that surrounds the fetus
d. The lower part of the uterus
e. Passageway from the uterus to the outside of the body that allows for menstrual flow and childbirth
f. Located in the pelvis on either side of the uterus; functions (1) to develop and expel the ova (eggs) and (2) to secrete hormones
g. Two trumpet-shaped muscular tubes that extend from the ovaries to the base of the uterus
h. The vascular structure in the uterus that connects to the maternal circulation and exchanges nutrients and wastes for the fetus
i. Release of an ovum from a vesicular follicle

26. Briefly describe the changes that occur during pregnancy in the following body systems:

   (a) Cardiovascular

   (b) Respiratory

   (c) Renal

   (d) Gastrointestinal

   (e) Skin

   (f) Musculoskeletal

27. How is a circulation problem or lack of oxygen to the fetus best monitored?
   a. by monitoring the blood pressure of the mother
   b. by checking fetal heart rate
   c. by checking the heart rate of the mother
   d. by measuring pulse oximetry on the mother's abdomen

28. What is the difference between a spontaneous abortion and a threatened abortion?

29. Risk factors for the development of an ectopic pregnancy include a history of: (Circle all that apply.)
    a. age younger than 15.
    b. pelvic inflammatory disease.
    c. previous ectopic pregnancy.
    d. tubal ligation.
    e. use of an intrauterine device.

30. Which obstetric problem is associated with the highest infant morbidity and mortality rates?
    a. multiple pregnancies
    b. premature or preterm labor
    c. third-trimester bleeding
    d. toxemia of pregnancy
    e. uterine rupture

31. Describe the pathophysiology of abruptio placenta.

32. Meconium-stained amniotic fluid is significant because:
    a. fetal asphyxia can occur.
    b. imminent delivery will occur.
    c. it indicates bleeding from the mother.
    d. placenta previa is likely to be associated.

33. Describe the prehospital treatment of the following labor complications:

    (a) Prolapsed umbilical cord

    (b) Breech (frank) birth

Match the stage of labor in Column 1 with its description in Column 2.

	Column 1	Column 2
34. ____	First stage	a. Complete cervical dilation to delivery of the baby
35. ____	Second stage	b. Birth to delivery of the placenta
36. ____	Third stage	c. Regular uterine contractions that gradually become more forceful and longer in duration

37. Identify three signs that delivery is imminent.

    (a)

    (b)

    (c)

38. Discuss basic principles that should be applied when field delivery is necessary.

39. Postpartum hemorrhage is best controlled by:

(a)

(b)

40. In addition to securing the airway and circulation, what is a primary concern in newborn care?

Answers to questions from chapter 37 can be found on page 478.

Chapter 38

Fever

OBJECTIVES

1. Describe the basic mechanisms for body temperature regulation.
2. Describe the function of the hypothalamus.
3. Define *normal body temperature* and *fever*.
4. List common causes of fever.
5. Describe the pathophysiology of fever.
6. Explain the effects of pyrogens on the body.
7. List appropriate history questions for the patient with fever.
8. Identify common signs and symptoms associated with fever.
9. Identify high-risk groups for the development of fever and sepsis.
10. Identify appropriate methods for measuring temperature and situations in which to use each.
11. Identify when fever is life threatening and describe how it is treated.
12. Describe how to care for a patient with a fever.

CASE PRESENTATION #1 (QUESTIONS 1-11)

You are dispatched to a residence for a "sick child" call. The only additional information provided by dispatch is that the patient is running a fever. On arrival, you are met at the door by a young mother; she is holding her 2-month-old infant who is bundled heavily in blankets. From what you can see at this point, the baby appears to be in no acute distress. She tells you that her baby has been very tired and has been feeding poorly for the past two days. As your partner prepares to examine the infant, you continue to elicit the child's history from the mother.

1. What additional history questions related to the patient's fever should you ask the mother?

As your partner puts on her gloves before performing a rapid assessment, the mother begins to cry. She asks, "Why are you afraid to touch my baby?"

2. What is an appropriate response from you and your partner?

The mother tells you that she has been checking the baby's temperature using temperature strips placed on his forehead. The temperature has been running about 102.8° F for 12 hours; she reports that she had just taken it again before you arrived. She also tells you that she has both baby aspirin and liquid Tylenol® available, but she did not administer either because she was not sure of the dosage.

3. Even though the mother reported a recent temperature reading, should you recheck the infant's temperature? If yes, explain what method you would use and why.

Your partner points out a purple skin rash that does not blanch under pressure and bulging fontanelles. There are no obvious signs of dehydration. The baby's heart rate is 180, and respirations are 60 and unlabored. You and your partner suspect meningitis.

4. What assessment findings related to the fever led you to suspect meningitis?

5. What are the correct medical terms for the infant's tiredness, poor feeding behavior, and skin rash?

6. What is the probable reason that your partner did not check for stiff neck, given that it is a specific sign of meningitis?

7. Is the infant's pulse rate within a normal range for his age? Why, or why not?

8. Why does the infant's age make him more susceptible to a serious disease like meningitis?

You administer blow-by oxygen to this patient and apply a pulse oximeter. With instruction from medical direction, you administer liquid Tylenol® to this patient. Your ETA to the hospital is approximately 5 minutes. While en route to the emergency department, your partner instructs the infant's mother on acceptable measures for fever reduction.

9. Explain why your partner instructed her to use acetaminophen (Tylenol®) and to avoid giving aspirin.

10. What explanation did your partner give the mother for avoiding ice, cold, and alcohol baths?

The patient's condition is unchanged on arrival at the emergency department. You turn the patient over to the emergency department staff and provide a report to the accepting physician.

11. Based on your patient report, what might you expect the physician to recommend for you and your partner?

CASE PRESENTATION #2 (QUESTIONS 12-18)

You are dispatched to a retirement community to transport a 65-year-old man to the local hospital. On arrival, the only history you can obtain is provided by the patient's wife. She informs you that her husband, who is normally alert and aware of his surroundings, has become progressively more confused over the past few days. She also tells you that he complained of chills yesterday and has been running a mild temperature. He has a history of diabetes, which is controlled with diet. Although the patient's airway is intact, he appears to be in mild respiratory distress.

12. Should any treatment be initiated at this time, or should treatment be withheld until after the assessment is completed?

13. What is your next assessment priority? Explain why this is so.

14. Why is cardiac monitoring especially important for this patient?

As your basic life support crew members administer high-concentration oxygen via a nonrebreather mask and connect the patient to the cardiac monitor, you quickly initiate an IV at a TKO rate. Your partner listens to breath sounds, which are congested with crackles, and reports the following vital signs: BP 130/90; pulse 92 and irregular; respirations 24 and shallow; temperature 100.8° F. The cardiac monitor shows sinus tachycardia with occasional premature atrial contractions.

15. Is this patient's temperature significant? Explain why, or why not.

Based on this patient's presentation, you suspect that he has pneumonia. You carefully monitor the patient while en route to the hospital. The risk factors that made this patient susceptible to pneumonia also put him at risk for developing septic shock.

16. Other than pneumonia, list this patient's preexisting risk factors for septic shock.

17. What signs and symptoms would indicate that this patient is developing septic shock?

18. How will your treatment be altered for this patient if he develops septic shock?

Within minutes after arrival at the emergency department, the patient's condition deteriorates. When you return approximately one hour later after another call, you follow up to find that the patient does have pneumonia. He was intubated, placed on antibiotics, and admitted to the ICU in serious condition.

CASE PRESENTATION #3 (QUESTIONS 19–23)

Late at night, you are dispatched to a dance club to treat a patient who is having a seizure. Upon arrival, you find a 25-year-old woman who is postictal and responds only to pain. According to her friends, the patient was smoking crack when she had a grand mal seizure that lasted about two minutes. Her vital signs are: BP 180/104; pulse 132 and regular; respirations 6 and shallow; temperature 104.2° F.

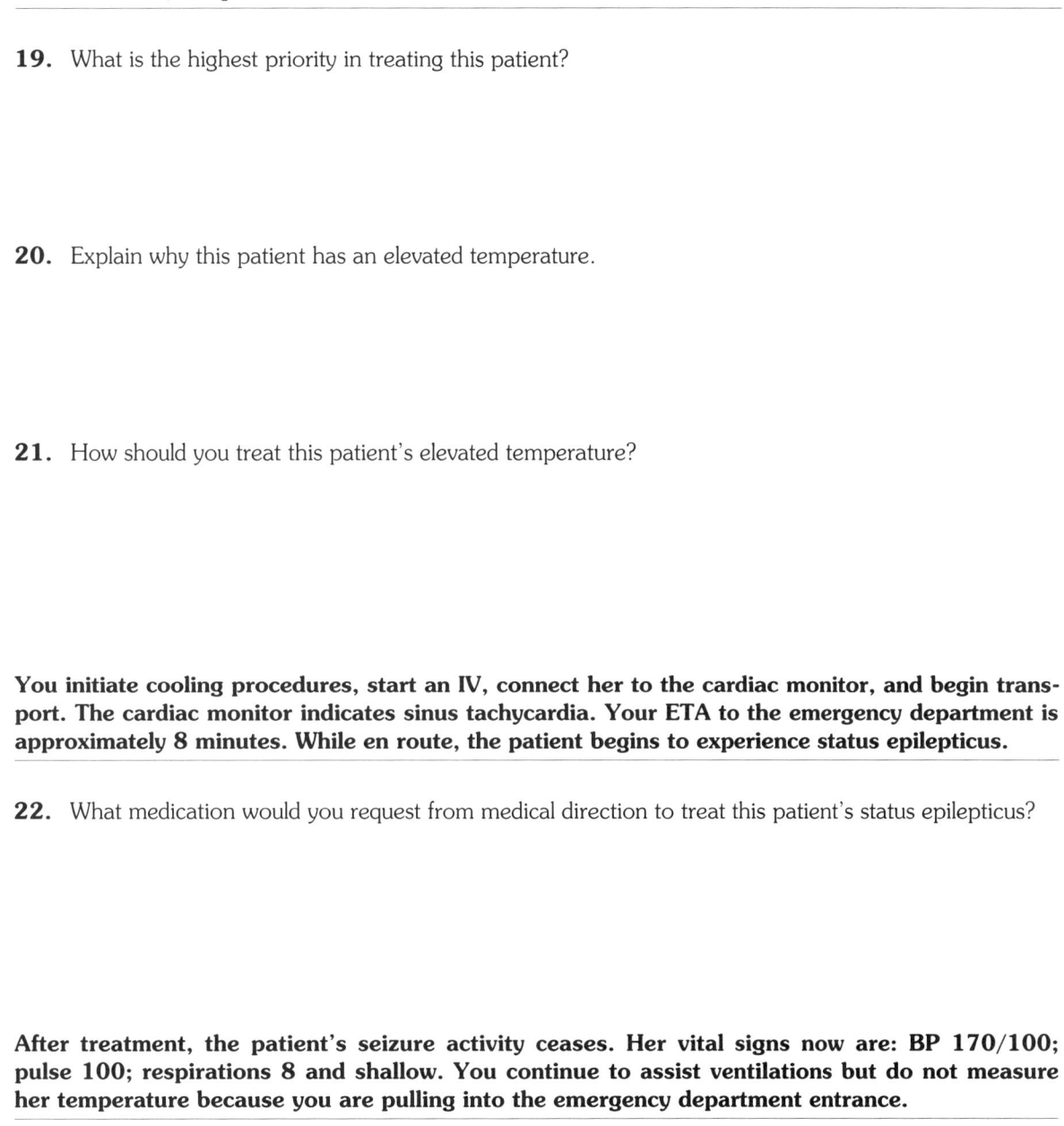

19. What is the highest priority in treating this patient?

20. Explain why this patient has an elevated temperature.

21. How should you treat this patient's elevated temperature?

You initiate cooling procedures, start an IV, connect her to the cardiac monitor, and begin transport. The cardiac monitor indicates sinus tachycardia. Your ETA to the emergency department is approximately 8 minutes. While en route, the patient begins to experience status epilepticus.

22. What medication would you request from medical direction to treat this patient's status epilepticus?

After treatment, the patient's seizure activity ceases. Her vital signs now are: BP 170/100; pulse 100; respirations 8 and shallow. You continue to assist ventilations but do not measure her temperature because you are pulling into the emergency department entrance.

23. What is a safer, quicker clinical method that you can use to estimate this patient's body temperature at this time?

General Review Questions

Fill in the blanks with the appropriate answers.

24. Body temperature is maintained by balancing heat _____ and heat _____.

25. The brain's primary control of body temperature and heat regulation takes place in the _____.

26. As the body attempts to maintain temperature at the higher set point through _____ and peripheral _____, the patient may experience chills.

27. The normal range for body temperature in Fahrenheit degrees is _____ to _____.

28. List four ways in which heat is lost from the body.

(a) _____

(b) _____

(c) _____

(d) _____

Match the normal body temperature in Column 2 with its location of measurement in Column 1.

	Column 1	Column 2
29. _____	Oral	a. 97.6° F
30. _____	Rectal	b. 98.6° F
31. _____	Axillary	c. 99.6° F

32. Define fever.

33. What is the most common cause of fever?

34. Explain how fever serves as a defense mechanism against intruding organisms.

35. Briefly explain why each of the following patients may present with fever.

   (a) a 55-year-old with acute onset of chest pain and shortness of breath

   (b) a 26-year-old who is experiencing weakness after jogging 10 miles on a hot muggy day

   (c) a 72-year-old who is complaining of right-sided weakness, difficulty talking, and nausea that developed suddenly

   (d) a 30-year-old who is complaining of dysuria and increased frequency of urination

36. What is the typical medical history that precedes septic shock?
   a. chest pain
   b. back pain
   c. recent infection
   d. trauma

37. Often the only sign of severe sepsis in an elderly patient is:
   a. a low-grade fever.
   b. altered mental status.
   c. a productive cough.
   d. nuchal rigidity.

38. Which of the following statements are TRUE about septic shock? (Circle all that apply.)
   a. Circulating bacteria release histamine.
   b. Peripheral vasoconstriction occurs.
   c. Venous return to the heart is decreased.
   d. It occurs most often in young adults.

39. Which of the following statements are TRUE about febrile seizures in children? (Circle all that apply.)
   a. They occur frequently in children between the ages of three and six years.
   b. They are characterized by a rapid rise in body temperature.
   c. Short-term management is aimed at treating the cause.
   d. Only children with a fever above 104° F are at risk.

40. Which of the following statements are TRUE about heat stroke patients? (Circle all that apply.)
   a. They usually have low-grade fevers.
   b. They usually are awake and alert.
   c. Skin usually is pale and diaphoretic.
   d. Rapid cooling with ice is essential.

For each of the following statements (41–43), circle the correct response, True or False. Briefly explain your answer.

41. Oral temperature readings may be altered by eating or drinking.

TRUE   **FALSE**

Briefly explain your answer: _____

_____

42. In most situations, axillary temperatures are taken in the prehospital setting.

TRUE   **FALSE**

Briefly explain your answer: _____

_____

_____

43. Oral temperatures should be assessed in patients who have a history of seizures.

TRUE   **FALSE**

Briefly explain your answer: _____

_____

_____

Answers to questions from chapter 38 can be found on page 480.

Chapter 39

Eye, Ear, Nose, and Throat Complaints—Medical

OBJECTIVES

1. Describe the basic anatomy and function of the following eye structures:
   a. Sclera
   b. Conjunctiva
   c. Cornea
   d. Retina
2. Describe the following eye conditions, including the management of each:
   a. Corneal abrasions
   b. Conjunctivitis
   c. Cataract
   d. Foreign body
3. Identify two assessment findings of the eye that constitute an emergency situation.
4. Discuss the basic pathophysiology, signs and symptoms, and complications of acute glaucoma.
5. Describe four conditions that may result in loss of vision or blindness.
6. Identify two functions of the ear.
7. Define and discuss the following conditions:
   a. Pharyngitis
   b. Otitis
   c. Vertigo
8. Identify potential causes, complications, and management of patients with epistaxis.
9. Discuss the clinical significance and management of a:
   a. Peritonsillar abscess
   b. Dystonis reaction
   c. Partial airway obstruction
10. Describe the appropriate assessment and significant findings for patients with complaints involving the eye, ear, nose, or throat.

CASE PRESENTATION #1 (QUESTIONS 1–4)

You are dispatched to a medical emergency at a long-term-care facility. You are greeted by a nurse, who takes you to an 85-year-old man who is awake, alert, and sitting up in a chair. His chief complaint is pain in his right eye. Your partner immediately tells the patient, "This is probably not an emergency, but we will check you out."

1. Could this patient's complaint be a true emergency? Briefly explain your response.

The patient's vital signs are: BP 154/90; pulse 106; respirations 18 and not labored. He tells you that he has been in pain for about 3 hours, and that it has become progressively worse. He is now feeling nauseated; he vomited just before your arrival. His medical history includes hypertension and a stroke that occurred 5 years ago.

2. What questions should be included in your focused history?

The patient does not complain of pain anywhere else, and there is no history of trauma. He states that he is having some trouble seeing you clearly, and that when he looks at lights, he sees halos. When you hold up your fingers at a 3-foot distance, the patient cannot discern the correct number of fingers. The sclera is not reddened, and there appears to be no pus in his eye.

3. Based on your findings thus far, what condition do you suspect? Briefly explain your response.

4. Describe what complication can result from the condition identified in Question 3.

You start a precautionary IV, contact medical direction, and prepare for transport. The patient arrives at the emergency department in stable condition. You are informed later that the patient had acute glaucoma and received pilocarpine; his vision then improved.

CASE PRESENTATION #2 (QUESTIONS 5–8)

You are dispatched to a medical emergency at the residence of a 66-year-old woman who lives alone. You find the patient sitting at the kitchen table holding a large handkerchief on her face. You immediately notice that it is saturated with blood. She is alert and appears to be very anxious.

5. Your initial step should be to:
   a. check her pulse and blood pressure.
   b. ensure that her airway is patent.
   c. determine the amount of blood loss.
   d. start an IV of Ringer's lactate.

The patient appears slightly pale. Vital signs are: BP 104/60; pulse 116; respirations 22 and shallow. She states that she is nauseated and has been vomiting blood. The nosebleed started about an hour ago, and she has not been able to stop it. Your partner pinches her nostrils and applies direct pressure to the nose.

6. What is the relationship between the patient's nausea and hematemesis and her nosebleed?

7. Your next step in the focused assessment is to:
    a. apply the ECG monitor.
    b. check for any allergies.
    c. determine the patient's medical history.
    d. examine the nose for foreign bodies.

You start an IV of Ringer's lactate, place the patient on a stretcher, and prepare for transport.

8. In what position should the patient be placed for transport? Briefly explain your response.

Shortly after arrival at the emergency department, the patient's condition begins to stabilize. She is admitted to the hospital because her platelet count is low, secondary to her Coumadin® therapy.

GENERAL REVIEW QUESTIONS

9. Which structure of the eye sends nervous impulses to the brain via the optic nerve?
    a. cornea
    b. lens
    c. retina
    d. sclera

Match the condition/term in Column 1 with its appropriate description in Column 2.

Column 1

10. _____ Corneal abrasion
11. _____ Conjunctivitis
12. _____ Cataract
13. _____ Otitis (media/external)
14. _____ Vertigo
15. _____ Pharyngitis

Column 2

a. The sensation that the world is spinning. It is caused by an abnormality of the inner ear balance organs or, rarely, of the brain.
b. Inflammation of the mucous membrane covering the anterior surface of the eyeball and the eyelids. It is caused by bacterial or viral infection, allergy, or environmental factors.
c. A condition that is characterized by high blood pressure.
d. Inflammation or infection of the ear.
e. Scrape of the convex, transparent, anterior part of the eye.
f. An infection of the throat that may cause difficulty swallowing.
g. An abnormal, progressive condition of the lens of the eye that is characterized by the loss of transparency.
h. A condition that is characterized by the presence of cerebrospinal fluid in the nose or ear.

16. The two primary functions of the ear are:

   (a)

   (b)

17. Which of the following emergency conditions typically can lead to loss of vision or blindness? (Circle all that apply.)
    a. acute glaucoma
    b. cerebral vascular accident
    c. conjunctivitis
    d. detachment of the retina
    e. retinal artery occlusion

18. What is the significance of a fixed and dilated pupil?

19. Which of the following conditions involving the throat is considered to be the most urgent?
    a. peritonsillar abscess
    b. pharyngitis
    c. strep throat
    d. tonsillitis

20. Describe two circumstances in which eye conditions are considered emergencies that warrant prompt transport.

    (a)

    (b)

21. You respond to a call involving a patient with breathing difficulty. On arrival, you find a 22-year-old woman who is sitting forward in a chair. She states that she is having difficulty swallowing and feels like she is going to swallow her tongue. The patient is drooling, and her jaw area feels stiff. You discover that she saw a physician earlier in the day, and he prescribed Haldol®. She says that the symptoms began about an hour after she took the medicine. She is likely experiencing a/an:
    a. allergic reaction.
    b. anxiety attack.
    c. conversion reaction.
    d. dystonic reaction.

For each of the following statements (22–25), circle the correct response, True or False. Briefly explain your answer.

22. Contact lenses should not be removed by the patient if a corneal abrasion is suspected.

    TRUE   **FALSE**

    Briefly explain your response: _____
    _____

23. At body temperature, normal saline is more appropriate than cold water for eye irrigation.

    TRUE   **FALSE**

    Briefly explain your response: _____
    _____

24. Topical anesthetics may be used for patients with a foreign body in the eye.

    TRUE   **FALSE**

    Briefly explain your response: _____
    _____
    _____

25. Uncontrollable epistaxis can compromise the airway.

    TRUE   **FALSE**

    Briefly explain your response: _____
    _____
    _____

26. List and briefly describe common causes of epistaxis.

27. Discuss the management of a patient with a partial airway obstruction.

Answers to questions from chapter 39 can be found on page 482.

Chapter 40

Nontraumatic Extremity Complaints

OBJECTIVES

1. Identify potential life threats associated with nontraumatic extremity complaints.
2. Describe the causes, pathophysiology, signs and symptoms, and potential complications of the following:
   a. Deep vein thrombosis
   b. Arterial occlusion
   c. Arthritis
   d. Compartment syndrome
   e. Sickle cell crises
   f. Hemarthrosis
3. Explain why a patient with a nontraumatic extremity complaint could possibly have a life-threatening or serious condition requiring physician care.
4. Given a patient with a nontraumatic extremity complaint, discuss the appropriate history and physical examination necessary for proper assessment.

CASE PRESENTATION #1 (QUESTIONS 1–7)

You are dispatched to a medical emergency. On arrival at the scene, the patient's mother anxiously greets you and leads you to her 19-year-old son's bedroom. He is lying in bed and is conscious, alert, and oriented to his surroundings. His chief complaint is pain in his left thigh. His vital signs are: BP 130/70; pulse 110; respirations 26.

1. What history information related to this chief complaint would be important to obtain initially?

History reveals that the patient fractured his left femur 4 weeks ago in a motorcycle accident. The fracture was surgically repaired with "pins," and he was released from the hospital 3 days ago. Examination of his thigh reveals that the area of complaint is swollen, red, and very warm to the touch. The pain is localized to this specific area.

2. After the initial examination, the next step in your physical examination should be to check for:
   a. distal pulses.
   b. the presence of Homans' sign.
   c. range of motion.
   d. sensation in the extremity.

The patient tells you that he was doing well until last night when this intense pain in his thigh started. It is now about 2:00 p.m. in the afternoon. He denies any chest pain or shortness of breath. He has been taking Tylox® for pain, but it has been ineffective for the past 24 hours. His physician also prescribed Coumadin®.

3. Coumadin most likely was prescribed for this patient to:
   a. control his dysrhythmia.
   b. eliminate excess fluid collection and swelling.
   c. lower his blood pressure.
   d. reduce the likelihood of blood clot formation.

On further physical examination, you find that his capillary refill time is less than 2 seconds, and distal pulses are present. He has extreme pain when the affected area is compressed mildly; he also has a positive Homans' sign.

4. Based on the history and physical findings of this patient, you most likely suspect:
   a. arterial occlusion.
   b. deep vein thrombosis.
   c. hemarthrosis.
   d. septic arthritis.

5. Explain your response to Question Number 4.

You prepare the patient for transport to the emergency department.

6. Describe the appropriate management of this patient.

7. A significant potential problem related to this patient's condition for which you should be alert is a(n):
   a. aortic aneurysm.
   b. heart attack.
   c. pulmonary embolus.
   d. ruptured heart valve.

CASE PRESENTATION #2 (QUESTIONS 8–12)

At 6:00 p.m., you are dispatched to a possible injured person. On arrival at the scene, you find a young woman (age 20) who is lying on the couch in her living room. She is awake and alert but in obvious distress from the pain in her right leg. Vital signs are: BP 150/76; pulse 120; respirations 28 and shallow.

8. What are some possible causes for her pain?

The patient tells you that she began feeling very ill at about 8:00 a.m. She has felt generalized aching all day, has a low-grade fever, and complains that she is experiencing excruciating pain in her right calf.

9. What history questions would be important to ask next?

The patient describes the pain as severe, aching, and localized to her right calf. She tells you that she has sickle cell disease and that she has had similar episodes of this type. She has taken her usual pain medication (Percodan®), which provided no relief. The leg is not swollen or discolored. Peripheral pulses are present, and capillary refill is normal.

10. Could her condition constitute an emergency situation? Explain your answer.

11. You are ready to transport. What is the IV solution of choice for this patient?
    a. D5W TKO
    b. Ringer's lactate wide open
    c. Normal saline TKO
    d. None; an IV solution is not indicated.

12. Briefly explain what causes extremity pain in patients with sickle cell crisis.

General Review Questions

Match the condition in Column 1 with its correct description in Column 2.

Column 1

13. ____ Arterial thrombosis

14. ____ Non-infectious arthritis

15. ____ Compartment syndrome

16. ____ Hemarthrosis

Column 2

a. A blood clot that forms in the larger veins of the legs, pelvis, or arms

b. Generalized single-extremity pain with diminished pulses and sensation. It is caused by an elevation of pressure within the fascial compartments of the extremity.

c. Occlusion of an artery by clot formation at the site of an atherosclerotic plaque

d. Joint pain with no history of trauma or swelling, and without fever, localized redness, or swelling at the site

e. Bleeding into a joint space with minimal or no apparent trauma

17. The most URGENT condition that causes generalized extremity pain is:
  a. arterial occlusion.
  b. deep vein thrombosis.
  c. hemarthrosis.
  d. septic arthritis.

18. What is the difference between a thrombus and an embolus?

19. Arterial emboli usually originate from the:
  a. abdomen.
  b. brain.
  c. carotid arteries.
  d. heart.
  e. upper extremities.

20. List five aspects of pain that the paramedic should evaluate in a patient with a complaint of extremity pain.

(a)

(b)

(c)

(d)

(e)

21. List four risk factors for the development of a deep vein thrombosis.

(a)

(b)

(c)

(d)

For each of the following statements (22–26), circle the correct response, True or False. Briefly explain your answer.

22. Patients who have weakness in the arm and leg on the same side of the body are likely to have experienced a cerebral vascular accident.

TRUE   **FALSE**

Briefly explain your response: _____

_____

23. In patients with extremity complaints, circulatory status is evaluated best by checking the distal pulses and capillary refill.

TRUE   **FALSE**

Briefly explain your response: _____

_____

24. The presence of a cool, pale extremity without a pulse most likely is caused by deep vein thrombosis.

TRUE   **FALSE**

Briefly explain your response: _____

_____

25. Cardiac ischemia may be associated with an extremity complaint.

       TRUE   **FALSE**

Briefly explain your response: _____

_____

26. Any available hospital is suitable for a patient with an extremity complaint.

       TRUE   **FALSE**

Briefly explain your response: _____

_____

_____

27. List the five "Ps" that are used in the assessment of an extremity complaint.

    (a)

    (b)

    (c)

    (d)

    (e)

Answers to questions from chapter 40 can be found on page 484.

Chapter 41

Poisoning and Overdose

OBJECTIVES

1. Describe the various routes by which toxic substances enter the body.
2. Identify characteristic findings of an opiate, and of an adrenergic and anticholinergic toxidrome.
3. Describe the general principles for assessing and managing patients who have overdosed or been poisoned.
4. Given a group of patients who have overdosed or been poisoned, describe the specific management for each.
5. Describe the action and indication for specific antidotes.

CASE PRESENTATION #1 (QUESTIONS 1-8)

You are dispatched to an apartment complex for treatment of a patient who possibly overdosed. On arrival, you are met by the patient's roommate, a young man in his early 20s. He tells you that he and his girlfriend, the patient, had been arguing. She locked herself in the bathroom and threatened to swallow a bottle of pills. She is still there. After you reassure the patient that you are there to help, she comes out of the bathroom and admits that she took approximately 20 pills. She is crying but otherwise appears to be in no acute distress.

1. Why is it crucial to determine what drug this patient has taken?

2. Why is it important to determine the approximate time of ingestion?

The patient is awake and alert; even though she is upset, she answers questions appropriately and is very cooperative. Her vital signs are: BP 124/80; pulse 92 and regular; respirations 20 and normal. Her skin is warm and dry. While you are assessing the patient, your partner finds a 50 pill-size bottle of Tylenol® in the bathroom that is half empty. The patient tells you that the whole thing was an accident and that she feels really foolish. She took the pills 10 minutes ago and thinks that if she were going to have any problems, she would have had them by now. She also tells you that, if she develops any problems, her boyfriend can take her to her private doctor.

3. Do you need to transport this patient to the emergency department? Why, or why not?

After you explain to the patient about the potential complications that can occur with the amount of Tylenol® that she ingested, she agrees to be transported by ambulance to the ED. You initiate a precautionary IV of normal saline at a keep open rate and connect her to the cardiac monitor. Your partner contacts medical direction and requests an order for activated charcoal. The physician orders Ipecac® instead and informs you that a specific antidote will be administered to this patient upon arrival at the ED. Your ETA is 20 minutes.

4. Why is Ipecac® an appropriate order?

5. What is the minimum amount of water that should be administered with Ipecac®?

6. What is the specific antidote that will be administered to this patient in the hospital setting, and when must it be administered?

7. Is it important to take to the hospital the bottle of Tylenol® that was found at the scene? Why, or why not?

Within minutes after administration of Ipecac® to this patient, she begins to vomit. The patient arrives at the ED in stable condition. Her vital signs are unchanged.

8. Why should you inspect the patient's vomit before you dispose of it?

CASE PRESENTATION #2 (QUESTIONS 9–13)

You are dispatched to a private residence for treatment of a pediatric emergency. While you are en route, dispatch tells you that the patient is a 3-year-old boy whose mother called 9-1-1 because she thinks her son ate at least six multiple vitamins approximately 5 minutes ago. He was asymptomatic at the time of the call.

9. It would have been helpful if dispatch had determined if the multiple vitamins that were ingested contained:
   a. calcium.
   b. folic acid.
   c. iron.
   d. thiamine.

On arrival, you see an active toddler who is running around the room. The patient appears to be in no acute distress, but his young mother is very upset. She explains that it is her fault for not recapping the bottle tightly. She thinks that there were only a few pills in the bottle, but she is not sure. The bottle label has worn off, and she does not remember the brand or type, only that they were multiple vitamins.

10. Which of the following principles should you keep in mind when you are preparing to examine this patient?
   a. Move as quickly as possible, and examine only what is necessary.
   b. Examine the patient while he is on the bed, and restrain him if necessary.
   c. Perform a thorough head-to-toe assessment.
   d. Separate the upset mother from the patient during the examination.

11. Describe the general guidelines that you should follow when interacting with this patient and his mother.

12. Why is it especially important for you to determine if this patient has vomited?

Your partner develops a good rapport with the toddler and performs the physical assessment. He finds nothing abnormal. The patient's pulse is 84 and regular, and respirations are 20 at rest. You contact medical direction, who advises you to transport the patient to the ED for evaluation. Your ETA is 4 minutes. Because details about the exact amount and type of multiple vitamins that were ingested by this patient are unclear, the physician orders no treatment at this time.

13. In your opinion, why did medical direction refrain from ordering activated charcoal or Ipecac® as part of the prehospital treatment for this patient?

While en route to the ED, the patient's condition remains unchanged.

Case Presentation #3 (Questions 14–20)

You are dispatched to a private residence in a new, affluent neighborhood for treatment of a 28-year-old woman who was found "passed out" in her bedroom by a friend. The same friend had just talked to the patient on the phone 15 minutes earlier. The friend also informed dispatch that, next to the patient, she found a handwritten note that expressed a feeling of hopelessness over financial difficulties and a partially empty pill bottle (labeled amitriptyline 50 mg).

14. Is this patient's level of consciousness consistent with an overdose of amitriptyline?

When you arrive, the patient appears to be unconscious and is lying across the bed. She responds only to deep pain stimulation. Her airway is open, but her breathing is slow at a rate lower than 10 per minute, and her gag reflex is diminished. A pulse is present. The blood pressure reading is 90/60.

15. Is intubation appropriate at this time? Why, or why not?

16. After airway management, what additional treatment is indicated immediately? Explain why.

17. How can you calculate the number of pills that this patient may have ingested?

Your more detailed examination reveals that this patient is experiencing severe tricyclic antidepressant intoxication. This manifests itself as an anticholinergic overdose.

18. What findings would you expect to obtain from your assessment of her pupils and skin?

As you are loading the patient into the ambulance for transport, you notice ECG changes on the cardiac monitor. Her QRS complexes have widened. You contact medical direction before leaving the scene for the ED. Your ETA is 7 minutes.

19. What medication would you expect medical direction to order because of the change in this patient's ECG?

20. You should be alert for what two additional, rapidly developing complications that are associated with tricyclic antidepressant intoxication? If they occur, how would you treat each of them?

The patient is delivered to the ED. Her condition is unchanged. An hour later, you return to the ED with another patient. You inquire about your previous patient. The nurse informs you that her condition steadily worsened. She went into full cardiac arrest and, despite aggressive treatment, did not recover.

General Review Questions

21. List the four routes through which a person can be exposed to a toxic substance.

(a)

(b)

(c)

(d)

22. Describe the three ways in which an antidote opposes the action of a poison.

(a)

(b)

(c)

List the toxidrome for each group of characteristic findings.

	Toxidrome	**Characteristic Findings**
23.	_____	dilated pupils, sweating, tachycardia, and hypothermia
24.	_____	pinpoint pupils, decreased respirations, hypotension bradycardia, hypothermia, and sedation
25.	_____	dilated pupils, flushed and dry skin, delirium or sedation, hyperthermia and tachycardia

For each of the following statements (26–30), indicate whether vomiting should be induced in each patient by circling Yes or No. Briefly explain your answer.

26. YES   NO   A 17-year-old who is extremely nervous after popping a few amphetamines so that he could be alert for an examination at school. He has vomited once since he took the amphetamines.

27. YES   NO   A 4-year-old who ingested 20 orange-flavored aspirin tablets 10 minutes before your arrival because he thought that they were candy.

28. YES   NO   A 25-year-old who is postictal because of a seizure that occurred after he swallowed 50 diet pills 15 minutes before your arrival.

29. YES NO A 30-year-old who, in a suicide attempt, drank an unknown amount of kerosene.

30. YES NO A disoriented 75-year-old who was found in bed; empty, unmarked pill bottles were found on her night stand.

For each of the following statements (31–37), describe the signs and symptoms for which you should be alert and the specific management of each patient.

31. A 60-year-old woman who has carbon monoxide poisoning from a faulty furnace.

Signs and symptoms:

Management:

32. A 26-year-old man who has taken an overdose of morphine.

Signs and symptoms:

Management:

33. A 35-year-old insect exterminator who has come in contact with organophosphate.

Signs and symptoms:

Management:

34. A 45-year-old worker in a chemical plant who is exposed to cyanide gas.

    Signs and symptoms:

    Management:

35. A 2-year-old who has swallowed dishwasher detergent.

    Signs and symptoms:

    Management:

36. A 45-year-old who has taken too many theophylline tablets.

    Signs and symptoms:

    Management:

37. A 19-year-old who becomes nervous after smoking cocaine for the first time.

    Signs and symptoms:

    Management:

38. Naloxone is used to reverse the effects of:
    a. barbiturates.
    b. benzodiazepines.
    c. ethanol.
    d. opioids.

39. Which of the following is effectively absorbed by activated charcoal?
    a. acetaminophen
    b. alcohol
    c. cocaine
    d. lye

40. Most poisonings that occur in children are related to:
   a. accidental ingestion.
   b. child abuse.
   c. drug abuse.
   d. neglect.

41. After you put on the appropriate protective gear, your first step in managing a patient who has inhaled poisonous gas is to:
   a. administer high-concentration oxygen with a nonrebreather mask.
   b. intubate and hyperventilate the patient.
   c. remove the patient from the toxic environment.
   d. transport the patient immediately to the nearest emergency department.

42. A delayed onset of symptoms may occur with ingestion of:
   a. camphor.
   b. cyanide.
   c. isoniazid.
   d. Lomotil®.

Answers to questions from chapter 41 can be found on page 485.

Chapter 42

Drugs of Abuse

1. Identify major life threats that need to be identified in the drug abuse patient.
2. Describe the physiological effects of cocaine.
3. List potential complications associated with cocaine use.
4. Describe the general effects of alcohol when combined with other drugs.
5. Identify the signs and symptoms and complications associated with acute alcohol intoxication and alcohol withdrawal syndrome.
6. Given a description of several patients with different clinical findings, identify patients suffering from acute alcohol intoxication and alcohol withdrawal, and describe the appropriate patient treatment for both conditions.
7. Identify commonly abused drugs, including their street names, and classify them according to category.
8. Given a description of several patients with different clinical findings, identify the drug of abuse and describe the appropriate patient treatment.

CASE PRESENTATION #1 (QUESTIONS 1–6)

You are dispatched to a dance club for treatment of a possible overdose patient. The dispatcher advises you that the caller said the patient is hallucinating and is very agitated and uncooperative.

1. While en route to the scene, you should be reviewing mentally what commonly abused substances that may result in hallucinations and agitation?

On arrival, you find an agitated 25-year-old male who is screaming, "Someone is out to get me!" His friends admit that they saw the patient sniffing cocaine in the restroom; since then, he has been acting strangely.

2. How should you approach this patient, and why?

As you attempt to take a history from the patient, you notice that he is grinding his teeth and his facial muscles are twitching. His pupils are dilated, and he is very diaphoretic. The patient's vital signs are: BP 160/90; pulse fast and weak; respirations 24 and unlabored. You administer oxygen, initiate a precautionary IV, and connect him to the ECG monitor. The ECG reveals sinus tachycardia at a rate of 160. There are no ectopic foci, and he denies any complaint of chest pain.

3. Was it appropriate to question this patient about the presence of chest pain? Why, or why not?

4. Why are the patient's vital signs elevated?

5. Should you have taken this patient's temperature? Why, or why not?

6. What classification of drugs would be useful in controlling this patient's signs and symptoms?

The patient is transported to the hospital with no further complications.

CASE PRESENTATION #2 (QUESTIONS 7-13)

You are dispatched to a private residence for treatment of an unconscious person. The caller was panicked and hung up after calling without providing any additional information. On arrival, the patient's boyfriend meets you at the door and tells you that his girlfriend was shooting up heroin and suddenly passed out. As you approach the patient, you note that she has slow, snoring respirations at a rate of fewer than 6 per minute.

7. What is the primary life threat for this patient? Describe the appropriate management of this patient.

8. What would you expect her pupils to look like?

9. Why should you be especially cautious when initiating this patient's IV?

10. What is the correct drug and initial dose that you should administer to improve this patient's condition?

11. What additional physical assessment finding might lead you to believe that this patient is a chronic heroin abuser?

12. If this patient is a chronic heroin abuser, why should you exercise caution in administering the drug identified in Question 10, and how should administration of the dose be altered?

After you administer to this patient the antidote for a heroin overdose, her respiratory rate increases to a rate of 16 per minute and she begins to moan when you call her name. About half way to the emergency department, her respirations decrease to a rate of 6 per minute, and she no longer responds to her name.

13. What should your action be now?

After additional treatment, the patient arrives at the emergency department in stable condition.

CASE PRESENTATION #3 (QUESTIONS 14–18)

In the early afternoon, you respond to a call from a homeless shelter to care for a patient who is seizing from an unknown cause. On arrival, you find a 60-year-old man who is actively seizing on the floor in the lounge.

14. In addition to airway maintenance, what are your main treatment priorities at this time?

After about 30 seconds, the patient stops seizing. He is postictal at this time. His airway is intact, and his respirations are adequate. Your partner reports that the patient's blood pressure and pulse are within normal limits. You continue your history and physical assessment. There are no signs of injury, and there are no other abnormal findings. You administer oxygen, initiate an IV, and monitor his cardiac rhythm, which is showing a normal sinus pattern. While you are administering treatment, some of his friends at the shelter tell you that the patient "stays drunk most of the time but has had a dry spell for about a day now."

15. Based on this information, you suspect that the patient's seizure activity is most likely due to:
    a. abrupt alcohol withdrawal.
    b. a closed head injury.
    c. acute alcohol intoxication.
    d. epilepsy.

16. In addition to Narcan®, what two drugs would be given routinely at this time, and in what order would they be given?

The patient's friends also tell you that in the past when the patient has gone without alcohol for several days, he became very shaky and confused about who or where he was.

17. During that time, the patient was most likely exhibiting signs and symptoms associated with:
    a. acute intoxication.
    b. delirium tremens.
    c. hallucinations.
    d. seizures.

Your transport time to the hospital is approximately 10 minutes. While you are giving your report to medical direction en route, the patient begins to seize.

18. What type of drug do you anticipate medical direction will order to control this patient's seizures?

After medication administration, the patient stops seizing. You continue to monitor him closely throughout transport. He is postictal and in stable condition on arrival to the emergency department.

General Review Questions

19. Hidden in the grid below are 16 street names for commonly abused drugs. Find all 16 names and circle them in the grid. Then, fill in the street names that correspond to the drug or drug category listed beneath the grid.

```
C  B  L  O  W  P  A  E  C
R  G  S  N  O  W  V  O  S
A  R  D  T  P  E  K  K  H
N  A  O  I  C  E  R  T  E
K  G  R  S  A  D  A  M  R
M  A  R  Y  J  A  N  E  O
P  F  L  A  K  E  C  P  I
F  L  P  P  S  Y  R  C  N
E  C  S  T  A  S  Y  P  Y
```

(a) cocaine _____

(b) amphetamines _____

(c) marijuana _____

(d) hallucinogenics _____

(e) narcotics _____

20. For each of the case scenarios presented below (a–e), indicate what type of drug was most likely abused.

(a) A 45-year-old woman was dismissed from the hospital after having a hysterectomy. She has been experiencing severe pain and took four times the prescribed dose of her pain control medication. You find her unconscious with an empty pill bottle on the bed. Her respirations are slow and snoring, and her pupils are constricted.

Drug of abuse: _____

(b) A 22-year-old man has taken a pill given to him by a friend at a party. His pupils are dilated, and he appears to be crying. As you take his vital signs, he keeps asking, "Why does your face look so flat and why are you talking so loud?" After you have been on the scene for approximately 5 minutes, he asks, "Why have you been here so long?"

Drug of abuse: _____

(c) A 10-year-old boy, who is clutching a plastic bag, appears to be drunk but denies any alcohol consumption. He is complaining of double vision and nausea. You detect a peculiar smell as you begin to perform your assessment.

Drug of abuse: _____

(d) A 32-year-old woman has taken three times the amount of a medication prescribed by her physician to help her sleep. Her speech is slurred, and she is disoriented. As you question her regarding the location of the medication bottle, she becomes more lethargic.

Drug of abuse: _____

(e) A 58-year-old unconscious man is found lying in the alley. He responds only to painful stimuli. The patient has an unkempt appearance. A police officer at the scene tells you that he thinks the patient is homeless. You find multiple empty mouthwash bottles lying beside him.

Drug of abuse: _____

21. Appropriate prehospital management for a conscious, alert adult who has taken an oral overdose of phenobarbital is to administer_____.

22. A patient who develops respiratory compromise after using a speedball can be treated by administration of _____.

23. A patient who is experiencing chest pain after using cocaine may benefit from the administration of _____.

24. When combined with other drugs, alcohol:
    a. often potentiates the drug's effects.
    b. usually increases tolerance of the drug.
    c. can cause an adverse or lethal reaction.
    d. a and c
    e. a, b, and c

25. Which of the following is *not* included in the narcotic category of abused drugs?
    a. Darvon®
    b. heroin
    c. morphine
    d. PCP
    e. Percodan®

26. Signs and symptoms of acute alcohol intoxication may include:
    a. ataxia.
    b. nystagmus.
    c. bradycardia.
    d. a and b
    e. a, b, and c

27. Which of the following drugs is a central nervous system stimulant?
    a. Ativan®
    b. barbiturate
    c. cocaine
    d. Dilaudid®
    e. methaqualone

Answers to questions from chapter 42 can be found on page 487.

Chapter 43

Environmental Emergencies

OBJECTIVES

1. Describe the pathophysiology, assessment, and prehospital management of patients who have been stung or bitten by an insect, reptile, or animal.
2. Describe the basic mechanism for body temperature regulation.
3. Identify individuals who are at high risk for developing heat- and cold-related illnesses.
4. Describe the pathophysiology, assessment, and management of patients who have heat-related illness.
5. Describe the pathophysiology, assessment, and management of patients who have been struck by lightning.
6. Describe the pathophysiology, assessment, and management of patients who have cold-related illness or injury.
7. Describe the pathophysiology, assessment, and management of patients who have high altitude illness.

Case Presentation #1 (Questions 1–4)

You are dispatched to a nature trail at the edge of town for a possible snakebite victim. On arrival, you find a 19-year-old alert man and his girlfriend sitting in a truck. They had been hiking away from the marked trail minutes earlier, when a brown snake bit the patient on the hand. They hiked back to the vehicle and called 9-1-1 on the mobile phone.

The patient's girlfriend proudly tells you and your partner about the action she initiated that she learned from watching television. While keeping the patient's hand elevated, she applied a rolled-up T-shirt as a tourniquet to his wrist; she also made an ice pack for his hand using ice from their soft drink cooler wrapped in a towel.

1. List history and physical findings that would assist you and your partner in determining that this patient's snakebite is envenomed.

2. Was the treatment that was rendered before your arrival appropriate? Explain your response.

You remove the ice pack to examine the patient's hand. It appears normal except for an imprint of the snake's jaw on the skin. The patient's vital signs are: BP 124/78; pulse 88; respirations 20. The patient's only complaint concerns a minor stinging sensation in the dorsal side of his hand where the bite occurred. Your partner contacts medical direction as you prepare the patient for transport. While continuing to keep his affected extremity elevated, you administer high-concentration oxygen using a nonrebreather mask, and you connect him to the cardiac monitor.

3. Describe any additional procedures that are appropriate for the management of this patient.

Your ETA at the hospital is 8 minutes. While en route, the patient and his girlfriend are very receptive to your explanation of current information from the medical community about the treatment of snakebites. The patient's condition is unchanged on arrival at the emergency department. The physician informs everyone that it is not likely that the patient was envenomed, but that he will be observed in the emergency department and given a tetanus immunization before discharge.

4. Did you make the right decision in transporting this patient? Explain your response.

CASE PRESENTATION #2 (QUESTIONS 5–8)

While stopped at a light on the way back to the station after a call, you are flagged down by a business man. He directs you to a landscape worker who is in front of an office complex. You jump out of the ambulance to assess the situation while your partner contacts dispatch. The scene appears safe, so you approach a young Hispanic man who is sitting on the ground, leaning against a tree. Two of his coworkers run toward you and anxiously attempt to explain in Spanish what happened.

You note that the patient is in moderate respiratory distress, with wheezing that is audible without a stethoscope. He, too, speaks and comprehends only Spanish. You and your partner are unable to effectively communicate verbally at this time. The patient points to an area on his arm that is red and swollen. You see what appears to be a stinger. His vital signs are: BP 100/64; pulse 110; respirations 26 and labored. You quickly conclude that the patient is having an allergic reaction caused by an insect sting.

5. In addition to wheezing, list three airway assessment findings in this patient for which you should be alert.

   (a)

   (b)

   (c)

6. You are unable to obtain an accurate history at this time. Should you, therefore, perform a more complete assessment before initiating treatment? Explain your response.

7. Describe the appropriate management of this patient.

The patient responds favorably to your treatment. By the time you reach the hospital 8 minutes later, his signs and symptoms are almost absent. An interpreter in the emergency department determines that this has happened to the patient once before after being stung by a bee, but this time the reaction began almost immediately.

8. What might be helpful for this patient in the event of future exposures? Explain your response.

CASE PRESENTATION #3 (QUESTIONS 9–14)

On a hot, humid day, you are dispatched to a low-income apartment complex for treatment of an unconscious person. While you are en route, dispatch informs you that the patient is a 70-year-old woman who has a history of chronic heart disease, but she is on no medications. Her elderly brother, who visits her every other day, found her lying on the sofa in front of the television. He called 9-1-1 when he was unable to wake her.

As you enter the apartment, you note that the temperature inside is extremely hot, and the patient is heavily clothed. On initial examination, the patient has a pulse and is breathing but is unresponsive to verbal or painful stimuli. A quick look with paddles reveals sinus tachycardia.

There are no obvious signs of trauma. Pupils are normal. As you measure her vital signs, you note that her skin is very hot and dry. Her vital signs are: BP 88/50; pulse 112 and weak; respirations 24 and shallow. Breath sounds are clear. Rectal temperature is 105.8° F. Your initial conclusion is that this patient is experiencing classical heat stroke.

9. Briefly describe the cause of classical heat stroke.

10. List the two most important distinguishing features of heat stroke that can be seen in this patient.

   (a)

   (b)

11. List additional physical assessment findings, including risk factors, that support your conclusion.

12. In addition to stabilizing the ABCs, what is the most critical management procedure that you should perform on this patient?

13. Describe appropriate management procedures for this patient and provide the rationale for each in each of the following areas:

   (a) Airway maintenance

   (b) IV fluid administration

   (c) Cooling measures

Within minutes, you have completed your initial interventions, and BLS assistance arrives. You contact medical direction and report that the patient's condition is unchanged. The physician instructs you to continue cooling measures, administer a 250-cc bolus of IV fluid, obtain a rapid glucose determination, and begin transport to the nearest hospital. Your ETA is four minutes.

14. While you are en route, for what complications should you be alert?

Case Presentation #4 (Questions 15–17)

You are dispatched to a homeless shelter for treatment of a 62-year-old man who is complaining of numbness of the fingers on both hands. Additional history provided by the caller reveals that the patient had been outdoors in the snow all day with his bare hands exposed. His fingers are white and covered with blisters.

15. Based on the information provided by dispatch, what do you suspect may be wrong with this patient? Explain your response.

Examination of the patient reveals that the caller's history and description of the patient's hands are accurate. Your initial assessment reveals no life-threatening findings. His vital signs are: BP 124/80; pulse 72; respirations 18. Rapid glucose determination is 120 dl. The patient admits that he drank a fifth of whiskey earlier in the day. His speech is slurred, but he is alert; he is refusing any further treatment, including transport to the hospital.

16. Does this patient have the right to refuse treatment? Explain your response.

While you are completing your report to medical direction, your partner convinces the patient to accept treatment. ETA at the receiving hospital is 6 minutes.

17. Management of this patient's frostbitten fingers should include:
    a. covering the skin with saline-soaked dressings.
    b. improving circulation by massaging the fingers.
    c. rewarming by placing his hands in warm water.
    d. transporting him with his arms in an elevated position.

General Review Questions

Describe appropriate prehospital management for each of the following patients (Questions 18–23). All patients have stable vital signs, and high-concentration oxygen and ECG monitoring have been established in all cases.

18. A 22-year-old woman who is complaining of pain in her left arm after she was stung by a yellow jacket 15 minutes ago. She is covered with hives and is scratching all over. Breath sounds are clear, and she denies any respiratory difficulty.

19. A 34-year-old man who is complaining of leg muscle cramps and nausea that began while he was running in a 10K marathon on the hottest day of the year. He is sweating profusely, and his skin is pale and moist.

20. Five minutes before your arrival, a 56-year-old man, while reaching for logs from the wood pile, was bitten on the right hand by a spider. He is complaining of severe pain that occured immediately at the site of the bite.

21. A 9-year-old who sustained a bite to his lower leg when he startled the neighbor's Doberman pinscher. The wound appears superficial, and there is minimal bleeding and swelling.

22. A 29-year-old woman, on her first ski trip, who developed a mild headache and fatigue that have lasted all day. Later that evening, when she and a group of friends ascended to a mountaintop restaurant via gondola for dinner, her symptoms became worse, and she began to experience mild shortness of breath and confusion.

23. A 34-year-old woman who was hit by lightning while playing golf. She is awake and alert but does not remember what happened. The only obvious injury is a superficial burn to her shoulder.

24. List four mechanisms that the body uses to dissipate excess heat.

   (a)

   (b)

   (c)

   (d)

25. List and explain the two initial physiologic responses that the body uses to produce heat and reduce heat loss in response to a lowering of body temperature.

   (a)

   (b)

26. Describe the general principles of management of a hypothermic patient who has a pulse and spontaneous respirations.

For Questions 27–32, place an E beside the signs and symptoms that are related to heat exhaustion, and an S by those that are related to heat stroke.

27. _____ Pale and clammy skin

28. _____ Coma

29. _____ Hot and dry skin

30. _____ Normal or slightly elevated temperature

31. _____ Narrowed pulse pressure

32. _____ Sweating

33. The J wave is a unique waveform that is frequently seen in Lead II of a patient's ECG as a result of:
   a. anaphylaxis.
   b. hyperthermia.
   c. hypothermia.
   d. lightning strike.

34. By what method should the core temperature measurement in a heat stroke victim be assessed?
   a. axillary
   b. oral
   c. rectal
   d. tympanic

35. Which of the following patients is at greatest risk for hypothermia?
   a. a 34-year-old asthmatic
   b. a 16-year-old unconditioned athlete
   c. a 12-year-old with cystic fibrosis
   d. a 44-year-old alcoholic

36. Local tissue necrosis is commonly associated with envenomation from a:
   a. black widow.
   b. brown recluse.
   c. fire ant.
   d. wasp.

37. The onset of fever, chills, muscle aches, and weakness several days after a bite by a domestic cat indicates the presence of:
   a. a normal reaction.
   b. anaphylaxis.
   c. infection.
   d. rabies.

38. A patient who is on which of the following medications is at increased risk for heat illness?
   a. aspirin
   b. digitalis
   c. lithium
   d. progesterone

39. Which of the following patients is the first priority in a mass casualty incident in which all were struck by lightning?
   a. The patient who is complaining of severe pain in the bottom of his foot where third-degree burns are present. BP 124/60; pulse 100; respirations 20.
   b. The unconscious patient with a weak, palpable pulse of 68 beats per minute and shallow respirations of 12 per minute.
   c. The patient with a detectable pulse who is actively seizing.
   d. The patient who is in respiratory arrest with a faint peripheral pulse.

40. Which of the following treatments usually is *not* withheld from a severely hypothermic patient until rewarming has been accomplished?
   a. ACLS drugs
   b. countershocks
   c. humidified oxygen
   d. pacing

Answers to questions from chapter 43 can be found on page 489.

Chapter 44

Aquatic Emergencies

OBJECTIVES

1. Distinguish between drowning and near-drowning.
2. List predisposing factors that lead to drowning and pressure-related diving injuries.
3. Differentiate between the pathophysiology of salt water and fresh water drowning, wet and dry drowning, and postimmersion and immersion drowning.
4. Identify factors that influence patient survival of a near-drowning episode.
5. Describe the pathophysiology, assessment, and prehospital management of near-drowning.
6. Describe the pathophysiology, assessment, and prehospital management of pressure-related diving injuries.
7. Given a description of several patients with different clinical findings, identify a patient with possible immersion syndrome, air embolism, or decompression sickness.

CASE PRESENTATION #1 (QUESTIONS 1–5)

At midnight you are dispatched to a private residence in an affluent neighborhood for a possible drowning. It is February, and the outside temperature has been in the low-20° range for the past two days with a wind chill factor of -10° F. On arrival, you are hurriedly led to the outdoor swimming pool area by a group of anxious teenagers. There you find a 15-year-old girl who is wet and unresponsive and is lying on the ground by the pool. As you immediately assess the patient, her friend tells you that she decided to have a party while her parents were out of town. The victim, who was intoxicated, had gone swimming in the undrained pool on a dare. She dove head-first into the pool and then floated to the surface, apparently unconscious. After struggling for about 5 minutes, her friends were able to pull her out, using a pole, just minutes before you arrived. The patient's skin is cold to the touch and cyanotic. You are unable to detect a carotid pulse or respirations. Her temperature is 84.4° F using a tympanic thermometer, and her pupils are dilated and nonreactive. You and your partner immediately begin CPR. Additional manpower is now en route to the scene.

1. What was a predisposing factor of this patient's condition? Briefly explain your response.

2. In your opinion, why did this patient became unconscious so quickly after jumping into the pool?

3. Describe how you should manage this patient's airway. Explain why.

You and your partner recognize the need for aggressive resuscitation. You direct your BLS-trained personnel to remove the patient's wet clothing, dry her, and apply blankets. As your partner is establishing an IV line of normal saline at a keep vein open rate, you perform a quick look with the cardiac monitor. The monitor shows that the patient is in asystole. Because you do not have standing orders for drug administration, you contact medical direction. The physician orders one course of ACLS drugs to be administered before transport is begun to the closest hospital. Your ETA is 4 minutes.

4. Explain the rationale for the physician's orders.

The patient's condition is unchanged on arrival at the emergency department. The emergency physician tells you and your partner that the patient's prognosis is poor, but he continues resuscitation measures for over an hour. Even with aggressive treatment, the patient is never revived.

5. Explain why the physician may have concluded that this patient's prognosis was poor, and why he continued aggressive resuscitation measures in spite of his prognosis.

CASE PRESENTATION #2 (QUESTIONS 6–12)

On a warm, muggy day, you are dispatched to a lake for treatment of an unconscious person. While you are en route, dispatch contacts you with the following additional information: Two 25-year-old men had been recreational scuba diving in shallow water. Within minutes after surfacing, one of the men complained of dizziness and a headache before suddenly losing consciousness.

6. Based on the information provided by dispatch, you suspect that this patient is experiencing a(n):
   a. acute stroke.
   b. air embolism.
   c. decompression sickness (DCS).
   d. subcutaneous emphysema.

7. What additional information related to the dive is important for you to ascertain?

On arrival, you find the patient lying on the boat ramp. His dive partner tells you that they were both certified last weekend and wanted to try out this new sport on their own. He also conveys that this was their first and only dive since completing the course. He mutters continuously, "I just don't understand how he could have gotten the bends, we were only down 15 feet for 20 minutes."

8. Explain why this patient is most likely *not* experiencing decompression sickness.

9. Explain what may have caused this patient's condition.

The patient moans and pulls his hand away when you pinch him. His airway is intact, and he appears to be in no respiratory distress. His vital signs are: BP 124/60; pulse 88 and regular; and respirations 20 and unlabored. Breath sounds are equal bilaterally, and pupils are equal but sluggishly reactive.

10. Calculate a Glasgow Coma Score for this patient.

You immediately manage the patient's airway by applying a high concentration of oxygen via nonrebreather mask. As you are preparing to establish an IV line and connect the patient to the cardiac monitor, your partner stresses the need to properly position the patient first. After your on-scene management is complete, you contact medical direction for a hospital destination.

11. Describe the proper position for this patient and the reason for the urgency.

12. You would expect the physician to direct you to transport this patient to what type of facility? Explain why.

CASE PRESENTATION #3 (QUESTIONS 13–16)

You are dispatched to the scene of a possible drowning at a private residence. On arrival, you are met by a screaming mother who apparently left her 1-year-old son unattended in the bathtub for approximately 5 minutes while she answered the phone. She removed the boy, who was floating face down in the water, from the bath and began mouth-to-mouth ventilation. The child is now conscious and is crying.

13. What factors associated with this event would lead you to believe that this patient will have a good outcome?

14. Which of the following techniques should you *avoid* when preparing to assess this patient?
   a. Allow him to get accustomed to you.
   b. Allow him to sit on his mother's lap.
   c. Examine him in private.
   d. Use your pen light to distract him.

Your assessment reveals no abnormalities. The patient is in no apparent respiratory distress, and breath sounds are clear bilaterally. His skin is warm, dry, and pink. He is moving all extremities, and pupillary response is normal. Vital signs are: BP 80 systolic by palpation; pulse is strong and regular at a rate of 140; respirations are 30 and normal; tympanic temperature is 98.8° F.

15. Even though this patient appears completely normal, explain why you should transport him to the hospital.

You contact medical direction while your partner is preparing the patient for transport. He has stopped crying and is tolerating blow-by oxygen well. Your ETA to the hospital is 4 minutes. The patient is delivered to the emergency department in stable condition. After you report the details of the event to the receiving physician, he asks you and your partner if you suspect child abuse.

16. Was this a valid question for the physician to ask?

General Review Questions

17. Differentiate between drowning and near-drowning.

18. Explain the physiologic reactions in the following classifications of drowning:

    (a) Wet

    (b) Dry

    (c) Postimmersion (secondary)

    (d) Immersion

19. List common signs and symptoms associated with barotrauma to the:

    (a) Ears

    (b) Sinuses

20. Describe the only appropriate time for resuscitation efforts to be attempted in the water.

21. Is it practical to administer mouth-to-mouth breathing to a victim who is still in the water? Explain your response.

22. Signs and symptoms of decompression sickness develop:
    a. days to weeks after a dive.
    b. immediately upon surfacing.
    c. two to three days after a dive.
    d. within 4 to 12 hours after a dive.

23. Factors affecting the clinical outcome of a submersion incident include:
    a. patient weight, water temperature, and depth of submersion.
    b. preexisting medical conditions, and salt versus fresh water.
    c. salt versus fresh water, length of submersion, and age of the victim.
    d. water cleanliness, length of submersion, and age of the patient.

24. Aspiration of salt water may result in pulmonary edema because salt water causes:
    a. destruction of surfactant.
    b. leaking of the alveolar capillary walls.
    c. shifting of intravascular fluid into the alveoli.
    d. shunting of blood to the body core as a result of peripheral vasoconstriction.

25. The most important physiologic consequence of a submersion incident is:
    a. acidosis.
    b. hypothermia.
    c. hypoxia.
    d. pulmonary edema.

26. When drowning occurs in fresh water, the water entering the lungs will:
    a. be pushed into the alveolar space.
    b. draw fluid into the lungs.
    c. be drawn rapidly into the bloodstream.
    d. remain in the lungs.

27. The best way to open the airway of an apneic near-drowning victim is:
    a. head-tilt.
    b. head-tilt, chin-lift.
    c. jaw thrust.
    d. tongue-jaw lift.

Answers to questions from chapter 44 can be found on page 491.

Chapter 45

Behavioral Emergencies

OBJECTIVES

1. Define the following behavioral terms and describe the characteristics and appropriate management of each:
   a. Situational crisis
   b. Maturation crisis
   c. Anxiety
   d. Psychosis
   e. Depression
   f. Manic behavior
   g. Bipolar disorder
2. Identify two conditions that are considered transient personality disorders.
3. Describe the appropriate interpersonal and intervention skills that should be used when assessing and managing a patient with a behavioral emergency.
4. Describe the five steps in a mental status examination.
5. Identify suicide risk factors using the SAD PERSONS mnemonic and describe the management of the suicidal patient.
6. Define *crisis intervention* and describe its four goals.
7. Discuss the impact of drug and alcohol abuse on behavioral emergencies.
8. Discuss the significance of the psychological component of illness and injury.
9. Describe the legal obligations that apply to behavioral emergencies.

CASE PRESENTATION #1 (QUESTIONS 1-7)

You are dispatched to a private residence for a medical emergency. A middle-aged woman greets you at the door and quickly informs you that she is concerned about her 24-year-old son, who is sitting in the kitchen. She states that he has really "flipped out" and might harm himself or her.

1. After ensuring that the scene is safe, how should you approach this patient?

Your partner continues to observe the patient and scene, while you begin the patient interview. You note that the patient is poorly groomed and appears to be talking to himself. As you introduce yourself, he gets up from the chair and starts pacing. He shouts, "I know they are going to kill me, can't you get me off this boat?" Immediately after he makes this statement, he starts mumbling about a war and then switches to discussing his garden in the backyard.

2. Given his delusional state, you should:
   a. acknowledge his statements without agreeing with the irrational thoughts.
   b. agree with him and politely ask him to sit down.
   c. discontinue the interview with him and just talk to the mother.
   d. tell him that he is acting bizarre and that he needs psychiatric help.

You perform a mental status examination while your partner talks to the mother. You observe that the patient is having auditory hallucinations, and that he shifts between talking to "the voices" and you. He is sporadically oriented, at which time he is responsive to your questions. He has expressed no suicidal thoughts but appears to be very sad. Meanwhile, his mother tells your partner that her son was diagnosed with schizophrenia as a teenager and has been taking Haldol® for 10 years. He has been hospitalized three times for similar episodes; otherwise, he has been able to maintain a job at a local factory. A month ago, his father suddenly passed away, and she has noticed increasing episodes of inappropriate statements and behavior.

3. Can a patient who is hallucinating be sporadically oriented? Explain your response.

4. Haldol is prescribed for which of the following conditions? (Circle all that apply.)
   a. anxiety
   b. bipolar illness
   c. depression
   d. psychiatric disorders

5. Is it possible that the patient's father's recent death led to an exacerbation of his current symptoms? Explain your response.

You explain to the patient in a firm but polite manner that he needs to go to the hospital. He does not resist this suggestion, but he begins to take off his clothes in preparation for leaving.

6. How should you handle this behavior?

His mother gets upset, which seems to agitate the patient. Eventually, you are able to reassure both of them successfully, and you transport the patient to the hospital. A few hours later, the patient is admitted to the acute psychiatric ward.

7. If the patient had not willingly agreed to go to the hospital, what course of action should you have taken?

Case Presentation #2 (Questions 8-12)

You are dispatched for treatment of a possible injured patient. You and your partner have made several calls to this apartment complex and are aware of the high crime rate in the area. You are immediately focused on scene safety, and you call dispatch to determine if the police have been dispatched also. Dispatch informs you that police are already on the scene. When you arrive, an officer informs you that the patient is an 18-year-old woman. She is holding a gun with the intent to kill herself, but she has not injured herself to this point.

8. What should be considering as you approach this situation?

9. What other resources can be available to assist you in such a situation?

The patient is crying and says, "Go away so I can finish this!" You learn that a friend called 9-1-1 and successfully kept her at bay until help arrived. The patient seems very agitated. Her friend tells you that the patient's boyfriend was killed during the past week in a motor vehicle collision. The patient has been very depressed and has been drinking heavily; she has isolated herself from family and friends. Police secure the gun at this point.

10. Given this additional information, how should you attempt to intervene?

11. Using the SAD PERSONS mnemonic, is this patient at high risk for suicide?

You are able to convince the patient that there are people who care about her and that she should seek help. She tells you that she feels better talking about her feelings to her friend and you, and that you can go now. She says that she will not harm herself.

12. What is your next step? Briefly explain your response.
   a. Agree to leave her if the friend will stay with her.
   b. Forcefully restrain her, and transport her to the hospital.
   c. Obtain a mental health "hold", and transport her to the hospital.
   d. Tell her that you are glad she is feeling better, and leave the scene.

Later, you learn that she was admitted to the psychiatric acute care unit for observation and treatment.

CASE PRESENTATION #3 (QUESTIONS 13-17)

You are dispatched to a private residence in an affluent area for a possible medical emergency. A middle-aged woman greets you at the door. As she leads you to the back porch where her husband, the patient, is located, she tells you that he was laid off about 3 weeks ago. He has had a difficult time since then, including some medical complaints. He is not aware that she has called 9-1-1 and gets upset with her when he sees you. He is alert and in no acute distress; he tells you, "I don't need any medical help."

13. How would you handle this situation?

14. The patient does not want help; therefore, would it be appropriate for you to leave the scene at this point? Explain your response.

The patient says that his stomach and back have been giving him trouble and that he has had difficulty sleeping. The trouble is described as generalized aches and distress. His vital signs are: BP 146/96; pulse 72; respirations 20. He begins to cry as you attempt to gain further information.

15. How should you respond to him at this point?

Meanwhile, your partner has been talking to the patient's wife in another room. She says that these symptoms started about a week after the job loss and have gotten progressively worse. She describes him as very depressed but not suicidal. Nothing significant is revealed in your medical evaluation of the patient, except that his blood pressure is a little high. He tells you that he appreciates your coming, but he does not want to see a doctor.

16. What is your next action?

You are unable to convince him to agree to transport to the hospital, and you prepare to leave the scene. He thanks you for your concern, and his wife assures you that he will not be left alone. You and your parrtner leave the scene.

17. Is there any resource that could be provided for this patient and his wife?

General Review Questions

Match the behavioral disorder listed in Column 1 with its correct description in Column 2.

Column 1

18. ____ Maturational crisis
19. ____ Anxiety state
20. ____ Psychoses (e.g., schizophrenia)
21. ____ Depression
22. ____ Situational crisis
23. ____ Manic behavior
24. ____ Bipolar disorder

Column 2

a. Characterized by high levels of worry and fear; one of the most common types of mental disorders; if severe, panic attacks or conversion disorder can occur.

b. May be caused by organic conditions, developmental factors, or stress. Associated with an impaired perception of reality, including hallucinations and delusions. Behavioral changes occur that are not consistent with stimuli present in the environment.

c. Severe disturbance in a person's emotions; little energy for self care; rarely dangerous to others, but may be to themselves.

d. Characterized by intense agitation, rapid, uncontrollable thinking, and emotional outbursts. Angry outbursts are common.

e. A psychologic disorder characterized by episodes of mania, depression, or mixed moods. One or the other phase may be predominant at any given time; one phase may appear alternately with the other, or elements of both phases may be present simultaneously.

f. Crises related to life-changing events, such as retirement, children, leaving home, menopause, divorce, and entering puberty.

g. Crises related to illness, injuries, disasters, death of a loved one, or loss of a job.

h. A persistent, irrational fear of some stimulus of humiliation or embarrassment.

25. Which of the disorders listed in Questions 18 to 24 are classified as "transient personality disorders"?

26. What is the first step in the assessment of a behavioral emergency?

27. Identify the steps/areas evaluated in a mental status examination.

28. Briefly describe the three main steps in the prehospital management of a patient's reaction to a crisis situation.

29. Behavioral emergencies frequently are associated with, or are a direct result of, alcohol or drug abuse. The main "additive effect" is an increased potential for _____, and a delay in patient management. Briefly discuss some ways that this can be addressed.

30. Briefly summarize the "psychological component of illness and injury" and its effect on the patient.

Answers to questions from chapter 45 can be found on page 493.

Section 4B

Patient Presentations—Trauma

CHAPTERS

46. Truncal Trauma
47. Head, Eyes, Ears, Nose, Mouth, and Throat Trauma
48. Orthopedic Injuries
49. Burn Injuries

Chapter 46

Truncal Trauma

OBJECTIVES

1. Describe anatomy of the chest and abdomen, including organs located in each area.
2. Describe and discuss mechanism of injury and potential organ damage for blunt and pentrating trauma.
3. Explain the significance of mechanism of injury in truncal trauma.
4. Describe the prehospital management of patients with truncal trauma, and identify the most important aspect of that management.
5. Describe the appropriate assessment of the chest and abdomen in a patient with truncal trauma.
6. Describe the correct procedure for chest decompression.
7. Describe the pathophysiology of the types of shock seen in truncal trauma and the appropriate field management of each type.
8. List five findings from recent studies regarding PASG use in the prehospital setting.
9. List the signs and symptoms, potential problems, and field management for the following:
   a. Impaled objects
   b. Open pneumothorax (sucking chest wound)
   c. Flail chest
   d. Pulmonary contusion
   e. Evisceration
   f. Suspected abdominal injury
   g. Pneumothorax
   h. Tension pneumothorax
   i. Cardiac tamponade
   j. Myocardial contusion
10. Define the following terms:
    a. Mediastinum
    b. Pleural space
    c. Peritoneum
    d. Deceleration injury
    e. Pneumothorax
    f. Flail chest
    g. Evisceration
    h. Hemothorax

CASE PRESENTATION #1 (QUESTIONS 1-5)

You are dispatched to a local bar for treatment of a possible victim of stabbing. On arrival, you find two patients. Both are alert and awake.

Patient #1: A 30-year-old man with multiple cuts and abrasions on both arms; no other apparent injuries; and warm and dry skin. His vital signs are: BP 136/70; pulse 100; respirations 16.

Patient #2: A 26-year-old woman who has two stab wounds in the left chest area. She is pale and somewhat sweaty. Her vital signs are: BP 100/60; pulse 130; respirations 28 and shallow.

1. After assessing scene safety and ABCs, your next priority is to:
   a. bandage the wounds on Patient #1.
   b. call for an additional ambulance crew to attend to Patient #1.
   c. prepare PASG for Patient #2.
   d. start an IV of Ringer's lactate on Patient #2.

You are preparing to transport Patient #2, who is complaining of increasing dyspnea.

Your partner quickly reevaluates the patient's blood pressure, and it is 80/50. You also note that the patient has distended neck veins and distant heart sounds. Breath sounds are equal.

2. Which of the following conditions should you suspect?
   a. flail chest
   b. open pneumothorax
   c. pericardial tamponade
   d. ruptured aorta

You administer oxygen to the patient.

3. Your treatment while en route includes all of the following *except*:
   a. apply and inflate the PASG.
   b. perform continued assessment.
   c. monitor the patient's breathing and pulse.
   d. start an IV of Ringer's lactate.

4. What universal precautions should you employ while you are managing this patient?

When you arrive at the emergency department, the patient's condition is the same, except that she is beginning to appear cyanotic. The emergency physician calls you to tell you that the patient did have cardiac tamponade, and that your assessment and management of the patient were appropriate.

5. Briefly describe what led you to this conclusion.

CASE PRESENTATION #2 (QUESTIONS 6–10)

You are dispatched to the scene of a motor vehicle collision. The incident occurred on a busy highway and involves a single vehicle that was traveling at a high rate of speed. The driver apparently lost control and crashed into the center median. The car is significantly damaged. There are no other passengers, and no other vehicles are involved. The driver, who was pinned by the steering wheel, is unconscious.

6. Your first priority on arrival is to:
    a. assure that the scene is safe.
    b. check the patient's breathing.
    c. control bleeding from the obvious head wound.
    d. package the patient for C-spine immobilization.

7. Describe the injuries to the truncal region that you would expect to see in a situation that involves blunt trauma, rapid deceleration, and a crushed steering wheel.

You quickly examine the patient, who responds to verbal stimuli. You detect the smell of alcohol on her breath. Examination of the chest reveals abrasions and bruising on the right side with paradoxical movement; breath sounds are decreased on the right side. She has sustained a large scalp laceration and an open fracture of the right tibia-fibia.

8. Treatment priorities at the scene include: (Circle all that apply.)
    a. assisting the patient's respirations.
    b. controlling the obvious bleeding.
    c. listening for the presence of bowel sounds.
    d. packaging the patient for C-spine immobilization.

Once you have extricated the patient and secured her in the ambulance, she arouses and states she that she does not want to go to the hospital. She is very disoriented; when you reassess her blood pressure, it is 80/50.

9. You continue patient treatment and transport based on the:
    a. concept of delegated practice.
    b. law of emancipated minor.
    c. Good Samaritan law.
    d. doctrine of implied consent.
    e. doctrine of informed consent.

10. Describe the appropriate treatment of this patient while en route to the hospital.

CASE PRESENTATION #3 (QUESTIONS 11–14)

You are dispatched to a private residence for treatment of an injured person. The patient is a 50-year-old man who fell about 20 feet from a ladder while working on the roof of his house. On arrival, you find that the patient is conscious and lying on his left side. He is complaining of severe abdominal pain in the left upper quadrant area. He has an open fracture of the left wrist and cuts on the upper arm area. He is able to move and has sensation in all extremities.

11. Based on the mechanism of injury and your initial assessment, you suspect what injuries to organs and structures?

His vital signs are: BP 94/50; pulse 112; respirations 22. There are bruises and scrapes on the left upper quadrant of the abdomen. The patient states that he is thirsty.

12. Signs of a possible abdominal injury include:
    a. bruising and scrapes to the abdomen.
    b. pain in the area.
    c. tachycardia.
    d. thirst.
    e. all of the above

13. You immobilize the cervical spine and prepare the patient for transport. What information about his history should you attempt to elicit?

14. While en route to the hospital, your assessment and treatment should include: (Circle all that apply.)
    a. assessing breath sounds and palpating the abdomen.
    b. bandaging and splinting the fractured wrist.
    c. continuing to monitor pulse and respirations.
    d. starting a dopamine drip if the patient's blood pressure drops.
    e. starting an IV of Ringer's lactate.

General Review Questions

Match the term in Column 1 with its corresponding definition in Column 2.

Column 1

15. _____ Evisceration
16. _____ Pleural space
17. _____ Hemothorax
18. _____ Flail chest
19. _____ Mediastinum

Column 2

a. Injuries that occur after falls from a significant height or ejection from vehicles

b. The protrusion of an internal organ through a wound or surgical incision, especially in the abdominal wall

c. A thorax in which multiple rib fractures cause instability in part of the chest wall and paradoxical breathing; the lung underlying the injured area contracts on inspiration and bulges on expiration.

d. An accumulation of blood and fluid in the pleural cavity, between the parietal and visceral pleura, usually as the result of trauma

e. A portion of the thoracic cavity in the middle of the thorax, between the sternum and the vertebral column, that contains all the thoracic viscera except the lungs

f. An extensive serous membrane that covers the entire abdominal wall of the body and is reflected over the contained viscera

g. The potential space between the visceral and parietal layers of the pleura

h. A collection of air or gas in the pleural space that causes the lung to collapse

20. The chest is separated into two areas. List the organs contained in each area.

   (a) Central Area

   (b) Lateral Area

21. The mechanism of injury in truncal trauma is:
   a. a reliable predictor of patient outcome in most cases.
   b. an important factor in determination of the risk and type of organ damage.
   c. assessed by the first responders and usually is not reevaluated by paramedics.
   d. typically not relevant because most injuries are apparent.

22. The most important factor in reducing mortality for patients with truncal trauma in the prehospital setting is:
   a. applying PASG as soon as possible on the scene.
   b. listening for breath sounds so that exact injuries can be determined.
   c. providing rapid transportation to a trauma center.
   d. starting at least two IVs to replace fluid loss.

23. Impaled objects in the truncal region should be:
   a. removed carefully to minimize additional bleeding.
   b. examined closely so that depth of penetration can be determined.
   c. left in place and carefully secured.
   d. ignored if the patient's vital signs are stable.

24. Describe appropriate field treatment for the following injuries:

(a) Sucking chest wounds

(b) Flail chest

(c) Evisceration

(d) Hemothorax

(e) Pulmonary contusion

25. Which of the following organs is most often injured in blunt trauma to the truncal region?
   a. intestines
   b. liver
   c. spleen
   d. stomach

26. The absence of breath sounds on *one* side of the chest most likely indicates _____.

27. Complications of a pneumothorax include:
   a. dyspnea.
   b. increased risk of tension pneumothorax.
   c. poor oxygenation.
   d. respiratory compromise.
   e. all of the above

28. Explain how a needle decompression is perfomed.

29. List two causes of the mechanical type of shock that occurs in patients who have sustained truncal trauma.

30. List two causes of cardiogenic shock in patients who have sustained truncal trauma.

   (a)

   (b)

31. Cardiac tamponade is most often caused by _____ trauma.

32. List five findings of recent studies regarding the use of PASG in the prehospital setting.

Answers to questions from chapter 46 can be found on page 495.

Chapter 47

Head, Eyes, Ears, Nose, Mouth, and Throat Trauma

OBJECTIVES

1. Describe the key anatomic structures of the head, eyes, ears, nose, and throat.
2. Describe the various mechanisms of head injury leading to unconsciousness and injuries to the head, eyes, ears, nose, and throat.
3. List signs and symptoms that may be detected on physical examination of a trauma patient with injuries to the head, eyes, ears, nose, and throat.
4. Calculate a patient's level of consciousness according to the Glasgow Coma Scale and the AVPU system.
5. Describe signs of increased intracranial pressure and cerebral herniation.
6. Describe measures that can limit or decrease intracranial pressure.
7. List three causes of altered mental status frequently found in trauma victims but not caused by trauma.
8. Describe how to manage injuries to the head, eyes, ears, nose, and throat.

CASE PRESENTATION #1 (QUESTIONS 1–7)

You are dispatched to the scene of a motorcycle accident on a country road, after the emergency is called in by a passing driver. A BLS-level fire department engine is first to arrive on the scene. Fire department personnel find an unhelmeted 19-year-old man who is lying in a supine position beside an overturned three-wheel recreational vehicle. He has a patent airway and a strong carotid pulse. The patient responds by opening his eyes and pulling his hand away when pinched, but he makes no verbal sounds. He has no obvious bleeding, and the only visible injury is a large hematoma on the forehead. His vital signs are: BP 150/90; pulse 60; respirations 16 and unlabored. While you are en route to the scene, the dispatcher informs you of the EMT's findings and describes the initial care provided, which included maintaining the patient's airway, administering oxygen via nonrebreather mask, and providing spinal immobilization.

1. Was the initial treatment provided by the EMTs appropriate? Explain your response.

2. Using the information provided by dispatch, calculate this patient's level of consciousness score using the Glasgow Coma Scale.

You and your partner arrive at the scene approximately 5 minutes later. The patient's condition has changed. He is now unresponsive to pain and has an unreactive, dilated right pupil. His vital signs are BP 200/110; pulse 54; respirations 8 and shallow.

3. How significant are the changes that have occurred in this patient's condition? Explain your response.

4. Is there any additional airway treatment that the EMTs could have initiated that would have possibly prevented further deterioration in this patient's condition? Explain your response.

You and your partner recognize the critical nature of this patient's condition and prepare for immediate transport. You quickly intubate and hyperventilate the patient (at a rate of 20 times per minute), connect him to the ECG monitor, and initiate an IV while en route. Your ETA to the local trauma center is 10 minutes.

5. Explain how intubation of this patient may prevent further complications.

While en route, you contact medical direction.

6. What is the single most important patient observation that is made by you that should be reported to the physician? Explain your response.

You arrive at the emergency department, and the patient's condition is unchanged. The receiving physician tells you that he suspects the patient has sustained an epidural hematoma, which will require immediate surgical treatment.

7. How would you have altered your treatment of this patient if you had been able to make this determination in the field?

CASE PRESENTATION #2 (QUESTIONS 8–12)

You are dispatched to the scene of a "domestic disturbance" at the request of police who are on the scene. On arrival, an officer leads you to the 25-year-old patient who is sitting on a bed holding a blood-soaked towel to her face. She reluctantly tells you that during an argument with her husband about an hour ago, he struck her in the face several times with his fist. When she removes the towel from her face, you note a distorted, edematous nose, which is actively bleeding, and a minor laceration to her lower lip. She hands you her front tooth, which was knocked out during the fight. Her only complaint is moderate pain to her nose and jaw. Your partner obtains the following vital signs: BP 130/94; pulse 104, strong and regular; respirations 20 and uncompromised.

8. The most appropriate treatment for suppressing the bleeding from this patient's nose is to:
   a. pack the nostrils with 4x4s.
   b. apply pressure by pinching the nose.
   c. instruct her to lean forward.
   d. insert a nasopharyngeal airway.

9. This patient's tachycardia may be the result of:
   a. her emotional upset.
   b. blood loss.
   c. catecholamine release.
   d. b and c
   e. a, b, and c

10. Describe treatment for her avulsed tooth.

Transport time is approximately 10 minutes. While en route to the hospital, the patient begins to complain of pain when clenching her jaw. You immediately suspect a mandibular facial fracture.

11. List additional signs and symptoms for which you would assess that are consistent with a mandibular fracture.

12. If this patient had been found unconscious, would she have been a candidate for nasotracheal intubation? Explain your response.

The patient arrives at the emergency department in stable condition. She is still experiencing pain to her jaw, but the bleeding from her nose has stopped completely.

GENERAL REVIEW QUESTIONS

13. Label the seven structures identified in Figure 47-1 by filling in the blank next to each letter, which corresponds with the same letter in the drawing.

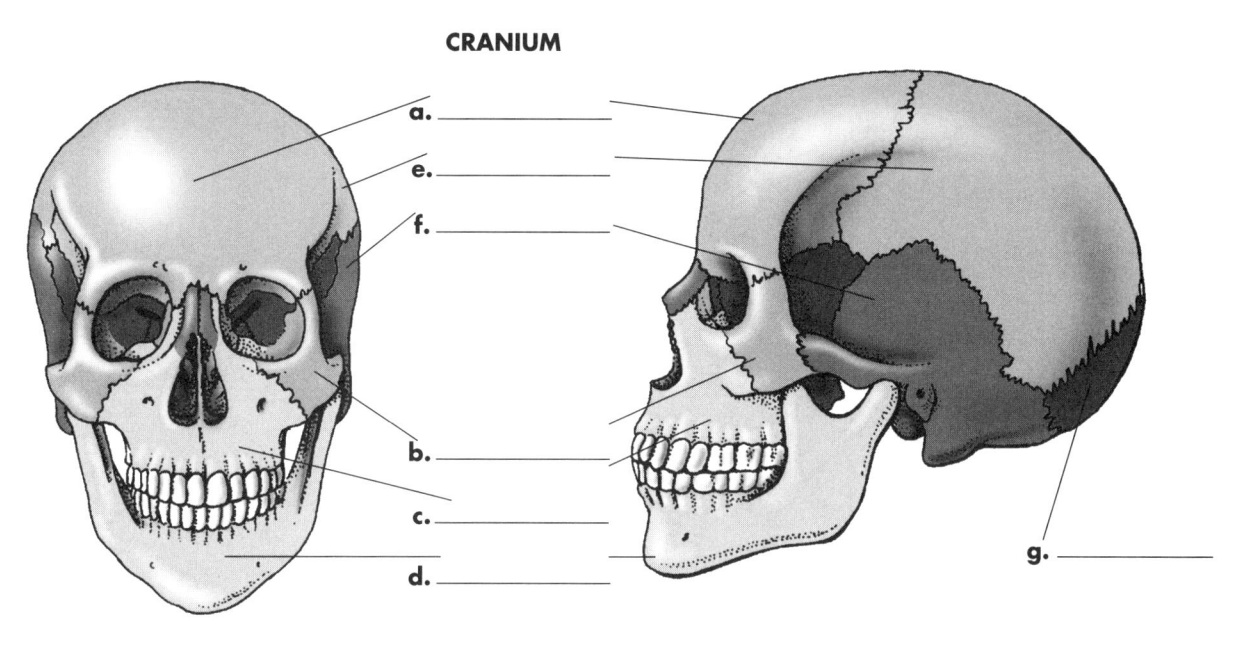

CRANIUM

a. _____
e. _____
f. _____
b. _____
c. _____
d. _____
g. _____

Figure 47-1

14. Label the seven structures of the ear identified in Figure 47-2 by filling in the blank next to each letter, which corresponds with the same letter in the drawing.

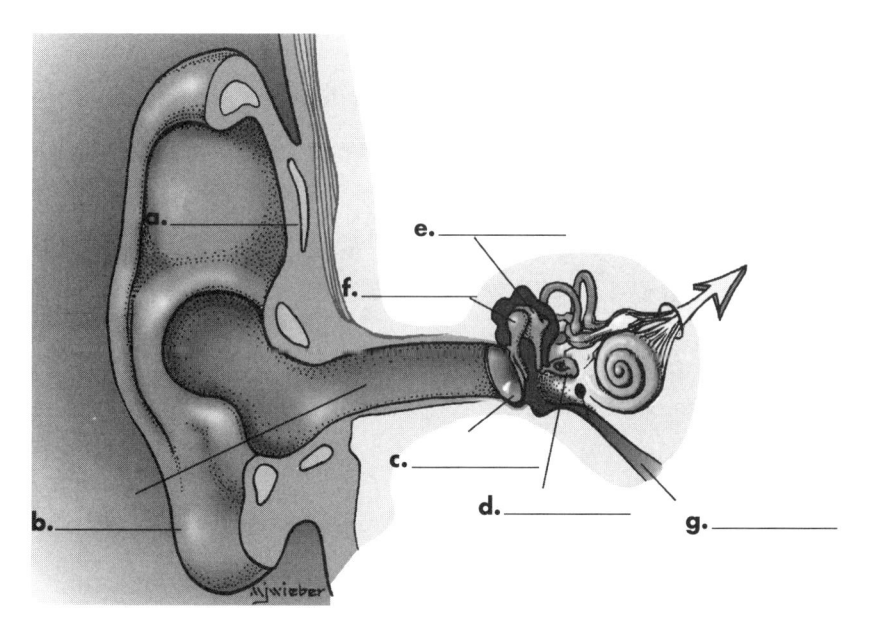

a. _____
e. _____
f. _____
c. _____
d. _____
b. _____
g. _____

Figure 47-2

15. Label the eight structures of the eye identified in Figure 47-3 by filling in the blank next to each letter, which corresponds with the same letter in the drawing.

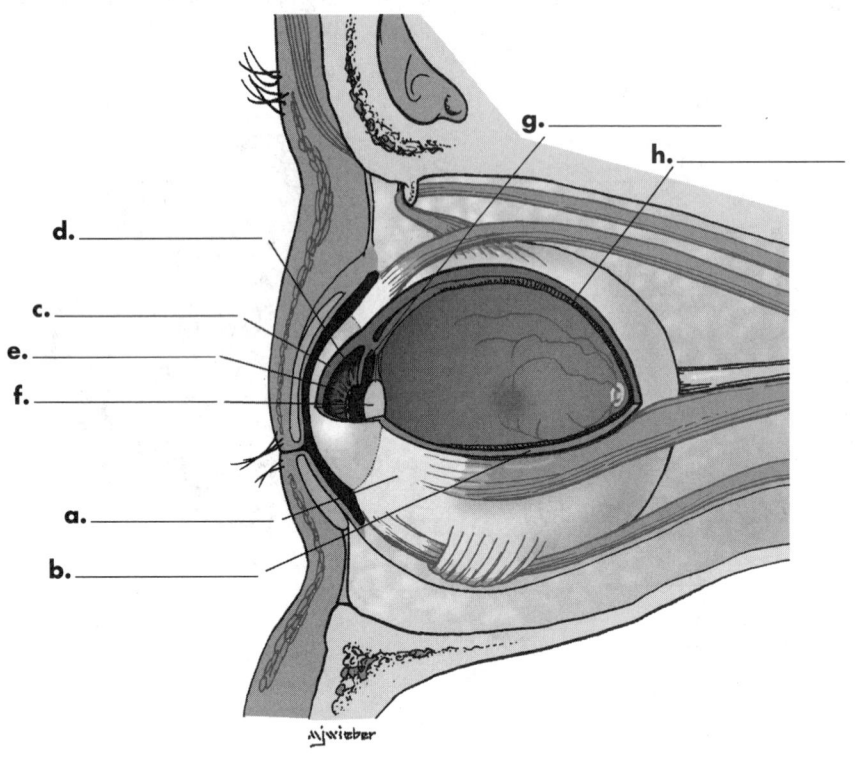

Figure 47-3 _____

16. Briefly explain how to prevent airway obstruction by the tongue in an unconscious patient with a head injury.

17. Briefly explain why it is important to remove dentures before endotracheal intubation in the unconscious patient.

18. Indicate what is abbreviated by each letter of the AVPU system of determining level of consciousness; fill in the blank next to it.

    A _____

    V _____

    P _____

    U _____

19. List the three parameters that are measured by the Glasgow Coma Scale.

    (a)

    (b)

    (c)

20. List three signs that may indicate the presence of a basilar skull fracture.

    (a)

    (b)

    (c)

21. List two medications that are used for diagnostic purposes in trauma patients with an altered mental status.

    (a)

    (b)

22. Next to each sign of increasing intracranial pressure listed below, indicate whether it is an early sign or a late sign.

    (a) unresponsive pupil _____

    (b) paralysis _____

    (c) changing mental status _____

    (d) posturing _____

    (e) changing level of consciousness _____

    (f) abnormal respirations _____

23. Describe specific treatment for each of the following injuries.

   (a) a bleeding scalp laceration with a depressed skull fracture

   (b) an impaled object in the head

   (c) cerebral spinal fluid leakage from the ear or nose

   (d) ruptured eye globe

24. A patient is considered to be in a coma with a Glasgow Coma Scale score of _____ or less.
   a. 5
   b. 7
   c. 8
   d. 10

25. Which of the following is TRUE about a subconjunctival hemorrhage?
   a. It causes serious disability.
   b. It results in external bleeding.
   c. It may result from simple coughing.
   d. It causes an abnormally shaped pupil.

26. Cushing's reflex is manifested by:
   a. hypotension and bradycardia.
   b. hypertension tachycardia.
   c. hypotension and tachycardia.
   d. hypertension and bradycardia.

27. What is the most rapid and effective intervention that is used to decrease intracranial pressure in a severely head-injured patient with clear signs of increasing intracranial pressure?
   a. glucose
   b. naloxone
   c. head elevation
   d. controlled hyperventilation

28. The most reliable indicator of increasing intracranial pressure is:
   a. unresponsive dilated pupils.
   b. nausea and vomiting.
   c. a change in the level of consciousness.
   d. posturing.

29. Causes of altered mental status that are often found in a trauma victim but are not caused by trauma include:
   a. alcohol abuse.
   b. narcotic overdose.
   c. hypoglycemia.
   d. all of the above

30. An intracranial hemorrhage that results from tearing of the middle meningeal artery is common with fractures of which portion of the skull?
   a. occipital
   b. temporal
   c. parietal
   d. frontal

Answers to questions from chapter 47 can be found on page 497.

Chapter 48

Orthopedic Injuries

OBJECTIVES

1. List the common signs and symptoms and complications associated with fractures.
2. Describe general principles of fracture management.
3. Describe how to assess a patient for potential spinal injury.
4. Explain the appropriate use of the common types of spinal immobilization devices and extremity splints, and list the advantages and disadvantages of each.
5. Describe airway management in patients with potential cervical spine injuries.
6. Describe the situation in which it is appropriate to attempt to realign an angulated fracture before splinting, and explain the correct method for doing so.
7. Describe the procedures used to determine the nerve and vascular function of extremities.

CASE PRESENTATION #1 (QUESTIONS 1–7)

You are dispatched to a rodeo arena for treatment of a rider who was injured when he fell off his horse. On arrival, you find a confused 26-year-old man who is lying on the ground and is unable to move. As you approach him, you observe that he is pale and diaphoretic. Your initial assessment reveals that his airway is intact and his respirations are not compromised. His pulse is rapid and weak at a rate of 96. There is no obvious external bleeding. Your partner informs you that his blood pressure is 112/70. You suspect that there are possible fractures based on a description of the fall by witnesses.

1. What is a priority of care for this patient and why?

2. Describe how to perform a neurologic examination on this patient to identify a possible spinal injury.

3. List the seven signs for which you would look when assessing this patient for a possible extremity fracture.

   (a)

   (b)

   (c)

   (d)

   (e)

   (f)

   (g)

Your continued assessment reveals an angulated fracture of the right upper leg. The skin is intact with moderate swelling at the injury site. You are unable to palpate a distal pulse, and the patient's foot is cool and pale.

4. Describe your next priority of care for this patient, and explain why it is so.

5. What type of splint is indicated for this patient's fracture?

After appropriately packaging the patient, you begin to transport. While en route to the hospital, the patient becomes more confused, and his rhythm changes from a sinus rhythm to a sinus tachycardia. Your partner informs you that the patient's blood pressure is now 88/50.

6. Is the change in this patient's condition a reason for concern? Why, or why not?

7. As you approach the emergency department, what should your course of action be with this patient?
   a. Remove his leg splint.
   b. Place him in Trendelenburg's position.
   c. Increase the IV fluid flow rate.
   d. No further treatment is necessary.

CASE PRESENTATION #2 (QUESTIONS 8–12)

You are dispatched to the scene of a motor vehicle and bicycle collision. The caller has informed dispatch that the driver of the vehicle is unhurt, but the bicyclist was thrown over the hood of the car onto the sidewalk 10 feet away. On arrival, you find an alert 22-year-old woman who is lying on her back and is complaining of pain to her right forearm and numbness to both legs. She is in no apparent respiratory distress; pulses are strong, and skin color is good. Her blood pressure is 122/90; pulse is 110; respirations are 20 and unlabored.

8. Based on this patient's presentation, in addition to administering oxygen, your treatment priority is to:
   a. splint the patient's elbow.
   b. check for orthostatic hypotension.
   c. log roll and palpate the vertebral spine.
   d. provide spinal immobilization.

9. Describe how to perform an abbreviated sensory assessment of this patient's lower extremities.

10. You have the choice of using an air splint, ladder splint, box splint, or vacuum splint on this patient's forearm. List the advantages and disadvantages (of each) that you would consider in deciding which one to use.

11. What three functions should you assess before and after you apply the splint to this patient's arm?

    (a)

    (b)

    (c)

You were on the scene for 20 minutes, and transport to the emergency department took 5 minutes. The patient's status did not change while en route.

12. Was your on-scene time appropriate? Why, or why not?

General Review Questions

13. Explain why it is important to limit the movement of fractured bones.

14. List two fracture sites that could lead to hypovolemic shock without obvious visual signs of hemorrhage.

   (a)

   (b)

15. In addition to airway management, the intervention of highest priority for the treatment of traumatized patients is immobilization of:
   a. dislocated joints.
   b. open extremity fractures.
   c. pelvic and femoral fractures.
   d. the spine.

16. The method of cervical immobilization that is used most often in the prehospital setting is:
   a. application of a halo-vest.
   b. application of sandbags and tape.
   c. a blocking technique using a rigid cervical collar.
   d. a blocking technique using a soft cervical collar.

17. A more controlled and reliable method of intubating a patient who is uncooperative, agitated, or not breathing is:
   a. bag-valve mask ventilation.
   b. endotracheal intubation.
   c. esophageal intubation.
   d. nasotracheal intubation.

18. The most appropriate procedure for maintaining cervical spine immobilization during airway management in patients with cervical spine injuries is _____ .

19. Describe how you would assess and treat a pelvic fracture.

20. Describe how you should manage cervical spine immobilization in a combative patient.

Answers to questions from chapter 48 can be found on page 499.

Chapter 49

Burn Injuries

OBJECTIVES

1. Identify high-risk groups and sources of burn injury.
2. Describe the structure and function of the skin.
3. Describe the pathophysiology and complications of burn injury in local and systemic responses.
4. Classify burn injury according to depth, extent, and severity based on established standards.
5. Identify measures that the paramedic should take to ensure personal safety and the safety of others at the scene of patients who have burn injuries.
6. Describe the assessment of the burn-injured patient.
7. Outline the prehospital management of the burn-injured patient.

CASE PRESENTATION #1 (QUESTIONS 1–8)

You are dispatched to the scene of a house fire in a residential neighborhood. Although the neighbor who reported the fire believes that the owner and her son are inside, there were no confirmed patients at the time of the call. As you approach the scene, you observe that the house is engulfed in flames.

1. When you position yourself at the scene, where should triage and patient care take place, and why?

As you get out of the ambulance, you see a firefighter who is using a plastic blanket to cover completely the charred body of a toddler-aged child. He tells you that the child is clearly a fatality, burned beyond recognition, and that firefighters are searching for the mother who is presumed to be inside still. Minutes later, the mother is removed from the house with her clothes still smoldering. She is conscious but disoriented and has extensive burns to the face and neck, anterior surface of the chest, and entire left arm. The burns appear red and glistening. She is in no apparent respiratory distress, although her nasal hair is singed and she has soot around her mouth. As your partner is administering a high concentration of oxygen to the patient using a nonrebreather mask, you remove her clothes.

2. Which of the following additional steps should be taken early during the initial assessment to stop the burning process?
    a. Apply cool, moist dressings.
    b. Apply ice packs.
    c. Remove all jewelry.
    d. Cover with a dry, sterile sheet.
    e. Apply petroleum gauze.

3. Why is it important to keep this patient covered after her clothes are removed?

4. What physical findings suggest to you that this patient may have possible inhalation injury?

5. At what point should you consider intubation?

While you are connecting the patient to the cardiac monitor, your partner reports that her blood pressure is 140/90 and her overall condition is unchanged.

6. Where should you place ECG pads, if they will not stick to her chest area?

7. Should you delay transport to the hospital so that an IV can be established? Briefly explain your response.

While en route, the patient's condition remains unchanged. As you approach the emergency department entrance, she begins to mumble incoherently. You reassure her. It is not until you are departing the hospital to respond to another call that you realize that she was asking about her son. For the remainder of your 12-hour shift, you are extremely anxious; several times, you are "short" with your partner as you relive the event in your mind.

8. Your behavior is probably the result of:
    a. conflict between you and your partner.
    b. sleep deprivation.
    c. posttraumatic stress.
    d. hallucinations.
    e. carbon monoxide poisoning.

CASE PRESENTATION #2 (QUESTIONS 9–12)

You are dispatched to a construction site to treat a patient who is injured from what the caller described as an "electrocution." On arrival, you are met by the job foreman, who begins leading you to the scene of the accident. He tells you that the patient is a 49-year-old man who received an electric shock of 120 volts, alternating current, for a duration of about one minute, from a power tool with a frayed electrical cord.

9. The most important aspect of this scene assessment is to determine:
    a. the location and condition of the patient.
    b. the potential hazards to you and your partner.
    c. the number of other possible patients involved.
    d. whether you need additional ambulances.

You determine that the power has been shut off. The patient is conscious and is sitting on the floor. He tells you that he was stunned when it happened and fell to his knees, but otherwise he feels okay. The palm of the hand that held the power tool appears burned and is covered with soot.

10. What is your immediate concern regarding life threats to this patient, based on the mechanism of his injury?

As your partner prepares to connect the patient to the cardiac monitor and measure his vital signs, the patient insists that he will be okay if he can just go home and rest.

11. Should you convince this patient to be treated and transported to the emergency department? Briefly explain your response.

The patient finally agrees to be treated and transported. You administer oxygen, initiate an IV, connect him to the cardiac monitor, and dress what appears to be a second-degree flash burn to his hand. His vital signs are: BP 130/88; pulse 92 and regular. The monitor shows normal sinus rhythm. He denies any respiratory difficulty or pain. Your continued assessment reveals no additional injury from the electric shock or the fall. There are three local hospitals of equal distance from the scene. Only one has a specialized burn unit.

12. According to the American Burn Association, this patient should be transported to which hospital? Explain why.

GENERAL REVIEW QUESTIONS

13. Match the layer of skin in Column 2 with its appropriate description in Column 1.

    Column 1

    _____ (1) Provides a layer of thermal insulation for muscles and bones

    _____ (2) Relatively thin, durable outermost portion of the skin

    _____ (3) Contains nerve endings, sebaceous glands, capillaries, sweat glands, and hair follicles

    _____ (4) Provides much protection to areas such as the soles of the feet and palms of the hands

    _____ (5) Burn injury to this layer is very painful.

    Column 2

    a. Epidermis
    b. Dermis
    c. Subcutaneous layer

14. List the four most common types of thermal burns.

    (a)

    (b)

    (c)

    (d)

15. Identify the two most common and well-recognized complications of fire-related accidents.

    (a)

    (b)

16. List the four areas of the body that are considered to be at "high risk" when burned.

(a)

(b)

(c)

(d)

17. The classification of burns assists you in making appropriate triage and _____ _____.

18. Hypovolemic shock, which occurs rapidly in a burn patient, is probably due to: _____ _____.

19. When a burn injury breaks the integrity of the skin, the victim may suffer disturbances in:
   a. appearance.
   b. fluid status.
   c. temperature.
   d. all of the above

20. Which of the following is *not* true regarding burns?
   a. Fires are the most common causes of fatal burns.
   b. Chemical burns are the most common type of burns.
   c. The largest number of burns occurs in children and the elderly.
   d. EMS providers can play a major role in burn prevention.

21. Early symptoms of carbon monoxide poisoning from smoke inhalation may include:
   a. headache, coma, and seizures.
   b. headache, dizziness, and nausea.
   c. nausea, wheezing, and dysrhythmias.
   d. dizziness, seizures, and cardiac arrest.

22. Which of the following is *not* considered when the severity of burns is determined?
   a. depth of the burn
   b. extent of the burn
   c. the patient's weight
   d. the patient's age
   e. the body part that was burned

23. Which of the following is *not* an injury that is commonly associated with electrical burns?
   a. flame injury
   b. blunt trauma
   c. cardiac dysrhythmia
   d. skeletal injury
   e. bacterial pneumonia

24. Pulmonary injury in the burn patient may result from:
   a. impaired oxygenation.
   b. aspiration of vomitus.
   c. inhalation of steam.
   d. a and c
   e. a, b, and c

25. Which of the following best describes a full-thickness burn?
   a. waxy with large blisters
   b. red, pink, and glistening
   c. red with clear blisters
   d. dry and paperlike

26. Exposure to which type of radiation is the most dangerous?
   a. alpha
   b. beta
   c. gamma
   d. ionizing

27. Pain medication is best administered to the burn patient:
   a. subcutaneously.
   b. intravenously.
   c. endotracheally.
   d. intramuscularly.
   e. orally.

28. For each of the following situations, classify the burn according to depth (first, second, or third degree), extent (body surface area), and severity (according to American Burn Association criteria). Identify those patients who meet the American Burn Association criteria for referral to a trauma or burn center.

   (a) A 40-year-old worker in a chemical plant who suffered burn injuries to the anterior surface of the upper legs when a flammable substance ignited. The burned skin appears charred and he is relatively pain free.

   Depth:

   Extent:

   Severity:

   Referral:

   (b) A 32-year-old who suffered a flash burn to his face and ears when lighting a barbecue grill. The burned skin appears reddened and is painful to the touch. He also has singed facial hair.

   Depth:

   Extent:

   Severity:

   Referral:

(c) A 4-year-old who pulled a pot of boiling water from the stove and suffered burns to the anterior surface of the chest and both legs. The burned skin appears pink with large serous blisters.

Depth:

Extent:

Severity:

Referral:

Answers to questions from chapter 49 can be found on page 500.

Section 5

SPECIAL SITUATIONS

CHAPTERS
50. General Principles of Rescue
51. Multiple-Casualty Incidents and Disasters
52. Hazardous Materials and Radiation Incidents
53. Air Medical Services
54. Rural EMS
55. Specialized Adjuncts for Therapy
56. Issues of Personal Violence
57. Death and Dying
58. Stress and Stress Management

Chapter 50

General Principles of Rescue

1. Discuss the significance of rescue safety.
2. Identify and discuss principles for scene evaluation and control as related to the following potential hazards:
   a. Traffic
   b. Environmental protection
   c. Fire
   d. Electrical
   e. Glass and plastic hazards
   f. Bumper and shock absorptions
   g. Unstable vehicle hazards
3. List the three general phases of rescue operations.
4. Describe appropriate methods for extrication of patients involved in motor vehicle collisions.
5. Identify the overall goal in the prehospital setting for patients in rescue situations.
6. Describe the following special rescue environments in terms of their potential hazards and principles of patient management:
   a. Wilderness
   b. Gunfire zones
   c. Water and ice rescue
   d. High-angle rescue
   e. Farm rescue
   f. Building collapse
   g. Confined space

Case Presentation # 1 (Questions 1-7)

You are dispatched to the scene of a motor vehicle collision. Upon arrival at the scene, you are informed that a car that was traveling at a high rate of speed struck a telephone pole. A bystander quickly points to downed power lines near the car. The driver and passenger are trapped in the car.

1. Your first priority in this situation is to:
   a. call for immediate assistance from the electrical company.
   b. establish a danger zone around the electrical hazard.
   c. look for signs that the power has been interrupted.
   d. initiate rescue of the trapped victims.

While taking appropriate precautions for your own safety, you approach the vehicle. You find the following: (1) the driver, who is conscious and moaning; (2) the front seat passenger, who appears to be unconscious.

2. What advice should you give to the driver immediately?

On closer inspection, you note that both doors are jammed and that fuel is leaking from the vehicle.

3. What precautions related to fire hazards are needed for both you and the patients?

4. To access the victim(s), it is preferable to enter the vehicle through the: (Circle all that apply.)
   a. front windshield.
   b. rear window openings.
   c. side windows.
   d. roof.

After you gain access to both victims, you determine that they are alive but are critically injured.

5. What should your next step be?

The victims are removed from the car within about 5 minutes, and the second unit transports the unconscious passenger. You are taking care of the driver. He is conscious and very disoriented and has a dilated right pupil. There is a large hematoma on the forehead. He also has chest abrasions and paradoxical movement of the chest on the right side. Vital signs are: BP 74/50; pulse 130, rapid and thready; respirations 28 and shallow.

6. Your overall goal in managing this patient is to:_____
   _____.

7. The patient is stabilized and prepared for transport. While en route to the hospital, your care includes:
   _____
   _____.

CASE PRESENTATION # 2 (QUESTIONS 8–12)

In the late afternoon, you are dispatched for treatment of an injured person at a mine explosion site. Dispatch informs you that the patient is apparently trapped and access is difficult.

8. While you are traveling to the scene, you recall the potential dangers of these situations, which include:

   _____

   _____.

As you arrive on the scene, you are told that the victim is buried under 25 feet of rock. You do have access to the victim. Your partner quickly puts on his protective head gear and says, "Let's go."

9. Your response to him is:
   a. "Determine if noxious gases are present, then we'll proceed."
   b. "Get my mask, too, then we'll go ahead."
   c. "Let's check with the foreman first."
   d. none of the above

You discover that specially trained rescue personnel are on site, and they are proceeding to rescue the patient. After 2 hours of standing by, the patient is finally located. He is unconscious but breathing, and he has a pulse. He has obvious crush injuries to the chest area, open fractures of both femurs, and second-degree burns on the face and arms. The patient's vital signs are: BP 60/40; pulse 130; respirations 6 and shallow. You are 90 miles away from the nearest trauma center.

10. Rank the following steps in terms of patient care priority:

    _____ Stabilize the femoral fractures.

    _____ Provide C-spine stabilization.

    _____ Start two IV lines of Ringer's lactate.

    _____ Assist ventilations and give oxygen.

    _____ Apply dressings to the burns.

    _____ Call for air medical transport.

The victim is extricated successfully from the mine. During the extrication, you, the patient, and the other rescuers have gotten very wet. You dry the patient off and cover him with blankets.

11. Explain why it is important to keep the patient dry and warm.

While waiting for air medical transport, you quickly establish two IVs, stabilize the femoral fractures, and monitor the patient closely. His vital signs improve. They now are: BP 100/70; pulse 100; respirations 20, with assistance.

12. The patient tells you that he is extremely frightened and is concerned that he is going to "lose his legs." What should be your response to him?

CASE PRESENTATION #3 (QUESTIONS 13–15)

You are dispatched to an explosion site. A male victim is located near the surface of the debris. He appears to be unconscious, but he responds to verbal stimuli. Vital signs are: BP 100/60; pulse 140; respirations 28. The extrication takes an hour and a half.

13. As the debris is removed, you recall potential problems that could occur, including:
   a. alkalosis.
   b. hyperkalemia.
   c. sudden cardiac arrest.
   d. b and c

14. What treatment should you provide at the scene while the patient is being extricated?

15. Because of his significant crush injury, what drug may be given to offset potential problems?

GENERAL REVIEW QUESTIONS

For each of the following statements (16–20), circle the correct response, True or False. Briefly explain your answer.

16. Protective gear (helmets, goggles, gloves, and other specialty equipment) is used only if time allows.

       TRUE   **FALSE**

Briefly explain your answer:_____

17. Shock-absorbing bumpers present potential hazards for rescuers.

TRUE   **FALSE**

Briefly explain your answer: _____
_____

18. In a life-threatening gunfire zone, removal of the patient from the area of danger may take priority over performance of a medical assessment, including ABCs.

TRUE   **FALSE**

Briefly explain your answer: _____
_____

19. The most dangerous aspect of a confined space rescue is the potential for both the reduced availability of oxygen and the presence of toxic gases.

TRUE   **FALSE**

Briefly explain your answer: _____
_____

20. Trench accidents that result in crush-type injuries to the chest or abdomen may be fatal.

TRUE   **FALSE**

Briefly explain your answer: _____
_____

21. The three phases of a rescue are: (a)_____, (b)_____, and (c)_____.

22. A unique challenge during a wilderness setting rescue is:
    a. appropriately managing the patient's airway.
    b. determining where to place the patient's IVs, once the patient is accessed.
    c. immobilizing the patient's cervical spine and packaging for transport.
    d. performing a continued assessment.

23. Significant concerns for the rescuer and the patient in water and ice rescue situations are: (Circle all that apply.)
    a. currents that may entrap people or boats.
    b. determining how to administer effective CPR in the water.
    c. swallowing large amounts of water, which could compromise the airway.
    d. dangerous water temperatures and possible hypothermia.

24. You are at the scene of a motor vehicle accident. A patient is trapped behind a steering wheel, and extrication is going to be prolonged. Should you start an IV before patient extrication is begun? Why, or why not?

25. List three possible confined space rescue situations.

(a)

(b)

(c)

Answers to questions from chapter 50 can be found on page 501.

Multiple-Casualty Incidents and Disasters

1. Define *multiple-casualty* incident.
2. Describe the differences in approach to patient care between single- and multiple-casualty incidents (MCIs).
3. Explain the steps of a systematic approach to an MCI.
4. Describe the actions required of the initial responder to an MCI.
5. List the roles of the first and subsequent responders to an MCI.
6. Differentiate between triage and treatment in an MCI.
7. Define and discuss examples of four patient triage categories: critical, urgent, delayed, and dead.
8. Define *START* and discuss how the four components are implemented.
9. Describe how transportation priorities are assigned to the victims of an MCI.
10. Describe the roles of physicians and hospitals in an MCI.
11. Discuss the importance of planning for an MCI and the role of critique sessions and drills in the planning process.
12. Briefly discuss the role of critical incident stress debriefing (CISD) as related to multiple-casualty incidents.

Case Presentation #1 (Questions 1–7)

At 11:00 p.m., on a cold and rainy night, your unit and a fire engine crew are called to the scene of a major accident. The location is on the cloverleaf of two interstate highways, and dispatch states that the incident could involve three or more vehicles. Your partner is sick, so you are riding with an EMT.

1. While en route to the scene, you should be considering:
   a. the mechanics of triage.
   b. potential multiple-casualty incident (MCI) principles.
   c. using the EMT as triage officer.
   d. a and b
   e. a, b, and c

2. Initial size-up reveals that four automobiles are involved; they are damaged heavily, and it appears there are eight to ten potential patients. There are no obvious immediate hazards at the scene. Which of the following should your assessment include? (Circle all that apply.)
   a. considerations for special resources at the scene and/or receiving hospital(s)
   b. the potential for special extrication needs
   c. the number of patients in each triage category
   d. the total number of victims involved in the incident

3. Once the scene is safe for entry, patients may talk to you and request help. For triage to be effective, it is important for the EMS provider to resist the temptation to: _____ _____.

4. Because there are multiple victims and additional assistance is needed, dispatch should be contacted immediately to: _____.

5. The EMT can be utilized best at this point to:
   a. direct incoming assistance.
   b. start CPR on a patient who is in cardiac arrest.
   c. start IVs where indicated.
   d. tag patients according to the size-up.
   e. both a and d

6. You find nine patients who are involved in the accident. Classify them according to the following triage categories: Dead, Delayed, Urgent, or Critical.

   (a) _____ an elderly male automobile driver with obvious severe head injuries, who has no pulse or respirations
   (b) _____ an 8-year-old girl who is crying and alert, and whose only apparent injury is a broken arm
   (c) _____ a middle-aged female automobile driver, who is alert and has severe chest contusions; she complains of dyspnea, and her pulse is strong.
   (d) _____ a young man approximately 20 years of age, who is unconscious with severe head injuries; pulse is barely palpable.
   (e) _____ a middle-aged woman who is found behind the steering wheel, with no vital signs
   (f) _____ a passenger who is barely conscious, with severe dyspnea and a weak pulse; there are no breath sounds on the right side. Other signs and symptoms indicate a possible tension pneumothorax.
   (g) _____ a young male patient (15 years of age) who is conscious and is complaining of severe leg pain; he is breathing adequately and has an obvious closed fracture of the tibia. There are no other apparent injuries.
   (h) _____ an 18-year-old passenger who is walking around; she has a severe head laceration but complains of no other pain.
   (i) _____ an elderly woman who apparently was thrown from the car and is found unconscious; her chest is markedly bruised. Radial pulse is palpable but very weak; respirations 8.

7. With triage completed, the additional ambulances on the scene should be directed to which three patients listed above?

Case Presentation #2 (Questions 8-13)

This call comes in as a report of a train accident. Because of the potential for multiple victims, dispatch sends four ambulances and fire personnel to the scene. You are the first EMS personnel to arrive. There is a derailment, and one car is on its side on fire.

8. Immediate scene considerations include:
    1. communication and command center location
    2. fire safety
    3. hazardous material spills
    4. possible electrical hazard
        a. 2 and 3
        b. 1 and 4
        c. all except 4
        d. all of the above

9. The purpose of the assessment phase is:

10. With more than 60 patients, your initial goal as triage officer is to:
    a. command all communications needed.
    b. contact all receiving hospitals about the incident.
    c. direct incoming units to severely injured patients.
    d. provide the most benefit to the greatest number of victims.

11. Your predetermined MCI plan for the community states that the senior fire department official is to be "commanding officer" of the scene. Two police units arrive and attempt to take over, thereby disrupting the flow of patients and communications. You should:
    a. allow them to continue their efforts.
    b. have them stop and assist your efforts.
    c. remind them briefly but firmly of the working plan.
    d. send them to the commanding officer for instructions.
    e. both c and d

12. Two emergency physicians arrive at the scene. Patients have been sorted: four are critical, three urgent, 20 delayed, and 33 dead. Some are ready to be transported. You send one physician to examine a patient with suspected tension pneumothorax. The other physician could assist *best* by:
    a. assisting the command officer.
    b. evaluating hospital availability and capabilities.
    c. reevaluating patients who are in the "delayed" category.
    d. re-triaging the patients.

13. Because many patients were killed in this incident and many horrifying injuries were observed, a critical incident stress debriefing (CISD) session is planned for EMS personnel. Describe how this session can be of benefit to scene personnel.

General Review Questions

14. A multiple casualty incident exists when the number of (a)_____ exceeds the number of (b)_____.

15. Rank order the following to develop a systematic approach to the treatment of patients in a multiple-casualty incident:
    a. Assessment (1) _____
    b. Command (2) _____
    c. Communication (3) _____
    d. Medical direction (4) _____
    e. Protection (5) _____
    f. Reassessment and treatment (6) _____
    g. Triage (7) _____

16. All of the following are true about communication and command centers EXCEPT:
    a. Each should have an incident commander.
    b. They help to minimize confusion.
    c. They notify and summon additional personnel.
    d. They should always be separated.

17. The designation of incident commander should be:
    a. determined by personnel who are first to arrive on the scene.
    b. determined by the police department.
    c. spelled out in advance in the MCI plan.
    d. assigned to the individual with the most experience.

18. The START plan follows the basic tenets of:
    (a)
    (b)
    (c)

19. START involves the *sequential* evaluation of:
    (a)
    (b)
    (c)
    (d)

20. Once patients are triaged and brought to the treatment center, the treatment officer:
    a. directs incoming ambulances.
    b. prioritizes treatment and resources.
    c. requests additional resources as needed.
    d. takes over communication from the command officer.
    e. b and c

21. Patients who are classified as "delayed" at a multiple-casualty incident can be employed to:

_____

_____

22. Most disasters occur unexpectedly. A community's efforts in handling a disaster can be promoted best by: (Circle all that apply.)
   a. defining mutual aid agreements.
   b. facilitating postincident critiques.
   c. predetermining the commanding officer's responsibilities.
   d. maximizing preplanning efforts and setting up practice drills.

23. Transport decisions and priorities at the scene:
   a. are classified differently from the categories of triage.
   b. are crucial to determine initially.
   c. are the same as triage categories.
   d. vary according to hospital capability.
   e. c and d

24. At some point after the multiple-casualty incident, it is important that all involved individuals:
   1. sit down and talk about the incident afterward.
   2. review specifics regarding patient care issues.
   3. discuss what went wrong, and how it could be improved.
   4. consider stress debriefing, if indicated.
      a. 2 only
      b. 1 and 3
      c. all except 4
      d. all of the above

25. Standard triage methods usually involve four categories of patients. Identify the category defined in each of the descriptions provided:

   (a) _____ patients who are salvageable with timely and appropriate intervention; these patients require early transport.

   (b) _____ patients who have been stabilized initially at the scene, or whose condition is anticipated to deteriorate without timely treatment

   (c) _____ patients who are salvageable, who do not appear to have life-threatening injuries, and who probably will not be harmed by delayed treatment

   (d) _____ patients who are dead, or those who are deemed nonsalvageable given the available medical resources and the number of patients on the scene who are in the critical or urgent category

Answers to questions from chapter 51 can be found on page 503.

Chapter 52

Hazardous Materials and Radiation Incidents

OBJECTIVES

1. Define the term *hazardous materials*.
2. Describe the means of identifying hazardous materials.
3. Describe the paramedic team's role at a hazardous materials incident.
4. Given an incident's scene diagram, label and describe the three safety zones in a hazardous materials response.
5. Identify the appropriate personal protective equipment required when responding to specific hazardous materials incidents.
6. Describe the signs and symptoms of exposure to hazardous materials that require intervention.
7. Describe the emergency management of patients who have been contaminated with hazardous materials.
8. List the resources for identifying and managing hazardous material situations.
9. Outline the appropriate response to a hazardous materials emergency.
10. Describe injuries caused by exposure to hazardous materials and radiation.
11. Describe the emergency management of patients who have been exposed to radiation.

CASE PRESENTATION #1 (QUESTIONS 1-10)

You are dispatched to the scene of a vehicle collision involving people with possible injuries. You are informed by police units on the scene that the collision involves a van and a cargo truck. There are several people involved, some of whom do not seem to be obviously injured.

1. What scene assessment issue should you be concerned with at this point?
   a. contents of the truck
   b. police qualifications and training
   c. patient gender
   d. traffic conditions

As you approach the scene, you see that the truck's cargo compartment has been torn open, and several cardboard boxes have been thrown to the ground. A white dusty powder is everywhere. Near the front of the cargo truck, you observe two conscious victims in the van; they are bleeding from head lacerations. A third victim, who has no obvious injuries, is lying on the ground near the rear of the cargo truck. The victim appears to be unconscious.

2. Your initial actions upon arriving at the scene include all of the following EXCEPT:
   a. surveying the vehicles for identifying placards.
   b. approaching the unconscious victim and checking ABCs.
   c. determining wind and weather conditions.
   d. notifying the dispatcher of the situation.

Your initial assessment of the scene reveals a placard on the side of the truck's cargo box. The placard is partially torn away, but you are able to see that it is white and has a number "6" at the bottom.

3. What resource book should be available on your EMS unit to assist in you identifying this hazardous material?

4. List three other pieces of information that may be found in this resource book.

5. If you are unable to determine the type of hazardous material involved, what actions should be taken by you and your partner?
   a. Withdraw to a safe distance, isolate the scene, notify the dispatcher, and request assistance from a hazmat team.
   b. Approach the unconscious victim, check ABCs, and move the patient to a safe location.
   c. Direct police to request aid from the health department, begin assessment and treatment of the victims, and request assistance from a hazmat team.
   d. Request fire department support, select appropriate personal protective equipment, and move victims from the scene to a safe location.

Upon arrival of the hazmat team, the area is cordoned off, and the unconscious patient is moved to a safe zone for treatment.

6. Your initial approach to this patient should include:
   a. initial patient assessment and patient history.
   b. assessment of ABCs and patient history.
   c. patient decontamination and continued assessment.
   d. assessment of ABCs, as well as spine evaluation and decontamination.

7. What precautions should you and your partner take before providing treatment to this patient, and why?

8. List the four steps that you and your partner should take when you perform gross decontamination of this patient.

   (a)

   (b)

   (c)

   (d)

The patient remains unconscious, but vital signs are stable. After decontamination, initial treatment, and patient packaging, you begin transport of the patient to the hospital. Upon arrival at the receiving facility, you are instructed to park in an area away from the emergency department. You are then instructed to enter through a door that is not typically used for emergency patients.

9. You believe that this instruction is being given for what reason?

10. Once the patient has been released to the hospital, what precautions should you and your partner take regarding the ambulance equipment?

CASE PRESENTATION #2 (QUESTIONS 11-15)

You are dispatched to treat an injured person at a local research laboratory. When you arrive, you are directed to a laboratory on the second floor. You are told that a worker fell off a ladder onto a worktable and broke several glass containers. The patient has been contaminated by a radioactive powder. You arrive at the door to the lab and see a sign indicating that radioactive materials are contained in the room.

11. What action should you take, and why?

When it is determined that it is safe to enter the room, you find a 41-year-old conscious man lying on the floor. He is bleeding moderately from a laceration to his hand and is unable to move because of severe hip pain. You see a powdery substance on his clothes and are told that this is the radioactive material. A container lying nearby, which contains a similar material, has a white label with the words "Radioactive I"; this indicates that there is almost no radiation associated with the spilled material. The patient also reassures you that this is the case.

12. After you assess ABCs, what is your next course of action with this patient, and why?

13. Describe the decontamination process for this patient.

14. Describe how you should "package" this patient for transport to decrease the possible spread of contamination.

The patient's condition remains stable while you are en route to the hospital. After release of the patient to the emergency department, you and your partner take several precautions to ensure that your equipment is free of contamination.

15. These precautions should include which of the following:
   a. Disinfect the ambulance with a mixture of chlorine bleach and antiseptic solution. You and your partner should shower and wipe down with an antiseptic solution.
   b. Take the ambulance to a certified radiation decontamination facility, where it can be dismantled and decontaminated. You and your partner should be decontaminated by certified laboratory personnel.
   c. Lock the ambulance and keep it at the hospital until it can be monitored for contamination. You and your partner should be monitored by a qualified health physicist.
   d. No precautions are necessary.

CASE PRESENTATION #3 (QUESTIONS 16–19)

You are dispatched to a football field to care for a possible stroke victim. On arrival, you find a middle-aged man who is staggering around a tractor. His assistant informs you that the patient began acting drunk after he finished spreading insecticides on the grass. The patient is awake but confused. He is sweating profusely and has a pulse rate of 48. His BP is 90/50; respirations are normal at 20 per minute. During your initial assessment, you note that the patient has pinpoint pupils and is salivating excessively. You suspect systemic toxicity from exposure to a hazardous material.

16. Based on this patient's presentation, it is most likely that he has been exposed to:
   a. carbon monoxide.
   b. cryogenic liquids.
   c. diesel fumes.
   d. organophosphates.

17. What drug should you anticipate administering to this patient as soon as possible, and why?

18. Describe the proper procedures that you and your partner should follow when decontaminating this patient.

Your field treatment for this patient has been completed, including decontamination. His pulse has increased to a rate of 80, and he is asking for a drink of water because his mouth is dry. Although the patient is stable at this time, you closely observe him during transport to the emergency department for any possible complications.

19. Why is it especially important that you monitor this patient's ECG rhythm?

General Review Questions

20. Identify two variables that must be considered when one is setting up a command post and staging area after a hazardous material incident, so that equipment and/or personnel will not come into contact with the hazardous material.

(a)

(b)

21. List four factors that you must take into consideration when selecting the proper level of personal protective equipment and clothing for protection from hazardous materials.

(a)

(b)

(c)

(d)

22. List three important precautions of decontamination in the field that should be taken during treatment of the patient with chemically contaminated skin.

(a)

(b)

(c)

23. Identify the method of decontamination of protective clothing and equipment that is used most often by the EMS system.

24. Identify two actions that EMS personnel should take when called to a scene where hazardous materials are burning and/or reacting with each other.

(a)

(b)

For each of the following statements (25–29), circle the correct response, True or False. Briefly explain your answer.

25. Hazardous materials are exotic chemicals or rare substances.

TRUE   **FALSE**

Briefly explain your answer: _____

_____

26. All containers, trucks, and rail cars must have a placard that identifies the hazardous material contained within.

TRUE   **FALSE**

Briefly explain your answer: _____

_____

_____

_____

27. EMS personnel are responsible for rescuing victims from dangerous chemical environments.

TRUE   **FALSE**

Briefly explain your answer: _____

_____

28. A hazardous material scene is considered safe when the hazardous material is contained within its shipping container.

    TRUE   **FALSE**

Briefly explain your answer: _____

29. Eyes that have been exposed to hazardous materials should be irrigated with normal saline or water.

    TRUE   **FALSE**

Briefly explain your answer: _____

30. Label Figure 52-1 and briefly describe each of the three safety zones (a–c) for a hazardous materials response.

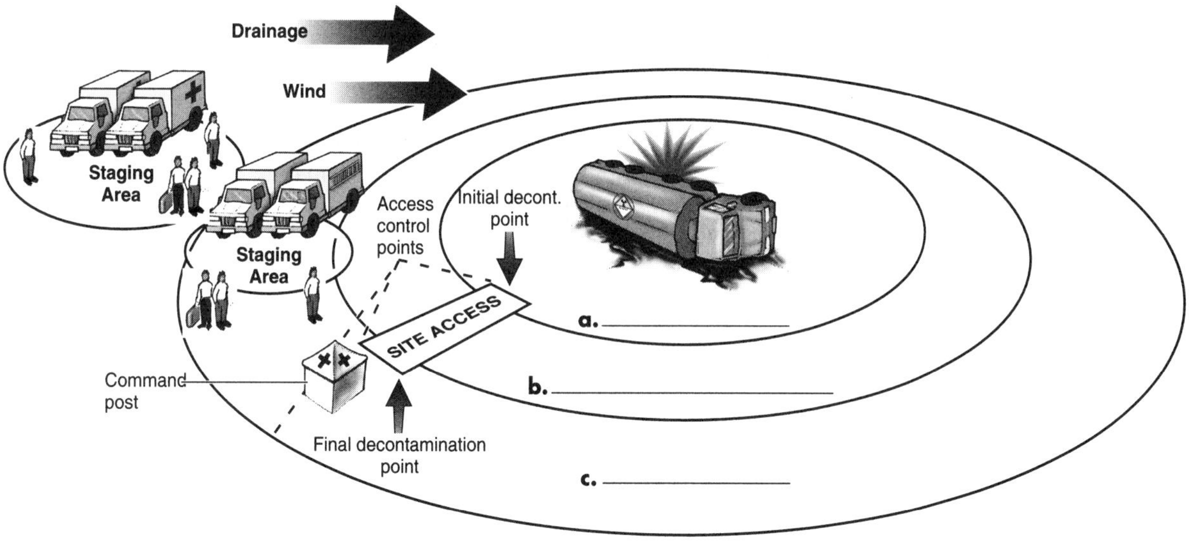

Figure 52-1 _____

(a) _____

(b) _____

(c) _____

Answers to questions from chapter 52 can be found on page 505.

Chapter 53

Air Medical Services

OBJECTIVES

1. Describe the role of the paramedic in air medical services.
2. List operational and clinical guidelines for using the helicopter in the prehospital setting.
3. Identify challenges related to patient assessment presented by the helicopter environment.
4. Describe the effects of altitude on the patient, the medical team, and equipment during air medical transport, and explain how to minimize these effects.
5. Describe the role of communications in air medical services.
6. Describe safety principles used for approaching the helicopter, loading the patient, and departing in a helicopter.
7. Describe how to select and safely prepare a helicopter landing zone.
8. Describe how to properly prepare a patient for helicopter transport.

CASE PRESENTATION #1 (QUESTIONS 1-10)

You are dispatched to the scene of a rollover motor vehicle collision involving a victim who is pinned inside the vehicle. On arrival, you find that the vehicle is upside down. Anticipating a lengthy extrication, you request a helicopter to transport the patient to the nearest trauma facility, which is 20 miles away.

1. Name two criteria that justify activating a helicopter for transport of this patient.

    (a)

    (b)

2. As you approach the scene, what should you anticipate to be a potential hazardous material problem due to the position of the vehicle?

3. List three items of protective clothing that you should wear during the extrication process.

   (a)

   (b)

   (c)

The patient is a teenager who is unresponsive to verbal or painful stimuli. Your initial assessment reveals that he has labored respirations at a rate of 20; a weak, rapid carotid pulse; bruising to the anterior chest; decreased breath sounds on the left; and tracheal deviation to the right.

4. Based on your initial assessment, what life-threatening airway injury do you suspect?

5. What specific treatment would you provide for this injury?

6. Why is it extremely important to treat this injury before air medical transport?

7. When establishing a suitable landing zone for the helicopter, you and your crew should consider all of the following safety guidelines EXCEPT:
   a. The area should be at least 50 by 50 square feet.
   b. The area should be completely free of trees, shrubs, rubbish, and other loose items.
   c. Any obstacles in the flight path should be identified for the pilot.
   d. The area should be flat with ground slope no greater than 8 degrees.

8. List five safety rules that you should follow when approaching the helicopter to assist in loading this patient.

   (a)

   (b)

   (c)

   (d)

   (e)

9. Describe the effect that altitude has on the following equipment, and explain how the air medical crew may compensate for these effects during flight.

   (a) oxygen administration apparatus

   (b) IV equipment

   (c) endotracheal tube

10. Identify two problems that the helicopter environment may pose for the air medical crew when patient reassessment is attempted during flight.

    (a)

    (b)

General Review Questions

11. Define the role of the air medical communication specialist.

12. Identify the most vital component of the communications center.

13. List four time and distance factors that are considered as guidelines by the National Association of EMS Physicians for using the helicopter in the prehospital setting.

    (a)

    (b)

    (c)

    (d)

Answers to questions from chapter 53 can be found on page 507.

Chapter 54

Rural EMS

OBJECTIVES

1. Describe the challenges facing rural EMS delivery systems.
2. List factors that affect communication in the rural EMS setting.
3. Explain how response times impact the delivery of rural EMS care.
4. Describe factors that can improve long response times.
5. List and describe the types of emergency situations most commonly encountered in the rural setting.
6. Describe protocol considerations that are unique to the rural setting.
7. Discuss the role of air medical transport in the rural setting.

In the following two case presentations, the EMS crew consists of two volunteers: one who has been trained as a paramedic, and the second who is an EMT-Basic. The ambulance service covers a 50-square-mile rural area that is largely mountainous and sparsely populated.

CASE PRESENTATION #1 (QUESTIONS 1–6)

You are dispatched to a private residence for a medical emergency. You and your partner arrive at the station approximately 12 minutes after the dispatch call comes in. Twenty minutes later, you and your partner arrive at the scene. The patient is an alert and oriented 68-year-old woman who is complaining of chest pain. She is apprehensive, diaphoretic, and short of breath. Her vital signs are: BP 102/60; pulse 110; respirations 26. She has no history of heart problems, and she is not taking any medications.

1. The closest hospital is 40 miles away. Your cardiac monitor and defibrillator apparently are not working properly. Would it be appropriate to consider air medical transport? Explain your answer.

You administer oxygen and attempt to start an IV on the patient. Your partner tells you that the helicopter is not available.

2. Your next course of action is to:
   a. allow the patient's husband to take her to the hospital using his private vehicle.
   b. continue to obtain a medical history from the patient.
   c. prepare for immediate transport by ambulance.
   d. try to contact the patient's physician by phone to obtain medical direction.

3. The patient's husband informs you that his bottle of nitroglycerin spray is available. Would it be appropriate to contact the patient's physician while en route to the hospital to obtain permission for the patient to take the nitroglycerin? Explain your answer.

About 20 miles from the hospital, the patient's skin color becomes ashen, and she loses consciousness. You cannot palpate a pulse, and she has agonal respirations.

4. Your next course of action is to:
   a. assist respirations using BVM, and ask your partner to drive faster.
   b. attempt to intubate while en route, and perform one-man CPR.
   c. begin one-man CPR, and continue until you reach the hospital.
   d. slow down the ambulance, attempt endotracheal intubation, and set up the automatic CPR device.

CPR is in progress with the automatic CPR device, and the patient is successfully intubated. You have standing orders to follow ACLS protocols for cardiac arrest.

5. Without knowing the rhythm, is it appropriate to administer IV epinephrine? Why, or why not?

Five miles from the hospital, the patient regains a pulse and begins moving around on the stretcher. Her vital signs are: BP 60 palpable; pulse 110 and weak; respirations are still assisted. The ECG monitor now is working properly, and the rhythm shows sinus tachycardia.

6. You should prepare to administer:
   a. adenosine.
   b. bretylium.
   c. dopamine.
   d. lidocaine.

CASE PRESENTATION #2 (QUESTIONS 7-9)

You and your partner are dispatched to a mining company for treatment of an injured worker. The terrain and road conditions make access to the scene very difficult. You arrive on the scene 20 minutes after the call is dispatched. The patient is a 35-year-old man who has fallen from a piece of equipment; his legs are trapped underneath the back wheel. He is awake and slightly pale and is in excruciating pain. There are no obvious injuries to the upper torso; both femurs have obvious open fractures. His vital signs are: BP 80/40; pulse 130; respirations 28 and shallow.

7. After you have secured the patient's ABCs and administered oxygen, your next priority is to:
   a. administer pain medication.
   b. bandage the open fractures.
   c. get the stretcher and apply PASG.
   d. take steps to extricate the patient rapidly.

The patient is now unconscious. His vital signs are: BP 70/40; pulse 150; respirations 28. The closest trauma center is 50 miles away. Air medical transport is available and can arrive at the preestablished location in 15 minutes.

8. Should you activate air medical transport or prepare for ground transport? Explain your answer.

9. Should you start an IV at the scene or while en route? Explain your answer.

GENERAL REVIEW QUESTIONS

10. List five factors that can hamper EMS service in the rural setting.

    (a)

    (b)

    (c)

    (d)

    (e)

For each of the following statements (11–18), circle the correct response, True or False. Briefly explain your answer.

11. Fatal traffic accidents rarely occur in rural areas.

      TRUE   **FALSE**

Briefly explain your answer: _____

_____

12. Farming and mining are hazardous industries that are located primarily in rural areas.

      TRUE   **FALSE**

Briefly explain your answer: _____

_____

13. Recreational accidents occur more frequently in the rural setting.

      TRUE   **FALSE**

Briefly explain your answer: _____

_____

14. Call volume is higher in rural areas than in urban settings.

      TRUE   **FALSE**

Briefly explain your answer: _____

_____

15. Community support is essential in establishing appropriate care for the rural setting.

      TRUE   **FALSE**

Briefly explain your answer: _____

_____

16. Response times are longer in rural areas and probably have the greatest impact on patient outcomes.

      TRUE   **FALSE**

Briefly explain your answer: _____

_____

17. Standing orders should be limited in the rural setting.

      TRUE   **FALSE**

Briefly explain your answer: _____

_____

18. Continuing education opportunities are limited in the rural setting.

      TRUE   **FALSE**

Briefly explain your answer: _____
_____

19. List five factors that affect communication in the rural setting.

    (a)

    (b)

    (c)

    (d)

    (e)

20. Which of the following can improve long response times? (Circle all that apply.)
    a. having first responders travel directly to the scene in their private vehicles
    b. training dispatchers to provide medical first aid directions over the phone
    c. using only ambulances for patient access
    d. upgrading street markers and maps for the defined rural area

21. Briefly describe special considerations in the rural setting for the following protocols:

    (a) Discontinuing CPR in the field

    (b) Providing trauma care (ALS) at the scene as opposed to en route

    (c) Making transport decisions

    (d) Role of air medical transport

Answers to questions from chapter 54 can be found on page 508.

Chapter 55

Specialized Adjuncts for Therapy

OBJECTIVES

1. Identify the types of patients who may have vascular access devices (VADs).
2. Describe three general categories of VADs and their appropriate uses in the prehospital setting.
3. Identify complications and emergencies that may be associated with the use of VADs.
4. Describe the steps for using VADs in the prehospital setting.
5. Identify potential emergencies experienced by hemodialysis patients and describe the proper prehospital management of those emergencies.
6. Describe the steps for using a dialysis device for vascular access in emergency situations.
7. Compare and contrast two types of tracheostomies.
8. Identify the most common complications associated with tracheostomy tubes, stomas, and mechanical ventilators, and describe the proper prehospital management of those complications.
9. Explain the purpose of enteral feedings and identify associated complications.
10. Describe the purpose of a ventricular shunt.
11. Identify the signs and symptoms of ventricular shunt occlusions and describe the appropriate prehospital management.
12. Describe the type of patient who may require an implanted automatic cardioverter defibrillator (AICD) and discuss the prehospital management of AICD emergencies.

CASE PRESENTATION #1 (QUESTIONS 1–4)

You are dispatched to a medical emergency at a private home. On arrival, you find a pale 48-year-old woman who is lying in bed. She is complaining of severe nausea and vomiting, which began 3 days ago following chemotherapy treatment for cervical cancer. When the patient attempts to sit up in bed, she becomes extremely dizzy. While your partner is initiating oxygen therapy and applying an ECG monitor for the patient, you obtain the following vital signs: BP 94/60; pulse 100, weak and irregular; respirations 20. Based on your assessment findings, you suspect that the patient is dehydrated.

1. What is the significance of the patient's dizziness?

Her ECG reveals sinus tachycardia with occasional premature ventricular contractions. As you prepare to establish an IV, the patient warns you that her veins are very fragile. She also states that blood that is drawn for laboratory tests and medications given for her cancer are passed through an implanted port in her chest. You are unsuccessful in establishing a peripheral IV on two attempts. You contact medical direction, who advises you to initiate fluid resuscitation using the patient's vascular access device (VAD).

2. Briefly explain why it is appropriate to use her VAD for IV fluid therapy.

3. List two procedures that you should perform after needle insertion into the VAD and before infusing fluid.

   (a)

   (b)

4. You notice that the flow of solution through the VAD is sluggish. You should:
   a. irrigate forcefully.
   b. increase the flow rate.
   c. aspirate using a syringe.
   d. transport for definitive care.

CASE PRESENTATION #2 (QUESTIONS 5-9)

You respond to an "unconscious person" call at a dialysis clinic. When you arrive, the nurse leads you to a waiting room, where you find a 45-year-old man who passed out after being dialyzed. You note that he is pale and diaphoretic. He has a rapid, weak pulse and is breathing approximately 6 times per minute. You also note that the patient has a shunt in his right arm.

5. Your first priority of care for this patient is:
   a. administering oxygen via nonrebreather mask.
   b. assisting his respirations with supplemental oxygen.
   c. connecting him to the ECG monitor.
   d. establishing an IV at a rapid rate.

6. Which arm should you use to measure his blood pressure? Explain why.

His blood pressure is 70 palpable. His ECG reading shows sinus tachycardia with peaked T waves. A quick secondary survey reveals no signs of trauma or other pertinent findings.

7. What is your first choice for an IV site in this patient? Explain why.

8. Name the solution of choice for fluid resuscitation in this patient.

While en route to the hospital, the patient begins to respond appropriately to verbal questioning. He has received 1500 mL of IV solution. You recheck his blood pressure, which is now 100/70.

9. Based on this patient's response to treatment, what most likely led to his unconsciousness?

Case Presentation #3 (Questions 10–12)

You are dispatched to the home of a 7-year-old girl who is complaining of headache and nausea. On arrival, you find that the patient does not appear to be in acute distress and her vital signs are stable. The patient's mother tells you that her daughter has a condition know as hydrocephalus. She also informs you that she pumped her daughter's ventricular shunt in an attempt to unplug it, but this time it did not seem to work.

10. Is this patient critically ill? Why, or why not?

In preparing the patient for transport to the hospital, you and your partner administer high-flow oxygen and establish an IV at a keep vein open (KVO) rate.

11. Explain why you should exercise caution when administering IV fluids to this patient.

12. List six additional signs and symptoms that would indicate that this patient's condition is deteriorating.

    (a)

    (b)

    (c)

    (d)

    (e)

    (f)

General Review Questions

13. In the prehospital setting, what types of patients might you encounter who have vascular access devices (VADs)?

14. Fill in the blanks with the appropriate VAD from the following list.
    Central venous catheters
    Peripherally inserted central catheters
    Implanted ports

    (a) These are often used for neonates, very young children, or patients who require only short-term therapy.

    _____

    (b) A Heuber needle may be inserted into a self-healing septum.

    _____

    (c) A small cap covers each catheter lumen and is filled with heparin or saline.

    _____

15. Following are the steps involved in the performance of venipuncture of a dialysis access device. Arrange them in the correct sequence:

    a. Using strict aseptic technique, briskly scrub the areas with several povidone-iodine pads.
    b. Identify the location and type of dialysis access device (e.g., graft, fistula, or shunt).
    c. Attach IV tubing, and secure it.
    d. Reassess the infusion site.
    e. Assess the site for redness, tenderness, swelling, or drainage.
    f. Insert a large, 14- to 16-gauge needle at a 15- to 20-degree angle, watching for a flashback.
    g. If additional distention of the vein is needed, apply a tourniquet.
    h. Aspirate slowly for a blood return and to remove heparin from the shunt.

    (1) _____
    (2) _____
    (3) _____
    (4) _____
    (5) _____
    (6) _____
    (7) _____
    (8) _____

16. Why might dialysate fail to drain from the peritoneal cavity, and what is the appropriate patient treatment when this occurs?

17. How do you select the proper-sized endotracheal tube for intubation through a tracheostomy?

18. For each of the following patients with a tracheostomy tube in place, identify associated complications that may be occurring, and list additional signs and symptoms that may develop.

    (a) a 65-year-old patient with excessive secretions

        Complication(s): _____

        Signs & Symptoms: _____

    (b) a 42-year-old patient with a temperature of 104° F

        Complication(s): _____

        Signs & Symptoms: _____

    (c) a 70-year-old patient with ecchymosis around the stoma

        Complication(s): _____

        Signs & Symptoms: _____

19. Management of tracheostomy complications is based on _____
_____.

20. The development of the automatic implantable cardioverter defibrillator (AICD) has reduced the death rate of high-risk patients with what two cardiac dysrhythmias?

    (a)

    (b)

For each of the following statements (21–24), circle the correct response, True or False. Briefly explain your answer.

21. The presence of an AICD is a contraindication for external countershock.

        TRUE   **FALSE**

Briefly explain your answer: _____
_____

22. Prehospital treatment is not necessary for a patient with minimal bleeding whose enteral feeding tube has been displaced.

        TRUE   **FALSE**

Briefly explain your answer: _____
_____

23. Tracheostomy tubes may be of single or double construction.

TRUE **FALSE**

Briefly explain your answer:_____
_____
_____

24. When treating a cyanotic patient whose mechanical ventilator alarm is sounding, you should first attempt to adjust the settings.

TRUE **FALSE**

Briefly explain your answer:_____
_____
_____

Answers to questions from chapter 55 can be found on page 509.

Chapter 56

Issues of Personal Violence

OBJECTIVES

1. Describe the management of violent patients.
2. Describe the indications and appropriate use of restraints.
3. Explain the psychosocial factors and psychological characteristics of child, adult, and elderly abusers.
4. Describe the physical signs and management of common injuries resulting from child, adult, and elderly abuse.
5. Identify typical responses that are demonstrated by the victims of child, adult, and elderly abuse.
6. Describe and demonstrate appropriate interpersonal skills in dealing with victims or perpetrators of personal violence.
7. Describe how to care for the victim and preserve evidence in cases of sexual assault.
8. Describe the medical and legal reporting requirements of child, adult, and elderly abuse, including proper record documentation.

Case Presentation #1 (Questions 1–7)

You and your partner are dispatched to an "injured person" call at a housing project. On arrival at the scene, you are met by a woman who says the patient is a friend of hers, and she will take you to her apartment. When you ask her what has happened, she says that the patient's husband has "beat her up again." The patient is unaware that her friend called 9-1-1.

1. Describe the safety factors that you should consider as you approach the scene and the patient.

You find the patient in her bedroom lying on the bed. She is crying and appears very startled when she sees you. Her face is bloody, and one eye is swollen shut.

2. What would be most important to communicate to her initially?

Although she is hesitant at first, she begins to relay her story. She is extremely frightened because her husband could return at any minute. She is fearful that he will hurt her again when he realizes that help was summoned. While you continue to reassure her, your partner performs a quick initial assessment that reveals the following: Airway is intact; BP is 150/94; pulse is 120; respirations are 28. She is awake but confused and disoriented.

3. Is her initial response typical of those associated with adult abuse situations? Briefly explain your response.

Focused examination reveals periorbital swelling to the right eye; large facial lacerations on her left cheek and the left side of her forehead; and a right pupil that is slow to react to light. There are red marks on her upper arms and old bruised areas on her abdomen. The patient begins to drift into and out of consciousness. Her friend tells you that this is the third episode of this type that she is aware of. The patient did not seek medical or other professional care after the previous beatings. You prepare the patient for transport.

4. You stabilize the patient's cerival spine, control the facial bleeding, and place her on a backboard. What other treatment should you provide while en route to the hospital? (Circle all that apply.)
   a. a detailed physical examination
   b. dopamine drip for her blood pressure
   c. an IV line of Ringer's lactate
   d. oxygen administration
   e. ventilation assistance

While en route to the hospital, the patient begins to talk more and is more lucid than she was at the scene. She tells you, "My husband will be sorry and he will promise not to hurt me again. This is what happened the other times, and I believed him."

5. Is the behavioral pattern described by the patient typical of that associated with spousal abuse? Briefly discuss your response.

Even though she realizes the seriousness of what has happened to her, the patient begs you not to tell anyone at the hospital about the incident.

6. What is the appropriate response to her request?

7. What is your legal obligation in this situation?

The patient is in stable condition upon arrival at the hospital. You report your findings to the emergency department personnel. On following up this case, you learn that she was treated and released, and that she and her two children went to a shelter for battered women.

CASE PRESENTATION #2 (QUESTIONS 8–12)

You are dispatched to a medical emergency at a private residence. On arrival, a teenaged girl ushers you into the home. She is crying and upset. In questioning her, you discover that her parents are not at home, and she is babysitting for her 3-year-old sister. She called 9-1-1 because she thinks her sister is hurt. You notice that the child is playing in the living room; she appears alert and is not in acute distress. The teenager is extremely frightened and concerned.

8. Before questioning the teenager about the situation, what should you say initially to reassure her?

She begins to calm down and tells you that she is concerned that her younger sister has been sexually abused by her stepfather. She noticed vaginal bleeding and bruises in her sister's genital area while giving her a bath, and she saw several "old bruises" on her back and legs. She tells you that her stepfather had forced himself sexually on her several times, and she never told anyone. However, when she saw her little sister's injuries, she decided that she must let someone know.

9. You and your partner briefly discuss the situation. What should you communicate to the teenager at this point?

10. Can you legally transport these two children to the emergency department without a parent's permission? Briefly discuss your response.

11. What is your legal obligation for reporting a suspected child abuse case?

You transport the children to the emergency department and report your findings to emergency department personnel. Later, you are informed that the parents are planning to bring suit against you for transporting the children without their permission.

12. Is this a concern for you and your department? Briefly explain your response.

CASE PRESENTATION #3 (QUESTIONS 13–16)

You are dispatched to a medical emergency at a private residence. When you knock on the door, nobody answers, but you hear a faint, female voice beckoning you to come in. The screen door is unlocked, and you can easily see inside. Lying on the couch in the living room is an elderly woman. The house is extremely unkempt, and several cats are running about. The odor of feces and urine is very strong. The patient's speech is slurred, and she says that her stomach hurts. Nobody else appears to be present in the home.

13. Describe your initial concerns about this situation.

The patient states that her husband died several years ago, and she now lives alone. She has severe arthritis, diabetes, and high blood pressure. Her daughter, who lives nearby, is her primary caretaker, but she has not checked on her for the past 3 days; usually, she comes by least once a day. The patient is upset because she doesn't know where her daughter is. You reassure the patient and begin your assessment. Vital signs are: BP 146/90; pulse 100; respirations 24. She is awake and oriented to place and time. Physical examination reveals bilateral bruises on her upper arms, wrists, and ankles. Her abdomen is soft and nontender.

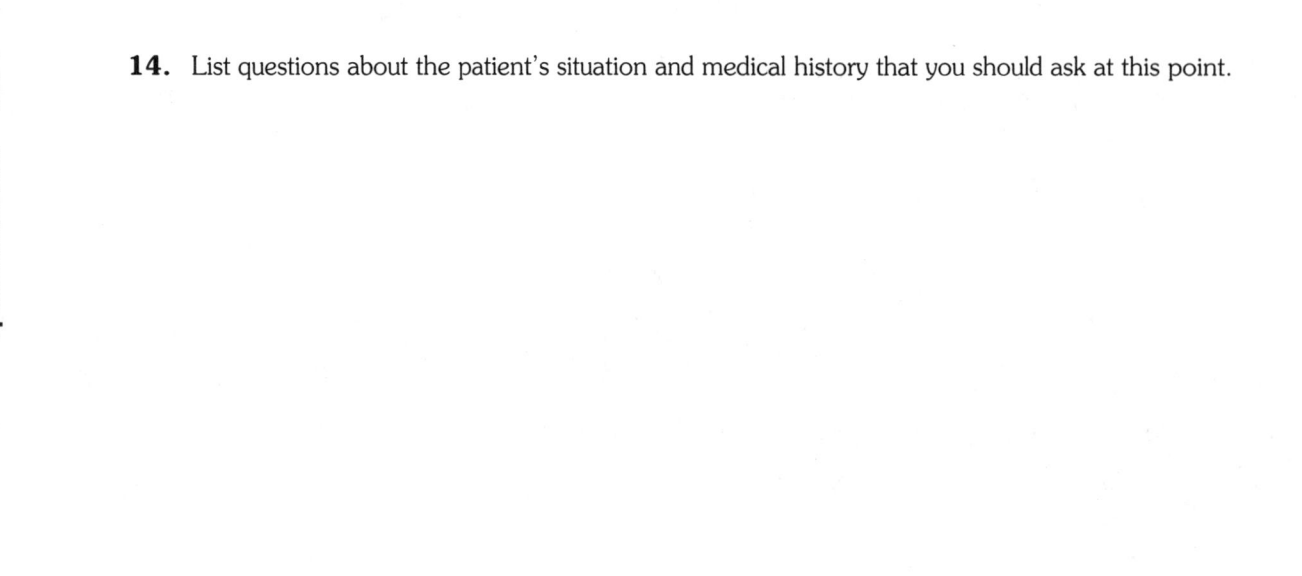

14. List questions about the patient's situation and medical history that you should ask at this point.

As you continue to interview and evaluate the patient, the front door swings open. The patient's daughter rushes in and screams, "What are you all doing here? My mother is fine!" She begins to scold the mother for calling 9-1-1; she tells you to leave and that she will take care of her mother.

15. How should you respond to the patient's daughter?

As you explain why her mother should seek medical attention, the patient suddenly begins yelling at her daughter, "Get out of my house! I will go to the hospital if I want to!" The daughter fails to persuade her mother otherwise. As she leaves the house, she says, "Mother, you'll be sorry for this!"

You transport the patient to the hospital and inform the receiving physician of your findings. Local protocol requires that you report situations like this to adult social services, which you do.

16. What should you document about this call on the prehospital care report?

General Review Questions

17. Statistically, who are the primary perpetrators of violence? Describe common behaviors that they demonstrate.

18. List four potential causes of altered mental status that should be ruled out when you are dealing with a patient who is exhibiting violent behavior.

   (a)

   (b)

   (c)

   (d)

19. Briefly describe the management of violent patients, including the use of restraints.

20. Before using restraints, the paramedic should ensure that one of three conditions exists. List these conditions.

   (a)

   (b)

   (c)

21. Describe the profile (psychosocial/psychological characteristics) of parents who abuse their children.

22. What is the most common type of burn injury that is associated with child abuse?
    a. flash burns
    b. radiation burns
    c. scalding with hot liquid
    d. thermal burns

23. What is "shaken baby syndrome"? What injuries are associated with it?

24. What is the leading cause of death in abused children?
    a. abdominal injury
    b. cardiac dysrhythmia
    c. extremity injury
    d. neurologic injury

25. Briefly discuss the characteristics of an environment in which adult abuse commonly occurs.

26. Describe how to preserve physical evidence at the scene of an alleged rape.

Answers to questions from chapter 56 can be found on page 511.

Chapter 57

Death and Dying

OBJECTIVES

1. Describe factors that influence reactions to death and dying.
2. Define the terms *bereavement, grief,* and *mourning.*
3. Describe the three general phases of mourning.
4. Identify how critical incident stress management applies to death and dying situations.
5. Compare and contrast typical family responses to a sudden versus an anticipated death situation.
6. Discuss important principles and appropriate methods to use when informing survivors about the death of a loved one.
7. Describe the paramedic's role in potential tissue or organ donation.
8. Describe the stages of death that a terminally ill patient typically experiences.
9. Explain the purpose of "hospice" and its role on behalf of terminal patients.
10. Define *DNR* and *living wills,* explaining their impact in the prehospital setting.

CASE PRESENTATION #1 (QUESTIONS 1–7)

You are dispatched to a private residence to assist a possible electrocution victim. An engine company also has been dispatched.

1. On arrival, you find a 40-year-old man who was apparently electrocuted while repairing faulty wiring in the attic. Your *first* priority is to:
   a. assess the safety of the area in which the patient is located.
   b. defibrillate at 200 joules.
   c. assess for the presence of pulse and respirations.
   d. start an IV.

2. After performing the initial step, you determine that the patient is in full cardiac arrest. The ECG monitors shows ventricular fibrillation. Immediate intervention should include:
   1. Apply an external pacemaker.
   2. Continue CPR.
   3. Defibrillate up to 360 joules.
   4. Secure the airway.
   5. Start an IV.
      a. 1 and 2.
      b. 2 and 3.
      c. 2, 4, and 5.
      d. all except 1.
      e. all of the above.

3. The patient is not responsive to initial treatment. The engine crew assists you in moving the patient to the ambulance. As you are leaving the scene, you notice the patient's wife and two teenaged children who are hovering together at the bottom of the stairs. You should:
   a. continue resuscitative measures.
   b. ignore the family and proceed with rapid transport.
   c. stop and speak with the family members.
   d. summon auxiliary personnel to provide the family with a progress report.
   e. a and d

4. You discover that the captain of the engine crew is available to talk with the family about the situation. This communication is particularly important because it:
   a. assists the family in beginning to grieve.
   b. assists in preparing the family for an undesirable outcome.
   c. eliminates grieving for the family.
   d. a and b
   e. a, b, and c

5. The patient's wife wants to accompany her husband in the ambulance to the hospital. What is an appropriate response to her request?

6. Your resuscitation efforts while en route to the hospital and those procedures performed in the emergency department are unsuccessful. The patient is pronounced dead by the emergency physician. You and your partner decide to go to the family waiting area to talk with the wife and children. In talking with the family about what has happened, you should do all of the following EXCEPT:
   a. Position yourself at eye level with those present.
   b. Ask those assembled about their relationship to the deceased.
   c. Avoid the words "dead" and "died."
   d. Display a compassionate attitude as you talk with them.

7. Important principles for the paramedic to recall when assisting the family in this situation include all of the following EXCEPT:
   a. Individuals react in a variety of ways to the news of sudden death.
   b. One should be nonjudgmental about the family's response, whatever it is.
   c. Survivors often display irrational behavior at this point.
   d. Survivors should be told that they will feel this way for only a few days.
   e. Contacting a neighbor or friend to assist the family is very appropriate.

CASE PRESENTATION #2 (QUESTIONS 8-11)

Late one Friday evening, you and an engine crew are dispatched to a residence for treatment of an unconscious patient. Dispatch tells you that the family states the patient is "dying of cancer" and has stopped breathing.

8. While en route to the scene, you should be considering: (Circle all that apply.)
    a. how best to mobilize the engine crew at the scene.
    b. the equipment that you may need.
    c. that because the patient's condition is terminal, there will be no need for resuscitation.
    d. your local protocols for managing cardiac arrest.

On arrival, you are led to a back bedroom by a hysterical man, who is approximately 22 years old. You find an elderly man in a hospital bed. He has no vital signs. You note that the patient has dependent lividity on the back of both arms and on his back. The person who took you to the room is the patient's son, who tells you that he left his father approximately 2 hours ago and came back to find him this way. You tell him politely but honestly that there is no need to begin resuscitation measures. The son becomes hysterical.

9. How should you initially respond to him?

10. The son wishes to view his father's body, but your partner doesn't think he should go back into the bedroom and see his father again because this will "upset him more." You should:
    a. cover the patient and prepare the son to see the body.
    b. discourage the son from going back into the bedroom.
    c. have someone accompany the son when he views the body.
    d. physically prevent him from viewing the body if he insists.
    e. a and c

11. You check the patient's driver's license; it reveals that he wanted to donate his eyes to the organ bank. You should: _____
    _____.

GENERAL REVIEW QUESTIONS

Match the term in Column 1 with its correct definition in Column 2. Use each answer only once.

Column 1

12. ____ Bereavement
13. ____ Mourning
14. ____ Living will
15. ____ Grief

Column 2

a. the socially patterned expression of the bereaved person's sorrow
b. an advance directive that is signed by a person of sound mental capacity well in advance of a life-threatening condition for the purpose of avoiding medical treatments
c. the spectrum of feelings that occur in response to loss
d. the state of loss
e. an order that has been signed by a physician for the purpose of eliminating resuscitation measures for a patient

16. Feelings and reactions to death and dying are influenced by an individual's:
    a. attitude about death.
    b. fear of death.
    c. own individual prejudices.
    d. personal experiences with death.
    e. all of the above

17. Briefly describe the following general stages of mourning:

    (a) Psychic pain spike

    (b) Feelings phase

    (c) Recovery

18. All of the following are appropriate to say to a family member who has experienced the death of a loved one EXCEPT:
    a. "I regret to tell you that your brother did not make it... he is dead."
    b. "Situations like this are always difficult for me, but I must tell you that your father has died."
    c. "Your mother has died... I am so sorry."
    d. "Your sister has passed on, but we know it was God's will for her."

19. If you are in the awkward position of deciding whether or not to resuscitate a terminal patient, the best course of action is:

20. For each of the following statements (a–c), circle the correct response, True or False. Briefly explain your answer.

   (a) DNR orders should be accepted at face value.

   TRUE   **FALSE**

   Briefly explain your answer: _____
   _____

   (b) The "family's wishes" in a situation involving a terminally ill patient and the decision whether or not to resuscitate take precedence in a questionable situation.

   TRUE   **FALSE**

   Briefly explain your answer: _____
   _____

   (c) Your actions can have a significant impact on families who are faced with a sudden loss.

   TRUE   **FALSE**

   Briefly explain your answer: _____
   _____

21. Discuss briefly how critical incident stress debriefing for an EMS provider may apply to death and dying situations.

22. Compare and contrast typical family responses for the following:

   Sudden death   **Anticipated death**

23. Describe the stages of death that a terminally ill patient typically experiences.

24. Explain the role of hospice on behalf of terminally ill patients.

Answers to questions from chapter 57 can be found on page 514.

Chapter 58

Stress and Stress Management

OBJECTIVES

1. Define the following terms:
   a. Stress response
   b. Eustress
   c. Critical incident
2. Describe the body's physiological response to stress.
3. Describe the three stages of the General Adaptation Syndrome (GAS) and the body's responses.
4. List the common causes and signs and symptoms of stress.
5. Discuss factors that affect an individual's response to stress.
6. Describe the three major types of stress response: acute, delayed, and cumulative.
7. Describe typical reactions of family, patients, and EMS personnel to the stress of an emergency.
8. Discuss stress related to paramedic education, training, and a paramedic's job.
9. Define *critical incident* and list examples.
10. Discuss critical incident stress management components and how they can be effective.
11. Discuss appropriate methods for coping with stress.

CASE PRESENTATION #1 (QUESTIONS 1–5)

You are dispatched to a residential area for a possible drowning. Hysterical family members meet you at the door and lead you to the pool in the patio area of their home. Lying face down on the side of the pool, you find a 2-year-old boy. He is not breathing, and he has no pulse.

1. Your first priority should be to:
   a. secure the victim's airway.
   b. oxygenate for the victim.
   c. perform cardiac compressions.
   d. obtain an ECG.

The child is unresponsive to your resuscitation efforts with continual CPR and ALS treatment measures. After nearly an hour of combined resuscitation efforts, he is pronounced dead in the emergency department. On the way back to the station, you find yourself thinking about your 2-year-old son, and you feel guilty that you were unable to "save" this child.

2. What type of stress reaction does this characterize: acute or delayed? Briefly explain your response.

3. Could this reaction also be a cumulative stress response? Briefly discuss why, or why not.

4. Briefly describe methods that could help you deal with this situation.

5. Signs and symptoms of an acute stress response can include: (Circle all that apply.)
   a. profuse sweating.
   b. rapid heart rate.
   c. guilt.
   d. blaming someone.
   e. fear.

CASE PRESENTATION #2 (QUESTIONS 6–9)

You are dispatched to a scene involving an injured person. On arrival, you find a 60-year-old woman who has tripped and hurt her foot. Your assessment reveals that there is no obvious fracture. The only apparent injury is a small laceration. Vital signs are stable, and the patient is neurologically intact. Your partner infers to the patient that she should not have called an "emergency" ambulance. He becomes verbally abusive to the patient. You quickly intervene, telling your partner to drive and you will take care of the patient.

6. Your partner's actions could be the result of acute/delayed/cumulative stress. Circle the correct response.

After the call, you approach your partner to discuss the incident. He is adamant that there was nothing wrong with his behavior on the call. As you continue to talk, he tells you that he is "sick of system abuse calls." He acknowledges that he has been having trouble at home and may be getting a divorce. You are also aware that he has missed a lot of work lately and has been having trouble with high blood pressure.

7. Considering his situation, which of the following indicate possible signs or symptoms of cumulative stress?
    1. hostile behavior with the patient
    2. denial that he acted inappropriately
    3. frequent absence from work
    4. negative attitude about the system
        a. 1 and 3
        b. 2 and 4
        c. all except 3
        d. all of the above

8. Individuals who demonstrate signs of cumulative stress usually (do/do not) acknowledge that a problem exists. (Circle the correct answer and explain your rationale.)

9. Briefly discuss how your partner's home situation could be a contributing factor to his current behavior.

CASE PRESENTATION #3 (QUESTIONS 10–14)

Your unit and four other ambulances are dispatched to the local airport for a possible airplane crash. A plane has requested an emergency landing because of engine failure. As the plane lands, you see the tail hit the runway and burst into flames. The emergency response team and crash vehicles are immediately activated, and they respond to the scene with you. On arrival, you see that bodies and wreckage are strewn in an area covering the size of a city block. Fifty-two of the 100 passengers are declared dead at the scene; 28 are critically injured, and 20 are classified as "walking wounded." You and your partner triage and tag patients for 2 1/2 hours. Finally, you are relieved for a break.

Answer the following questions, which are related to the above situation, by indicating whether each is True or False.

10. _____ The drama and intensity of this event classify it as a critical incident.

11. _____ Although you are overwhelmed by what you have just seen and done, you tell yourself that you "must go on." This is a typical and sometimes necessary response for emergency personnel.

12. _____ Critical incidents are often accompanied by acute or delayed stress reactions.

13. _____ When you arrive back at your duty station, there is still 10 hours left on your shift. You are totally focused on the events that you just experienced and are quite upset. The station officer says that he is relieving you of your duties. This is an appropriate action for the officer to take.

14. _____ Critical incident stress debriefing is an appropriate procedure for emergency personnel who participated in this call.

GENERAL REVIEW QUESTIONS

15. What is "eustress," or good stress? Briefly discuss its benefits, and give an example.

16. The organ and/or physiologic responses of the body to stressors include:
   a. the cortex of the brain, which processes and interprets the data based on previous experience.
   b. the midbrain's response, which attaches an emotional interpretation.
   c. stimulation of the sympathetic nervous system.
   d. aldosterone secretion, which leads to increased blood pressure.
   e. all of the above.

17. List the three stages of the general adaptation syndrome (GAS), and provide a brief explanation of what occurs in the body during each stage.

   (a)

   (b)

   (c)

18. Stress can result from: (Circle all that apply.)
   a. changes in work status.
   b. boredom or inactivity.
   c. nutritional imbalance.
   d. negative self image.

19. List three factors that may affect the magnitude of the stress response.

   (a)

   (b)

   (c)

Indicate whether each of the following statements is True or False.

20. _____ Delayed stress can occur days, weeks, months, or years after an event.

21. _____ Nightmares or flashbacks are signs of delayed stress.

22. _____ Paramedic school usually is not a source of stress for most students.

23. _____ EMS personnel are typically action-oriented "risk takers."

24. _____ A characteristic of EMS personnel is that they frequently express emotion.

25. List five events that are classified as critical events that may require CISD intervention:

(a)

(b)

(c)

(d)

(e)

26. The most common type of emergency call for which a request for debriefing is initiated involves _____.

27. Circle all the TRUE statements. Critical incidents:
  a. are sudden and unexpected.
  b. disrupt one's sense of control.
  c. are often associated with provider guilt.
  d. may involve feelings of emotional loss.
  e. overwhelm one's ability to cope.

Answers to questions from chapter 58 can be found on page 516.

Answers

Chapter 1: Overview of EMS

1. **c** Dispatchers have various levels of capability. Emergency medical dispatch training is a specialized course that includes instruction in telecommunications, caller interrogation, pre-arrival instructions, and call prioritization. **(Objectives 3, 10, and 11)**

2. EMD training is desirable. A tiered response requires that all providers be designated according to their capability and that dispatch policies specify the appropriate responders for each type of call. **(Objectives 3, 9, and 11)**

3. Nearby responders can begin patient stabilization while awaiting the arrival of higher trained, but more distant, providers. In some areas, basic life support ambulances respond together with advanced units and transport less serious patients, keeping advanced life support available for more serious emergencies. Air ambulances also may respond together with ground ambulances. **(Objectives 3, 9, and 10)**

4. **b** In cardiac arrests and other true emergencies, the few minutes saved through this communication can mean the difference between a viable patient and one who suffers hypoxic brain death. First responders are particularly important in rural areas with long ambulance response times. The condition of the patient on arrival is most valuable to convey, in terms of potential patient prognosis. **(Objectives 3 and 10)**

5. ALS providers are able to provide early invasive care under direct or indirect medical direction. The scope of practice varies among states, but ALS includes capabilities for defibrillation, invasive airway techniques, application of antishock garments, and administration of intravenous fluids and medications. **(Objectives 3, 9, and 10)**

6. **b** The medical director authorizes the medical practice of the EMS providers and takes responsibility for the quality of health care provided. **(Objectives 3 and 4)**

7. Treatment protocols are the standards of practice for an entire EMS system and the yardstick by which all actions are measured. These standards apply to all segments of the system, including on-line physicians and prehospital personnel. Medical treatment can often be provided without direct, on-line medical guidance. Standing orders are used in many areas to authorize medical procedures that must be performed before base hospital contact is attempted. Treatment protocols are overseen by the EMS medical director. In addition, medical directors oversee other areas, including standard operating procedures, continuing education, and quality assurance. A paramedic is directly responsible to the system's medical director. **(Objectives 3 and 4)**

8. Mutual aid agreements provide for emergency response from another jurisdiction by an ambulance service closer to the scene, or for back-up during multiple calls. During significant medical incidents or disasters, mutual aid agreements may provide for the provision of additional units to the affected area, as well as for coverage of areas left uncovered by initial response to the incident. **(Objectives 8 and 9)**

9. **No.** COBRA law states that the "transferring physician certifies that personnel transporting the patient are appropriate for the care needed during transport." **(Objective 6)**

10. **Yes.** If the patient is unstable or requires treatment not specifically approved for EMS by the state, a physician or other medically qualified hospital staff member should accompany the patient during transfer. **(Objectives 3, 6, and 10)**

11. **I.** Levels II, III, and IV would not have *all* of the immediate services that are available at a Level I center. **(Objective 10)**

12. A trauma center is a specialized hospital with the capability to treat victims of traumatic injury. These facilities are categorized as Level I, II, III, or IV, according to standards developed by the American College of Surgeons. **(Objectives 3 and 10)**

13. A trauma system should be planned so that it includes the number of trauma centers needed to ensure efficiency, effectiveness, and appropriate management of the patient. When such a system is in place, patients in the prehospital setting can be transported to a facility that can expediently manage their injury. **(Objectives 3, 9, and 10)**

14. Preresponse, prehospital, hospital, critical care, and rehabilitation. **(Objective 2)**

15. The White Paper served as a needs statement for the national effort to improve emergency care. Among its findings were: ill-designed equipment, generally inadequate supplies, lack of an accepted standard for the competence and training of ambulance personnel, and poor communication between ambulances and hospital emergency departments. Emergency facilities of most hospitals were found to be poorly equipped and inadequately manned; ordinarily, they were used for only limited numbers of seriously ill persons or for charity victims.

    The significance of the White Paper is that it called for an organized response to the inadequacies that it described, similar to the intense efforts that have been made to conquer cancer, heart disease, and mental illness. Two federal programs were enacted to overcome the perceived problems in EMS. **(Objective 1)**

16. The NHTSA is responsible for setting patient care standards through the development of training curricula for prehospital providers (EMS Dispatchers, First Responders, Basic EMTs, Intermediate EMTs, and EMT-Paramedics). Through grant monies provided to each state, the NHTSA also has funded ALS program development, advances in the design of ambulances and communications equipment, and other EMS system improvements. **(Objective 6)**

17. Manpower, training, communication, transportation, adequate facilities, critical care units, public safety agencies, consumer participation, access to care, patient transfer, coordinated patient record keeping, public information and education, review and evaluation, disaster linkage, and mutual aid. **(Objective 3)**

18. **False.** EMS may be funded by any or all of the following: general tax revenues, special district revenues, subscription services, and health insurance (e.g., Medicaid, Medicare, and private health insurance). **(Objective 5)**

19. **True.** Regulations may be found in EMS acts, medical and nursing practice acts, hospital licensure laws, and other sources. The amount of direct control exercised by state and regional EMS organizations over system participants varies from state to state. **(Objective 6)**

20. **True.** These standards (known as the KKK 1822C standards) reflect the minimum standards for ambulance operations and include lighting and patient compartment specifications. **(Objectives 7 and 10)**

21. **True.** COBRA is a federal law that mandates requirements for both transferring and receiving physicians regarding the transfer of a patient from one facility to another. **(Objectives 6 and 10)**

22. **False.** Some states accept another's licensure as proof of competency to practice, and they do grant reciprocity; others require further written and/or skills testing. **(Objective 8)**

23. An effective EMS system requires the participation of numerous independent organizations, including public safety agencies, ambulance services, and hospitals. Interdependence of these organizations is necessary for the best possible patient care to be provided; however, this requires organization, standardization, and a plan for leadership within the system. **(Objectives 9 and 10)**

24. **R**egional **EMS O**rganization. This is a community council on EMS that brings together the leaders who provide such care, for the purposes of planning, education, and funding. It is responsible for the coordination of all system participants. **(Objective 6)**

25. The state's health department or an equivalent organization. Most states also have an EMS advisory committee, often appointed by the governor, that provides both professional and consumer input to the administrative agency. **(Objectives 6 and 9)**

26. **d (Objective 7)**

27. Tiered response, response times, advanced life support, early defibrillation, and mutual aid and disaster medical response. **(Objective 9)**

28. *System access*: a simple, reliable method by which an individual can access the EMS system. Most states employ the 9-1-1 system.

    Dispatch centers: centers that communicate with, and direct, all emergency medical service units within a system. These centers should dispatch the closest, most appropriate unit to the scene.

    Trained dispatchers: individuals who are trained in both telecommunications and medical techniques. They should be able to elicit adequate information from the reporting party and, based on medically acceptable standards, should determine the appropriate response and provide pre-arrival instructions.

    Dispatch and medical communications systems: The EMS system should have the capability of linking dispatch to the actual EMS unit, the EMS unit to the hospital, and so forth. This requires specialized equipment and knowledge of the latest communication techniques. **(Objectives 3 and 11)**

29. Research is necessary to validate current EMS treatment modalities and to identify new methods that will benefit the patient. Clinical trials should be conducted for the purpose of evaluating new procedures or treatments. Research can yield new system configurations and new responsibilities for providers. **(Objective 12)**

Chapter 2: Roles and Responsibilities

1. **c** Your fundamental responsibilities are to conserve life, to alleviate suffering, to promote health, to do no harm, and to encourage the quality and equal availability of emergency medical care. Therefore, you are responsible for the care of both of the patients. **(Objective 1)**
2. **b** You are responsible for providing services based on human need, with respect for human dignity, unrestricted by consideration of nationality, role, creed, or status. **(Objective 1)**
3. **b (Objective 3)**
4. **a (Objective 3)**
5. **c (Objective 3)**
6. **c**
7. **f**
8. **g**
9. **h**
10. **h**
11. **e**
12. **d** and **e**
13. **b**
14. **a**
15. **c** and **f**
16. **d (Objective 4)**
17. Spinal immobilization; airway management; control of bleeding. **(Objective 4)**
18. The White Paper set the stage for an organized system that would ensure continuity of emergency care, thereby reducing morbidity and mortality among trauma victims. **(Objective 2)** (See also Answer 15 in Chapter 1.)
19. Any of the following: American Ambulance Association (AAA); American College of Emergency Physicians (ACEP); National Association of EMS Physicians (NAEMSP); National Association of EMTs (NAEMT); National Association of Search and Rescue (NASAR); National Association of State EMS Directors (NASEMSD); National Council of State EMS Training Coordinators (NCSEMSTC); National Flight Paramedic Association (NFPA) **(Objective 6)**
20. A national registry agency prepares and administers standardized national testing materials for three levels of prehospital providers: EMT-Basic, EMT-Intermediate, and EMT-Paramedic. **(Objective 8)**
21. **c**
22. **d**
23. **b (Objective 7)**
24. Helps keep the paramedic competent; helps keep the paramedic up-to-date on current information. **(Objective 5)**

Chapter 3: The EMS Call

1. Advanced life support **(Objective 2)**
2. CPR instructions **(Objective 1)**
3. The number of patients needing treatment; patient accessibility; scene safety; EMS role assignments; condition of the patients; required equipment and medications **(Objective 7)**
4. Because you have a higher level of training than the First Responders, you should establish leadership and assign roles to each member of the team so that patient care can be maximized. **(Objective 5)**
5. **c (Objective 5)**
6. **a** Written and verbal reports about the patient's condition should be given to the nurse or physician, not to the admitting clerk. **(Objective 6)**
7. Restock and clean the vehicle, perform equipment maintenance, review the call. **(Objective 7)**
8. Police and fire departments, the gas company, and the hazardous materials team. **(Objective 2)**
9. **No.** The scene should not be approached until it has been determined to be safe; if you become a patient, the available resources at hand will be decreased. **(Objective 5)**
10. During assessment. **(Objective 5)**
11. **d (Objective 5)**
12. **No.** Because the patient is stable and the hospital is a relatively short distance away, the risk of using the helicopter does not outweigh the benefit. In addition, the expense is not justified by the patient's condition. **(Objective 5)**
13. **e** Notes should not be taken. **(Objective 7)**
14. (a) **X** (b) **X** (c) **Z** (d) **Y** (e) **Z (Objective 5)**
15. Information gathering, EMS contact, prehospital instructions, coordination of supportive public safety services, mutual aid requests, and disaster response **(Objective 2)**
16. First aid training; CPR training. **(Objective 1)**
17. **c** Sometimes little specific information about the medical complaint is available. **(Objective 3)**
18. **e (Objective 5)**
19. Scene safety; patient accessibility; scope of the incident; environmental factors; leadership and other EMS roles; available communications equipment and anticipated needs; scene control requirements. **(Objective 4)**

Chapter 4: Medical Accountability

1. Having input into: (1) dispatch protocols and priorities, (2) disaster management, and (3) the direction of continuing education for EMS personnel. **(Objectives 2, 3, and 4)**
2. **c** Standing orders may be used in any system as they are set forth by the EMS medical director. They are not implemented on a case-by-case basis; nor are they followed only when medical direction cannot be contacted. **(Objectives 2 and 5)**
3. Hospital designation, particularly in the care of the trauma patient, is a complex issue in most communities. Having input into destination policies is an important role of the medical director; this input identifies for the EMS provider which facility is most appropriate for the care of a given emergency. **(Objectives 2, 4, and 6)**
4. Most systems with strong medical direction have medical protocols. These usually include standing orders, triage of the trauma patient, disaster plans, and hospital destination policies. All of these items are illustrated in Case Presentation #1. **(Objectives 2, 3, 4, and 5)**
5. **a** A check of breath sounds would have indicated that the patient had fluid in his lungs. Because this condition can result in poor oxygenation, a high concentration of oxygen should have been administered. Any abnormalities found in capillary refill, pupil size and reaction, or extremity strength would not affect treatment decisions. **(Prerequisite Chapter Objective)**
6. Medical accountability involves both on-line and off-line medical direction. Off-line medical direction occurs before and after patient care situations. In this case, the medical director contacts the paramedic after patient care to discuss how patient assessment and treatment could have been performed differently. **(Objectives 2 and 4)**
7. **Both.** Retrospective medical direction focuses on how the system is providing care and what can be done to improve the care given. Prospective medical direction ensures that the components are in place for providing quality care, one of which is continuing education. Thus, both aspects are being addressed by the medical director. **(Objectives 3 and 7)**
8. **a** For most paramedics, the authority to care for patients occurs through this legal concept. It means that the paramedic renders care as a physician surrogate, acting under the physician's license; the physician, in turn, agrees to supervise the care provided by the paramedic. **(Objective 1)**
9. **e** In concurrent medical direction, the physician is available to assist the paramedic at the actual patient encounter. Because the physician is physically present to give orders, this case also constitutes on-line medical direction. **(Objectives 2 and 3)**
10. **c** Although all others listed share aspects of responsibility, the medical director is ultimately responsible for patient care. **(Objectives 2 and 4)**
11. **d** The procedure for designating which hospitals should receive emergency patients involves a cooperative effort between hospital administration and EMS system officials. The primary role of the medical director is to understand the capabilities of the hospitals served by the EMS agency so that clear and equitable policies regarding patient distribution can be established. **(Objectives 2, 6, and 7)**
12. **d (Objective 5)**
13. **a (Objective 3)**
14. **c (Objective 2)**
15. **b (Objectives 2, 3, and 7)**
16. **d** Providing professional and public accountability for medical care in the prehospital setting is the purpose of medical direction. Standing orders and run reviews are components of medical direction, and the number of physicians required varies from system to system. **(Objectives 2, 3, 4, and 7)**
17. Written/operational. These are both important areas for involvement of medical directors, so that quality patient care and system improvement can be ensured. **(Objective 4)**
18. **d** Although all of these are aspects of quality improvement, improvement of patient care is its goal. **(Objective 7)**
19. Quality assurance and improvement are vital to an effective EMS system. System research feeds into this process by evaluating whether practices are necessary and appropriate. Because some aspects of prehospital practice have not been studied in terms of efficacy, this process must continue. Paramedics can be a part of this endeavor; their field expertise adds an essential component to the research process. **(Objective 8)**

CHAPTER 5
Legal Accountability

1. **c** Identifying any life-threatening conditions is always a priority in patient assessment. **(Prerequisite Chapter Objective)**
2. **d** It is preferable to conduct the assessment in toe-to-head order in infants and children younger than school age because small children usually do not like strangers poking at their faces. **(Prerequisite Chapter Objective)**
3. **c** The patient is in pain and needs medical care; the parents' permission to treat is not needed because it is implied under the circumstances of an emergency situation. **(Objective 6)**
4. **Yes.** Failure to restrain this patient from removing his elbow splint could result in a stable injury becoming an unstable injury. **(Objective 9)**
5. **Yes.** Most states have statutes that mandate reporting of suspected child abuse. The paramedics need to have only reasonable suspicion about the circumstances and are not required to believe that child abuse has in fact occurred. **(Objective 4)**
6. **No.** Disclosure extended to other persons who are not involved in the patient's care is considered a breach of confidentiality. **(Objective 5)**
7. **Yes.** The competent adult has a right to refuse treatment; therefore, the paramedic must defer to a competent patient's refusal of care, even if the paramedic believes that the patient's choice may result in further illness. **(Objective 6)**
8. **d** A claim of battery can arise if the paramedic uses force on a patient. False imprisonment is the intentional and unjustifiable detention of a person against his will. **(Objective 9)**
9. **c** The paramedic must educate the patient as to the risks and consequences of refusing treatment so that the refusal can be informed. **(Objective 8)**
10. Act consistently with the local protocol, which often mandates contact with medical direction; conduct a physical assessment; solicit additional information from bystanders. **(Objective 8)**
11. **b** The paramedic has a duty to continue to provide care until relief of the responsibility is provided by the patient or by another medically qualified person, or until care is no longer needed. **(Objective 7)**
12. Failure to immobilize this patient properly could cause a stable spinal injury to progress to a debilitating neurologic injury, which could be grounds for negligence.

    Elements required to prove negligence include:

    The patient was injured.

    The action or inaction of the paramedic caused, or contributed to the injury.

    The paramedic violated his duty to care for the patient.

    The paramedic acted in an unusual, unreasonable, and imprudent way.

    (Objective 2)
13. **No.** Based on the mechanism of injury and his presentation, this patient should have had proper spinal immobilization. A cervical collar alone was inadequate. **(Objective 3)**
14. **b** **(Objective 1)**
15. **a** **(Objective 1)**
16. **d** **(Objective 1)**
17. **c** **(Objective 1)**
18. **f** **(Objective 1)**
19. *Implied* consent occurs when a patient is unconscious and appears to have a life-threatening injury.

20. *Involuntary* consent occurs when permission to treat is granted by the authority of law, such as a statute or a court order, regardless of the patient's desire.
21. *Expressed* consent is the voluntary, unequivocal expression by the patient of desire and willingness to be treated, which is made either verbally or in writing.
22. *Implied* consent to treat a minor occurs when the child is suffering from what reasonably presents as life-threatening injury or illness. The child need not be unconscious. **(Objective 6)**
23. **c** Cancer is not considered a situation in which resuscitation efforts should be withheld, according to American Heart Association guidelines. In such circumstances, the paramedic should be deterred from initiating resuscitation only when clear and unequivocal information reflects the patient's desires. **(Objective 10)**
24. Abuse of elderly persons; rape; gunshot wounds; contagious disease; child abuse. **(Objective 4)**
25. Are restraints necessary?

    What type of restraint is suitable?

    Are restraints necessary for the duration of the patient contact?

    Does the patient have any injuries or illnesses that must be considered either before or while restraints are used?

    (Objective 9)
26. Disturb as little as possible in any potential crime scene; inform appropriate law enforcement personnel if objects had to be moved or altered during the process of patient care; adequately document pertinent information on the patient care record. **(Objective 11)**
27. The paramedic's decision to withhold or stop resuscitation procedures should be based on clear, physician-directed protocols or standing orders, or should result from on-line medical direction. **(Objective 10)**

CHAPTER 6: Medical Terminology

1. **e (Objective 5)**
2. **b (Objective 5)**
3. **c (Objective 5)**
4. **f (Objective 5)**
5. **d (Objective 5)**
6. **a (Objective 5)**
7. **h (Objective 5)**
8. **C (Objective 6)**
9. **B (Objective 6)**
10. **F (Objective 6)**
11. **D (Objective 6)**
12. **E (Objective 6)**

13. **A (Objective 6)**
14. **b (Objective 1)**
15. **b (Objective 1)**
16. **c (Objective 1)**
17. **a (Objective 1)**
18. **b (Objective 1)**
19. **d (Objective 1)**
20. **d (Objective 1)**
21. **b (Objective 1)**
22. **a (Objective 1)**
23. **b (Objective 1)**
24. **d (Objective 1)**
25. **e (Objective 1)**
26. **a (Objective 1)**
27. **c (Objective 1)**
28. Acute myocardial infarction **(Objective 7)**
29. Cancer **(Objective 7)**
30. Congestive heart failure **(Objective 7)**
31. Chronic obstructive pulmonary disease **(Objective 7)**
32. Cerebral vascular accident **(Objective 7)**
33. Diabetes mellitus **(Objective 7)**
34. Hypertension **(Objective 7)**
35. Transient ischemic attack **(Objective 7)**
36. Tuberculosis **(Objective 7)**
37. ETOH **(Objective 1)**
38. gtts **(Objective 1)**
39. fx **(Objective 1)**
40. hs **(Objective 1)**
41. ICP **(Objective 1)**
42. lac **(Objective 1)**
43. OB **(Objective 1)**
44. p **(Objective 1)**
45. unc **(Objective 1)**
46. You are dispatched to a private residence for an elderly F who **POPTA**. On **PE**, she is **AOX3**. Her **c/c** is **bilat** hip pain, although she can **MAE** with ease. Her **PERL; VS** are **WNL**, except for a **BP** of 200/110. She has a **Hx** of **HTN**, but takes no **Meds**. In addition to providing spinal stabilization, you administer the following **Tx** before transport to the **ED** by **MICU**: **O₂** at 4 **LPM**; **ECG** monitoring; **IV** with **NS** at a **TKO** rate. **(Objective 1)**
47. You are dispatched to a park to evaluate a 52-year-old man who is having **dyspnea** after having been stung by a bee. He also complains of **dysphagia** and that his **pharynx** is closing off. You note that the patient has **circumoral cyanosis** and **tachycardia**. His medical history includes **tonsillectomy** and a heart problem for which he takes an **antiarrhythmic**. After receiving treatment for an allergic reaction, the patient is **asymptomatic**. **(Objective 1)**

48. **a.** Anterior surface of the chest, medial to the right nipple.
    b. Anterior surface of the left arm, proximal to the wrist.
    c. Medial aspect of the left ankle.
    d. See "X" on the diagram.
    e. See "Y" on the diagram.
    f. See "Z" on the diagram.

    (Objectives 3 and 4)

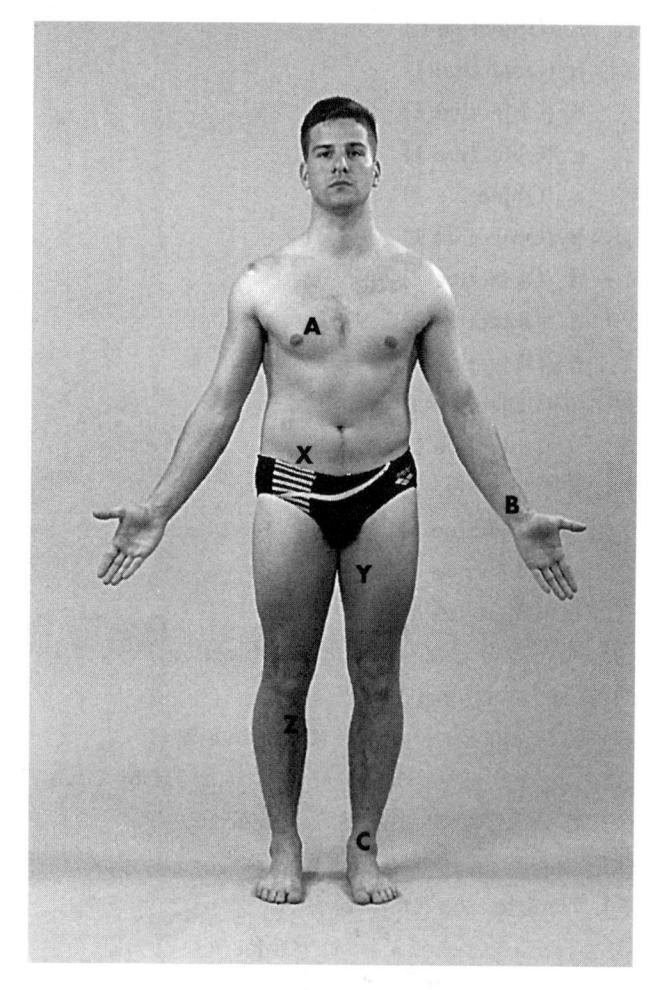

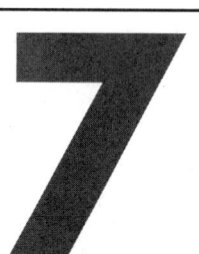

CHAPTER 7 Basic Body Systems

1. Low. Hemoglobin, an iron compound that carries oxygen, will be less saturated as a result of this patient's inadequate oxygen intake. **(Objective 6)**
2. Active. The patient is having to work actively at exhaling the lungs' contents through narrowed and partially obstructed lower airways. **(Objective 6)**
3. Intercostal muscles within the chest wall, and the sternocleidomastoid muscle in the neck. Assessment finding: muscle retractions between the ribs and in the neck. **(Objective 4)**
4. Sympathetic nervous system. Assessment finding: fast and bounding pulse. **(Objective 4)**
5. Anaerobic metabolism, which is inefficient. Oxygen is needed by the body's cells to convert nutrients to usable energy. Without oxygen in the tissues, energy can be obtained only briefly and inefficiently. **(Objective 6)**
6. This patient's dyspnea is primarily caused by bronchoconstriction that results from her asthma attack, which restricts movement of air into and out of her lungs. Epinephrine affects the air passages in the respiratory system by causing brochodilation. This, in turn, reverses the primary cause of her dyspnea. **(Objective 6)**
7. Adrenergic **(Objective 5)**
8. The action of epinephrine increases heart rate and the strength of cardiac contractions. **(Objective 5)**

9. **Yes.** Based on the mechanism of injury, this patient could have sustained damage to the central nervous system. To avoid aggravating any potential injury, the patient should be turned as a unit, keeping his head and spine in alignment. **(Prerequisite Objective)**
10. **Yes.** The fluid may be cerebrospinal fluid. Cerebrospinal fluid surrounds the brain and spinal cord, both of which are completely encased in bone. Leakage of cerebrospinal fluid to the outside may indicate a break in the bone structure. **(Objective 5)**
11. **No.** Although the primary function of the spinal cord is to serve as a transmitter of information to and from the brain, occasionally it creates reflex pathways that do not require processing by the brain. These reflex pathways are created when afferent (sensory) neurons, which receive information from inside or outside of the body, send messages directly to efferent (motor) neurons to elicit a response. In addition, some neurons (connector or interneurons) conduct impulses or messages directly between afferent and efferent neurons. The patient's leg movement could have been elicited from such a reflex response. **(Objective 6)**
12. You can conclude that the scene is safe because the police were assessing the patient inside the vehicle, and there was no additional information from dispatch to lead you to believe otherwise. You can conclude that the patient is conscious based on his ability to provide a history of the incident to police at the scene. **(Prerequisite Chapter Objective)**
13. Femur **(Objective 4)**
14. Lungs, heart, liver, spleen. **(Objective 4)**
15. In the hospital setting, urine output is one of the key measurements for determining whether a patient is suffering from shock. Based on consideration of his known and potential injuries, the occurrence of shock is a distinct possibility for this patient. **(Objective 5)**
16. One and one half to two liters of urine are produced in an average day. This is equivalent to about 70 ml per hour. **(Objective 5)**
17. Nervous; respiratory; circulatory; lymphatic; endocrine; reproductive; muscular; urinary; digestive; skeletal; integumentary. **(Objective 3)**
18. **(a)** brain, spinal cord; **(b)** cranial nerves, spinal nerves **(Objective 4)**
19. **(a)** plasma, **(b)** erythrocytes, **(c)** hemoglobin, **(d)** leukocytes, **(e)** platelets **(Objective 2)**
20. **(a)** Inhalation: As the diaphragm contracts, the base of the lungs is drawn downward, which expands the respiratory container and creates an inflow of air into this reduced-pressure environment.

    (b) Expiration: Typically a passive process, this requires only the relaxation of the respiratory muscles.

    (Objective 6)
21. The lymphatic system helps to restore fluids and filters out waste from the body. **(Objective 5)**
22. Hormones are delivered to their target organs via the bloodstream. **(Objective 6)**
23.

	Target	Action
a.	Kidney	increases water absorption
b.	Uterus	increases uterine contractions
	Mammary gland	increases milk secretion
c.	Bone	increases rate of bone breakdown
	Kidney	increases vitamin D synthesis
d.	Heart	increases cardiac output
	Blood vessels	increases blood flow to skeletal muscles, heart
	Lungs	bronchodilates
	Liver	increases the release of glucose and fatty acids into the blood
	Fat cells	prepares for physical activity
e.	Kidneys, intestines, sweat glands	increases rate of sodium transport into the body; increases rate of potassium excretion; secondarily favors water retention
f.	Liver, skeletal, fat tissue	increases uptake and use of glucose and amino acids
g.	Primarily liver	increases breakdown of glycogen and release of glucose into the circulatory system

(Objective 6)

24. **5** a.
    3 b.
    2 c.
    7 d.
    6 e.
    1 f.
    4 g. **(Objective 4)**
25. **2** a.
    7 b.
    3 c.
    6 d.
    8 e.
    4 f.
    1 g.
    5 h. **(Objective 4)**
26. **d**
27. **c**
28. **b**
29. **a**
30. **e** **(Objective 6)**
31. **a**
32. **d**
33. **c**
34. **e** **(Objectives 1 and 2)**
35. **c** **(Objective 4)**
36. **d** **(Objective 4)**
37. **a** Heart sounds are produced by closing of the heart valves. The autonomic nervous system helps to regulate heart rate. The left side of the heart is its most heavily muscled side. **(Objective 4)**
38. **d** **(Objective 6)**
39. **d** Acetylcholine is used as a neurotransmitter by the parasympathetic nervous system. The sympathetic nervous system creates an adrenergic response and opposes cholinergic response. **(Objective 5)**
40. **(a)** cerebral cortex; **(b)** hypothalamus; **(c)** midbrain; **(d)** cerebellum; **(e)** medulla; **(f)** spinal cord **(Objective 4)**
41. **(a)** skull; **(b)** clavicle; **(c)** sternum; **(d)** ribs; **(e)** humerus; **(f)** vertebra; **(g)** radius; **(h)** ulna; **(i)** pelvis; **(j)** femur; **(k)** patella; **(l)** tibia; **(m)** fibula **(Objective 4)**

Chapter 8: Principles of Pathophysiology

1. **b** Evaluating airway and respirations is the first priority. **(Prerequisite Chapter Objective)**
2. **a (Objective 21)**
3. The patient's respiratory rate is 6. In respiratory acidosis, carbon dioxide is retained for some reason; usually, there is hypoventilation resulting from respiratory depression that occurs with some overdoses, or from chronic pulmonary disease such as emphysema. **(Objective 21)**
4. **Low.** When the concentration of hydrogen ions go down, pH drops. **(Objective 17)**
5. The respiratory system. **(Objective 19)**
6. The kidneys; hours or days, in some cases **(Objective 19)**
7. **a** In the prehospital setting, the key to acid-base balance is management of airway and ventilation. The best method by which to rid the body of excess carbon dioxide is to establish a patent airway and hyperventilate the patient. Reducing the level of carbon dioxide is as important as increasing the oxygen level. **(Objectives 18 and 20)**
8. Determination of the patient's blood gas status can indicate how well airway management was performed in the field, which may help guide future treatment of patients with similar presentations. **(Objective 18)**
9. **a** Checking for allergies, obtaining the medical history, and preparing the patient for transport are secondary to management of airway and oxygenation. **(Prerequisite Chapter Objective)**
10. Autonomic **(Objectives 22 and 23)**
11. Sympathetic. When a stressor or insult to the body occurs, the body attempts to create energy. The sympathetic branch responds (known as *fight or flight response*) to promote blood flow to the vital organs (heart and brain). **(Objectives 23 and 24)**
12. **a.** Beta **(Objective 25)**

    b. Beta 2 **(Objective 25)**

    c. Alpha **(Objective 25)**

    d. Both **(Objective 25)**
13. Patients with heart disease often take potassium. It is necessary for the transmission and conduction of nerve impulses, the maintenance of normal cardiac rhythms, the contraction of skeletal and smooth muscle, and the conduction of cardiac rhythms. **(Objective 12)**
14. **No.** History and physical examination findings provide no indication of volume loss. An IV TKO for drug administration is indicated. **(Objectives 10, 11, and 15)**
15. D5W or Ringer's lactate would be appropriate at a TKO rate. **(Objective 16)**
16. Crystalloid. Crystalloids are the fluids of choice for volume replacement in both prehospital and hospital settings. They are also used as vehicles for drug administration. Crystalloids are classified according to their tonicity. The three primary crystalloids most often used in fluid replacement are 0.9% normal saline, RL, and D5W. **(Objective 14)**
17. Underhydrated / does. The patient has been vomiting blood for two hours, which easily could lead to volume loss. Additionally, she demonstrates signs of shock (pale, sweaty, dizzy, with tachycardia and hypotension); this supports a conclusion of underhydration and the need to replace fluids. **(Objective 10)**
18. Acidotic. The patient's condition indicates signs of shock, which typically is accompanied by acidosis. **(Objective 21)**
19. A crystalloid volume expander—Ringer's lactate or normal saline. These tend to stay in the vascular space and increase intravascular volume. **(Objectives 14 and 15)**
20. Sympathetic nervous system activation: increased pulse and respirations; pale, sweaty skin. **(Objectives 23, 24, and 25)**

21. **a.** respiratory—delivery of oxygen to the cells and exchange of carbon dioxide
    b. nutritional—delivery of the substances needed for cellular metabolism (glucose and other carbohydrates, amino acids, fatty acids, vitamins, minerals, trace elements)
    c. regulatory—delivery of substances such as electrolytes and hormones
    d. excretory—removal of cellular debris and waste products, such as those of cellular metabolism (carbon dioxide, water, acids)
    e. protective—defense against injury and invading microorganisms
    (Objective 2)
22. **f (Objective 3)**
23. **g (Objective 1)**
24. **e (Objective 1)**
25. **b (Objective 1)**
26. **d (Objective 1)**
27. **c (Objective 1)**
28. **a (Objective 3)**
29. Of the lymphoid organs, the spleen is one of the most important. Its major function is to filter and cleanse the blood. The spleen also serves as a reservoir, storing about 300 mL of blood that can be made readily available to the body when needed. **(Objective 1)**
30. **b (Objective 4)**
31. blood / immune **(Objective 5)**
32. Lymphoid organs serve as a link between the blood and the immune system. The two primary functions are: (1) the return to the circulation of excess proteins and fluid volume from the tissue spaces; (2) the immunologic defense of the body. **(Objective 5)**
33. **d (Objective 6)**
34. Approximately 85% to 95% of all Americans are Rh positive. Antibodies to the Rh factor do not occur naturally and must be acquired as a result of exposure to Rh-positive blood. Rh-negative mothers must be given a vaccine after each birth to prevent the formation of antibodies to any subsequent Rh-positive fetuses. **(Objective 7)**
35. **c (Objective 8)**
36. **(a)** Intracellular
    (b) Extracellular
    (c) Interstitial
    (d) Plasma
    (Objectives 1 and 9)
37. **a** Dehydration is a common condition and can occur gradually. It is often associated with electrolyte loss. Overhydration occurs infrequently. It may be associated with a sodium imbalance, excessive water ingestion, or administration of too much intravenous fluid. **(Objective 10)**
38. **(a)** Sodium is the most abundant extracellular cation and is especially important in the regulation of body water. **(Objective 12)**
    (b) Potassium is necessary for the transmission and conduction of nerve impulses, the maintenance of normal cardiac rhythms, and the contraction of skeletal and smooth muscle. **(Objective 12)**
    (c) Calcium is necessary for strengthening the structure of bones and teeth. It also functions as an enzyme cofactor for blood clotting, and is required for hormone secretion and muscle contraction. **(Objective 12)**
    (d) Magnesium activates the enzyme that is essential for normal cell membrane function; it is the energy source for the sodium-potassium pump. **(Objective 12)**
39. **c (Objective 12)**
40. **b (Objective 14)**
41. **d (Objective 14)**
42. **e (Objective 14)**
43. **a (Objective 13)**
44. **c (Objective 13)**

45. **b, c,** and **d**
46. **a** and **e**
47. **b, c,** and **d**
48. **b, c,** and **d**
49. **a** IV fluid choice depends on the underlying condition or illness.
50. **b** and **d** **(Questions 45–50: Objectives 11, 14, and 15)**
51. 7.35 to 7.45 **(Objective 17)**
52. **a** The kidneys and respiratory system are also buffers, but they are back-up systems. **(Objective 19)**
53. **c** Most patients in the field with acid-base abnormalities either are hypoventilating or are in respiratory arrest. **(Objective 21)**
54. Respiratory acidosis. The patient's respiratory rate is 6. In respiratory acidosis, carbon dioxide is being retained. Hypoventilation, secondary to respiratory depression, is a common cause. Head injuries can cause pressure on the respiratory center, which may lead to respiratory depression. **(Objectives 17 and 21)**
55. Metabolic acidosis. Abnormal metabolism that results in excess acid production causes metabolic acidosis. This patient exhibits signs of diabetic ketoacidosis, which causes acidosis from abnormal fat metabolism. **(Objectives 17 and 21)**
56. Respiratory alkalosis. Although respiratory alkalosis is typically a compensatory mechanism, "pure" forms occur with hyperventilation syndrome, secondary to anxiety, or upon rapid ascent to a high altitude. This patient has been upset and is experiencing tachypnea; there is no other pertinent medical history. **(Objectives 17 and 21)**
57. Respiratory and metabolic acidosis. With no respirations and retained carbon dioxide, respiratory acidosis is inevitable. If the heart stops, decreased circulation leads to anaerobic metabolism, the accumulation of acids, and resulting metabolic acidosis. **(Objectives 17 and 21)**
58. **c** Blood pressure and pulse evaluation relate directly to overall cardiovascular status; the respiratory system, however, is involved immediately when an acid-base disturbance occurs. **(Objectives 18 and 20)**
59. Vagus nerve/slow **(Objective 24)**
60. **C** — increases contractility

    A — increases automaticity

    R — increases rate

    D — dilates coronary arteries

    I — increases irritability

    O — increases oxygen demand

    (Objectives 24 and 25)

CHAPTER 9 Shock

1. **a** Checking the airway is the first assessment priority. **(Prerequisite Chapter Objective)**
2. **Yes.** Even without vital sign information, there are factors that indicate the possibility of shock. They include: the mechanism of injury, evidence of possible abdominal injury (and internal bleeding), pale skin, and the patient's complaint of thirst. **(Objectives 6 and 9)**
3. Rapid pulse and respirations and normal blood pressure are typical vital signs seen in early shock. **(Objectives 6 and 10)**

4. **a** Whenever the body senses a fall in cardiac output, baroreceptors trigger the adrenal glands to release epinephrine and norepinephrine, the major chemicals of the autonomic nervous system. The central, reticuloactivating, and voluntary nervous systems serve other purposes in the body. **(Objective 12)**

5. **e** Given your suspicion of internal bleeding, volume expanders such as 0.9% normal saline and Ringer's lactate are appropriate. Five percent dextrose and 0.45% normal saline do not stay in the vascular space as long, and they are not typically used for fluid replacement. **(Objective 13)**

6. **e** The mechanism of injury, physical examination findings, and patient's complaint suggest the possibility of intraabdominal injury and internal bleeding. Assessment findings do not indicate that there is a chest injury; such an injury could be a type of cardiogenic shock. Vital signs indicate compensation (early), not progressive or irreversible signs (late). **(Objectives 10 and 13)**

7. If compensatory efforts are successful, the body maintains perfusion, and blood pressure remains within normal limits. The alpha effect to the peripheral blood vessels (vasoconstriction) is one of the primary reasons this occurs. **(Objective 11)**

8. **Yes.** There are a wide variety of conditions that can lead to shock; however, of all the signs, decreased blood volume due to hemorrhage is the most common (hypovolemic shock). Knowledge of this fact is important because it increases one's index of suspicion for the presence of hemorrhage or hypovolemia. **(Objectives 6 and 14)**

9. **a** Chest pain is the most common symptom in cardiogenic shock that occurs secondary to a myocardial infarction. Determination that the patient experienced chest pain before collapsing would supersede information about his medical history, medications, and allergies. **(Objectives 9 and 13)**

10. **Late.** The patient's level of consciousness and vital signs are consistent with late shock: BP: 74/50; pulse 64 and weak; respirations 14 and labored. Additionally, the patient is pale, and cyanosis can be noted around the nail beds, mouth, and extremities. **(Objectives 6, 10, and 13)**

11. Cardiogenic. When an infarct occurs, the heart muscle often malfunctions and is unable to pump to its full capacity. This complication is seen less often than dysrhythmia following an acute myocardial infarction; however, it can occur, and it is associated with a high mortality rate. **(Objective 14)**

12. **(a)** distended neck veins, and **(b)** the presence of pulmonary edema (detected by assessment of both breath sounds and degree of difficulty breathing) **(Objective 14)**

13. **a** When compensatory mechanisms fail, tissue hypoxia is inevitable. With this, a byproduct of the anaerobic metabolism is acid that builds up in the blood, which results in profound metabolic acidosis. If alkalosis were to occur, acid level would be diminished, which is not the case. Respiratory acidosis would be present if respiratory effort were suppressed, which it is not at this point. **(Objective 10)**

14. **Slow.** With this type of shock, treatment is aimed at treating rate and rhythm, and possibly administering medications for improvement in blood pressure. If his lung sounds are clear, a "fluid challenge" of Ringer's lactate or normal saline could be ordered. Local protocols should be followed. **(Objectives 13 and 14)**

15. Potential problems include dysrhythmias (which occur frequently in this condition), decreased respirations, falling blood pressure, and possible cardiac arrest. **(Objectives 10, 13, and 14)**

16. Respiratory status. With breathing difficulty and stridor, maintenance of the airway is of primary concern. **(Objective 14)**

17. **b** The patient's medical history supports this conclusion; there is no history of asthma, and no indication of heat exhaustion, neurogenic shock, or a vasovagal episode. **(Objective 14)**

18. **c** Epinephrine is indicated to address his breathing problem and potential circulatory collapse. Benadryl will be used eventually, but is secondary to epinephrine. The same is true for dopamine and steroids; potentially, they could be used for his condition but would not be the first priority. Some systems are also considering the use of albuterol for respiratory compromise due to allergic reactions. **(Objective 14)**

19. **Yes.** With anaphylaxis, there is severe respiratory and circulatory compromise, secondary to massive vasodilatation (leading to shock) and smooth muscle constriction (which closes the airway). **(Objectives 10 and 14)**

20. Prepare to transport the patient. With his potentially life-threatening condition, the doctrine of implied consent would apply. **(Prerequisite Chapter Objective)**

21. **e (Objective 1)**

22. Chemoreceptors are specialized cells that are sensitive to the concentrations of oxygen, carbon dioxide, and hydrogen ions within the body. When an acid-base disturbance is indicated, they stimulate the medulla to adjust the rate and depth of ventilations. **(Objective 3)**

23. The size of the vessels, and the amount of blood flow to the vessels. **(Objective 2)**

24. **d** Functioning together, the venules regulate the capacity of the vascular system and serve as a blood reservoir. **(Objective 2)**

25. **e** Patients with in-dwelling catheters are more prone to septic shock. The man who fell (a) is likely to be hypovolemic. The patient stung by a bee (b) is likely to be in anaphylactic shock. The man with chest pain (c) is likely to be in cardiogenic shock, and the 43-year-old woman with diarrhea and vomiting (d) is likely to be hypovolemic. **(Objective 14)**

26. Maintain arterial pressure; oppose the effects of gravity on blood flow in the arteries; and accomplish selective distributions of flow according to needs throughout the body **(Objective 2)**

27. **a, b, d,** and **e** Parasympathetic influence occurs primarily to the vagus nerve, and not directly to the blood vessels themselves. **(Objectives 4 and 11)**

28. **i**

29. **a**

30. **b**

31. **h**

32. **c**

33. **f**

34. **e**

    (Questions 28–34: Objectives 3 and 5)

35. **(a)** In elderly patients, the compensatory mechanisms are less efficient; thus, deterioration may occur more quickly in response to shock.

    (b) Children tend to compensate longer, but they also deteriorate more quickly when compensatory mechanisms fail. **(Objective 7)**

36. The young and the elderly; victims of trauma; those with a history of ulcers or gastrointestinal bleeding, acute myocardial infarction, or allergic reactions; those with in-dwelling tubes such as Foley catheter, shunts, or venous access devices; diabetics; drug abusers; and those with compromised immune systems **(Objective 8)**

37. **d** Because all of the other factors may vary, and they are not always easily measurable, the most reliable sign is the patient's presenting signs and symptoms. **(Objective 9)**

38. **a** Cyanosis occurs later in the shock process. Pale skin, rapid respirations, and tachycardia are all earlier signs. **(Objectives 10 and 11)**

39. Hypoxia, hypoxemia, ischemia, and acidosis all lead to relaxation of the precapillary sphincters; the postcapillary sphincters contract, resulting in pooling of blood within the capillaries. Venous return is diminished; cardiac output and blood pressure fall. High levels of acid in the blood reduce its oxygen-carrying capacity. Cyanosis begins, usually around the nose, mouth, and ear lobes, and in the extremities. **(Objective 10)**

40. **b** This has the greatest influence on mortality associated with shock; the other interventions may be appropriate. However, it is clear that early recognition of the condition increases the likelihood of patient survival. **(Objectives 9 and 13)**

41. **d** All other types of shock are accompanied by a fast pulse, with sympathetic compensation. **(Objective 14)**

42. **e** Closed head injury in the adult patient is not likely to cause hypovolemia or signs associated with it; myocardial infarction leads to failure of the pump, or cardiogenic shock. **(Objective 14)**

43. Shock that occurs when the heart is unable to pump efficiently because of traumatic injury is mechanical or obstructive shock. Cardiac tamponade and tension pneumothorax are common causes. **(Objective 14)**

44. **(a)** The nervous system may lose sympathetic control of vascular resistance, or **(b)** massive stimulation of the parasympathetic system can occur (as in drug overdose or poisoning). Circumstances seen in the field that are associated with neurogenic shock include spine injury, blunt trauma to the back of the head, and overdoses affecting the central nervous system. The most common cause is spine trauma. **(Objective 14)**

45. The vascular effects of capillary dilation and permeability result in a shock-like condition of the patient, because vasodilation leads to venous pooling and a fall in cardiac output. Additionally, the permeability causes a loss of fluid from the intravascular space into the tissues, which results in edema (seen in the face, eyelids, and so forth) and a fall in blood pressure. Bronchoconstriction (smooth muscle constriction) is evidenced by tightness in the throat, shortness of breath, and wheezing. **(Objective 14)**

46. Advanced or very young age, hypothermia, use of a pacemaker, and intake of drugs such as alcohol and beta blockers. **(Objective 15)**

Chapter 10: Infection Control

1. **b** Needlestick exposure from a hepatitis B patient carries a 6% to 35% chance of disease transmission. **(Objective 5)**
2. **No.** Contaminated needles should not be recapped. The most common preventable bloodborne pathogen exposure is a puncture injury that occurs during needle recapping. A no-recapping policy is an integral part of an EMS system's exposure control plan as mandated by OSHA. **(Objectives 4 and 8)**
3. Hepatitis B vaccination. The OSHA bloodborne pathogen standard requires that employers provide, at no cost to the employee, hepatitis B vaccine for those who are occupationally exposed to blood or other potentially infectious materials. **(Objective 5)**
4. Discrimination against the disabled. Under the Americans with Disabilities Act (PL 101-366), tuberculosis is classified as a disability, and failure to provide care for individuals afflicted with this disease may constitute discrimination. **(Objective 7)**
5. **b** Droplets produced by coughing are the principal mode of transmission of tuberculosis. Therefore, the best way to protect yourself from infection is by placing a mask on the patient. **(Objective 5)**
6. Maximum **(Objective 5)**
7. **d** Subtitle B of the Ryan White Act is intended to protect prehospital care personnel from communicable disease by requiring that they be notified "routinely" or by "request." a, b, and c fall under "routine" notification. **(Objective 7)**
8. **j** **(Objective 2)**
9. **g** **(Objective 1)**
10. **f** **(Objective 1)**
11. **b** **(Objective 1)**
12. **k** **(Objective 1)**
13. **a** **(Objective 1)**
14. **h** **(Objective 1)**
15. **i** **(Objective 1)**
16. **c** **(Objective 1)**
17. **d** **(Objective 2)**
18. **True** Many victims with communicable diseases are completely asymptomatic, particularly during the window, incubation, or carrier phase. **(Objective 5)**
19. **False** The first step is to wash the equipment with soap and water to remove any obvious body fluid or tissue. Disinfection is then performed with an Environmental Protection Agency (EPA) approved "hospital disinfectant" chemical germicide or with a solution of chlorine bleach 1:100 with water. **(Objective 9)**
20. **False** Linen should be changed after each patient use. Contaminated linen should be placed in appropriately labeled leakproof bags or containers; it should not be sorted or rinsed before laundering. **(Objective 9)**
21. **False** National Federal Protection Agency (NFPA) infection control standards state that "protective clothing, station/work uniforms or other clothing shall not be taken home" for laundering. According to OSHA, if a uniform is intended to act as PPE, the employer must "provide, clean, repair, replace and/or dispose of it." **(Objective 9)**
22. **False** TB bacteria are difficult to kill; a commercial disinfectant labeled "tuberculocidal" is required. **(Objective 9)**
23. **False** Under BSI, *all* body fluids and tissues are considered potentially infectious. **(Objective 6)** TB testing should be offered annually. **(Objective 8)**

24. **b** People at high risk for tuberculosis include HIV victims, alcoholics, immigrants from countries with a high prevalence of tuberculosis, nursing home or institutionalized patients, and indigent elderly men in urban settings. **(Objective 5)**

25. **a, b,** and **c** Centers for Disease Control (CDC) guidelines, as modified by the United States Fire Administration, recommend that personal protective equipment for emergency childbirth should include a gown, disposable gloves, protective eyewear, and a mask. **(Objective 9)**

26. **a**

27. Incubation period **(Objective 1)**

28. Window phase **(Objective 1)**

29. Seroconverted **(Objective 1)**

30. Direct **(Objective 3)**

31. Indirect **(Objective 3)**

32. Treat all victims as potentially infectious; use appropriate PPE when providing medical care; wash hands after every patient contact. **(Objective 1)**

33. The purpose of PPE is to prevent the patient's body fluids from contacting the providers' skin or mucous membranes. **(Objective 9)**

34. Hepatitis A: foodborne/fecal (oral)

    Hepatitis B: bloodborne/sexually transmitted

    Hepatitis C: bloodborne; rarely sexually transmitted

    Tuberculosis (TB): airborne/respiratory transmission

    Human immunodeficiency virus (HIV): bloodborne/sexually transmitted

    (Objectives 4 and 5)

35. Tetanus; diphtheria; measles; mumps; rubella; polio.

    Before being assigned to emergency response duties, all paramedics should receive any necessary immunizations as part of proper infection control practice. **(Objective 8)**

36. From mother to fetus; by inoculation of HIV-positive blood products through the skin or onto damaged mucous membranes; by sexual contact with an HIV-positive person. **(Objective 5)**

CHAPTER 11 General Pharmacology

1. **a** Respirations are 8 and shallow and require assistance. Airway is always a priority over obtaining further history, starting an IV, or inducing vomiting. **(Prerequisite Chapter Objective)**

2. Overdose **(Objective 7)**

3. **d (Objective 7)**

4. **a (Objective 7)**

5. **c (Objective 17)**

6. Side effects/narcotic analgesics **(Objective 16)**

7. The generic name is the name of the drug that is unique to that particular chemical. It often serves as the official, standard name. All U.S. Government–approved drugs have a generic name and are listed in the U.S. Pharmacopeia. **(Objective 1)**

    The trade name is the name given to a generic drug by the company that manufactures it. Many generic drugs have several trade names. **(Objective 1)**

8. **c** The FDA has complete control over the safety and effectiveness of drugs in human subjects. **(Objective 2)**

9. The DEA enforces the Controlled Substances Act, which places certain restrictions on drugs such as narcotics, sedatives, and stimulants. Use of these drugs requires special paperwork and high accountability, to verify legitimate use and to detect diversion. **(Objective 2)**

10. **(a)** drug effect (therapeutic effect); **(b)** target organ; **(c)** absorption; **(d)** distribution; **(e)** metabolism; and **(f)** elimination. **(Objectives 3 and 4)**

11. **(a)** Factors affecting absorption are: **(1)** the route of administration, which affects the rate of absorption; and **(2)** the patient's physiologic condition. **(Objective 4)**

    (b) Factors affecting distribution are: **(1)** the chemical makeup of the drug (fat or water solubility); the drug's ability to pass through the cell membrane; and **(3)** blood flow to certain organs. **(Objective 4)**

12. The basic site of drug interaction. Receptors regulate normal physiologic functions.

13. A drug that stimulates (switch-on) a receptor.

14. A drug that binds to a receptor but will not initiate the effect, it blocks other chemicals (that can turn on the receptor) from binding.

15. The relationship between the dose of a drug and its effect.

16. The margin between a drug's therapeutic effect and its toxicity. **(Questions 12–16: Objective 5)**

17. The lock and key theory is the theory that a drug or chemical messenger must have a very specific shape to activate a receptor. Many medications used in the prehospital setting produce their effects as agonists or antagonists at receptor sites in the autonomic nervous system. **(Objective 6)**

18. A major function is to detoxify and convert (metabolize) chemicals and drugs so they can be eliminated easily by the kidney. Normal function of the liver is necessary to adequately remove drugs from the body; however, function may be affected significantly by aging or disease. **(Objective 3)**

19. The kidney serves as a "filtering system" that eliminates unnecessary or potentially harmful substances. As with the liver, this process may be hampered by aging or disease. **(Objective 3)**

20. **f**
21. **d**
22. **b**
23. **a**
24. **c**
25. **k**
26. **h (Questions 20–26: Objective 7)**

27. 10
28. Liter
29. Meter
30. Gram
31. **e**
32. **b**
33. **d**
34. **c**
35. **a (Questions 27–35: Objective 9)**

36. 1,000
37. 1
38. 2,000
39. 65,000
40. 750
41. 1
42. 2.2

43. .065
44. 256,000
45. .045 **(Questions 36–45: Objective 10)**

A. <u>Ratio/Proportion method:</u>
How supplied and solve for X.

B. <u>Desired dose vs. Dose on hand</u>
$$x = \frac{\text{dose ordered (D)} \times \text{volume on hand (Q)}}{\text{dose on hand (H)}}$$

46. $\dfrac{10\ mg}{2\ mL} = \dfrac{6\ mg}{X\ mL}$

   $\dfrac{10\,x}{10} = \dfrac{12}{10}$

   $x = \dfrac{12}{10}$

   $x = 1.2\ mg$

   $x = \dfrac{6}{10} \times 2$

   $x = \dfrac{12}{10} = 1.2\ mg$

47. $\dfrac{50\ mg}{1\ mL} \times \dfrac{25\ mg}{X}$

   $\dfrac{50\,x}{50} = \dfrac{25}{50}$

   $x = \dfrac{25}{50}$

   $x = \dfrac{1}{2}$ or .5 mg

   $x = \dfrac{25}{50} \times 1$

   $\tfrac{1}{2} \times 1$

   $x = \tfrac{1}{2} = .5\ mg$

48. $\dfrac{100\ mg}{10} \times \dfrac{75\ mg}{X}$

   $\dfrac{100\,x}{100} = \dfrac{750}{100}$

   $x = \dfrac{750}{100}$

   $x = 7.5\ mg$

   $x = \dfrac{75}{100} \times 10$

   $x = \dfrac{750}{100}$

   $x = 7.5\ mg$

(Questions 46–48: Objective 11)

49. Step 1 Convert pounds to kg (1 lb = 2.2 kg)
    50 lbs / 2.2
    = 22.7

    Step 2 Multiply weight in kg × dose per kg
    22.7 × .01 = .227 or .28 mg

   (Objective 12)

Formula: **What physician orders × drops/mL**
$$\dfrac{}{60}$$

50. $\dfrac{150 \times 15}{60} = \dfrac{2250}{60} = 37.5$ drops/min (38)

51. $\dfrac{250 \times 10}{60} = \dfrac{2250}{60} = 41.66$ drops/min (42)

52. 1000 mL over 8 hours = 125 mL/hr

    $\dfrac{125 \times 10}{60} = \dfrac{1250}{60} = 20.83$ drops/min (21)

(Questions 50–52: Objective 13)

53. The physician orders a dopamine drip to run at 5 mcg/kg/min. Your patient weighs 154 lb. You mix 200 mg in 500 mL of D5W. How many gtts/min do you run your IV?

    154 lbs = 70 kg
    200 mg/500 mL = 400 mcg/mL
    $\dfrac{70 \times 5 \times 60}{400} = 52.5$ gtts/min

54. You have a dopamine drip concentration of 800 mcg/mL. Your minidrip is running at 40 gtts/min on your 75-kg patient. How many mcg/kg/min is this patient receiving?

    (HINT: Work this one backward in the formula.)

    ? = 7 mcg/kg/min $\dfrac{75 \times ? \times 60}{800} = 40$

    (Questions 53–54: Objectives 12 and 14)

55. **d**
56. **e**
57. **a**
58. **f**
59. **c**
60. **a** and **h**
61. **b**
62. **i**
63. **g**

    (Questions 55–63: Objective 15)

64. Intravenous / oral **(Objective 15)**

65. **(a)** verify the order; **(b)** patient; **(c)** dosage; **(d)** label; **(e)** calculate; **(f)** drug; **(g)** route; **(h)** precautions; **(i)** side effects **(Objective 8)**

66. Digitalis (Digoxin®). The patient has doubled his dose 2 days in a row. With this group of drugs (cardiac glycosides), there is a very narrow range between the therapeutic dose and the toxic dose. Symptoms of nausea, fatigue, weakness, and dizziness are common with digitalis toxicity.

67. **d** (an antidysrhythmic)

68. **b**

69. **b** **(a)** applies to coronary vasodilators, **(d)** refers to anticoagulants, and **(e)** pertains to diuretics. One of the main therapeutic actions of digoxin is to slow the heart rate, not increase it.

70. **(a)** diuretic; **(b)** remove excess fluids from the body; **(c)** CHF; **(d)** hypertension.

71. **Therapeutic action:** Slows heart (sinus) rate; decreases conduction of impulses through the AV node; lowers blood pressure

    Examples: propranolol (Inderal®), nadolol (Corgard®), atenolol (Tenormin®), metoprolol (Lopressor®)

72. **Therapeutic action:** Slows conduction through the AV node; slows ventricular response with atrial tachyarrhthmias; relaxes vascular smooth muscle

    Examples: diltiazem (Cardizem®), verapamil (Calan®, Isoptin®), nifedipine (Procardia®, Adalat®), amlodipine (Norvasc®), nicardipine (Cardene®)

73. **Therapeutic action:** Dilates blood vessels; decreases myocardial oxygen demand

    Examples: nitroglycerin (NTG®), isosorbide dinitrate (Isordil®), isosorbide mononitrate (Ismo®)

74. **Therapeutic action:** Acts with a clothing protein to help dissolve blood clots

    Examples: streptokinase (Streptase®), tissue plasminogen activator [TPA] (Activate®)

75. **Therapeutic action:** Vasodilates arterial smooth muscle; decreases arterial pressure

    Examples: methyldopa (Aldomet®), clonidine (Catapres®), prazosin (Minipress®), minoxidil (Loniten®)

76. **a, b,** and **c** Chronic depression, eating disorders, and panic attacks are frequently treated with antidepressants. They are *not* effective for psychotic conditions or seizure disorders.

77. **c** Narcotics alter pain, antidepressants treat depression, and sedatives induce sleep.

78. **d** *Mellaril* is a major tranquilizer (antipsychotic).

79. g
80. i
81. k
82. h
83. l
84. c
85. f
86. d
87. b
88. e
89. j
90. m
91. a

(Questions 66–91: Objectives 16 and 17)

Chapter 11a — Appendix: Prehospital Medications

1. Administering oxygen, initiating an IV, and applying a cardiac monitor are always appropriate actions in the treatment of an emergency cardiac patient. Supplemental oxygen increases the amount of oxygen in the blood that is flowing to ischemic tissue. Vascular access is important for providing pain control and for administering emergency cardiac medications when they are needed. Because this patient is at risk for developing life-threatening cardiac dysrhythmias, it is essential that he be monitored. **(Prerequisite Chapter Objective)**

2. Aspirin blocks the formation of a substance that causes platelets to clump together; it is indicated for patients with chest pain that is consistent with myocardial infarction. Although aspirin is also effective as an analgesic, it is not used in the prehospital setting for this purpose. **(Objectives 2 and 3)**

3. Procardia® is a calcium channel blocker; it lowers blood pressure by relaxing vascular smooth muscle. **(Objectives 1 and 2)**

4. **Yes.** This patient's blood pressure is stable, and he has no history of CNS hemorrhage to contraindicate the administration of nitroglycerin. **(Objectives 2 and 3)**

5. Nitroglycerin causes systemic arterial and venous dilation, which reduces the workload and oxygen demand on the heart. **(Objective 2)**

6. Headache, syncope, facial flushing, and nausea. **(Objective 2)**

7. **Two.** The usual dosage of nitroglycerin by sublingual tablet is one tablet every 5 minutes to a maximum of three administrations. **(Objective 2)**

8. Although both medications increase blood pressure, norepinephrine increases myocardial oxygen demand and produces myocardial ischemia. This is an adverse reaction that could make this patient's condition worse. Norepinephrine also causes vasoconstriction of kidney and mesenteric blood vessels as opposed to dopamine, which dilates kidney and mesenteric vessels at low doses. **(Objective 2)**

9. Any patient who makes the statement, "I feel like I'm going to die," should be taken seriously. The fact that patients who are experiencing an acute myocardial infarct may experience an impending sense of doom has long been acknowledged. **(Prerequisite Chapter Objective)**

10. **Yes.** The patient, using a patient-regulated demand valve, controls the amount of gas that is administered. You should not attempt to hold the mask in place. Dosing is totally controlled by the patient, who may choose to stop at any time. The duration of administration is determined by the timing and effectiveness of pain relief. **(Objectives 2 and 3)**

11. Morphine sulfate; IV push. **(Objectives 2 and 3)**

12. Lidocaine should be administered first, then, procainamide; procainamide is given for the treatment of ventricular dysrhythmia that is unresponsive to lidocaine. **(Objectives 2 and 3)**

13. 1:10,000 In adult cardiac arrest, 1 mg (10 ml) 1:10,000 IV push is indicated. **(Objective 2)**

14. Streptase® is a thrombolytic agent. Thrombolytic agents are absolutely contraindicated in patients who have undergone prolonged CPR of longer than 5 to 10 minutes. **(Objective 2)**

15. Dextrose 50% and naloxone. This patient has signs and symptoms that indicate the use of both medications to determine the cause of his unresponsiveness. The initial dose of dextrose 50% is 25 gm. The initial dose of naloxone is 2 mg. **(Objectives 2 and 3)**

16. Thiamine. Thiamine deficiency is common among alcoholics because it often is not provided in a normal diet. Administering glucose to a thiamine-deficient patient can precipitate a severe neurologic condition called Wernicke's encephalopathy. **(Objectives 2 and 3)**

17. This patient is at risk for developing seizures. Ativan® and Valium® are equally effective in controlling seizures, but Ativan® has a longer duration of action than does Valium®. Thus, Ativan® may be more beneficial for this patient because of the 20-minute transport time. **(Objectives 2 and 3)**

18. Respiratory depression or arrest, periods of excitement, hypotension, confusion, prolonged coma. **(Objective 2)**

19. **Yes.** Alcohol may worsen CNS and respiratory depression. **(Objective 2)**

20. **No.** Lights and sirens could precipitate seizures in this patient. He is already at risk for the development of seizures based on his history alone. **(Prerequisite Chapter Objective)**

21. Patency is assessed by auscultating to confirm adequate air movement in the lungs and by determining if there is equal and sufficient expansion of the chest wall. **(Prerequisite Chapter Objective)**

22. Maintenance of the airway and administration of high-flow oxygen. **(Prerequisite Chapter Objective)**

23. Epinephrine, 0.01 to 0.03 mg/kg 1:1,000 subcutaneously (SQ) (to a maximum dose of 0.3 mg); then, Benadryl, 1 to 2 mg/kg IM or IV. **(Objectives 2 and 3)**

24. Applying a constricting band proximal to the site; injecting 0.1 to 0.2 ml of the same 1:1,000 epinephrine solution at the site. **(Objectives 2 and 3)**

25. Steroids may have been ordered additionally because they decrease the inflammatory response and reduce edema in many tissues. **(Objectives 2 and 3)**

26. **f** **(Objective 2)**

27. **d** **(Objective 2)**

28. **i** **(Objective 2)**

29. **b** **(Objective 2)**

30. **e** **(Objective 2)**

31. **c** **(Objective 2)**

32. **a** **(Objective 2)**

33. **h** **(Objective 2)**

34. Activated charcoal **(Objective 3)**

35. Atropine sulfate **(Objective 3)**

36. Calcium chloride **(Objective 3)**

37. Sodium bicarbonate **(Objective 3)**

38. Naloxone **(Objective 3)**

39. Naloxone **(Objective 3)**

40. Dose: 0.04 mg/kg diluted in 1 to 2 ml normal saline

    Route: endotracheal **(Objective 2)**

41. Dose: 0.01 to 0.03 mg/kg diluted in 2 ml of normal saline

    Route: delivered by handheld or mask nebulizer **(Objective 2)**

42. Dose: 0.01 mg/kg

    Route: IV push, IM or SQ **(Objective 2)**
43. Dose: 0.1 mg/kg to 0.3 mg/kg

    Route: slow IV push **(Objective 2)**
44. **d (Objective 2)**
45. **d (Objective 2)**
46. **e (Objective 2)**
47. **b (Objective 2)**
48. **b (Objective 2)**
49. **d (Objective 2)**
50. **b (Objective 3)**
51. **d (Objective 3)**
52. **a (Objective 3)**
53. **b (Objective 3)**

CHAPTER 12: Basic Rhythm Interpretation

1. Third degree; there is no relationship between the P waves and QRS complexes. **(Objective 13)**
2. **(a)** Rate — What is the rate?

    (b) Pattern — Is the rhythm regular or irregular? If irregular, is there a pattern?

    (c) QRS width — Is it normal (less than 0.12 second in duration) or abnormal?

    (d) Atrial activity — Is there atrial activity? If so, what is it?

    (e) Relationship — Is there a relationship between the atrial activity and the QRS complexes? **(Objective 5)**
3. The QRS complexes are narrow, less than 0.12 second, which indicates that the impulses originated above the ventricles. In this patient's form of heart block, all atrial activity is blocked from conduction to the ventricles, and the QRS complexes arise from junctional escape activity. **(Objectives 9 and 13)**
4. Electrical capture will be indicated by abnormally wide QRS complexes. **(Objectives 9 and 14)**
5. **c** This patient's clinical presentation, including an acute onset of chest pain radiating down the left arm, abnormal vital signs, abnormal breath sounds, anxiety, and confusion, suggests cardiogenic shock from an acute myocardial infarction. **(Prerequisite Chapter Objective)**
6. Because standard electrode placements are very sensitive to patient motion and ambulance vibration, they are not practical for field monitoring. A modified lead II is the solution and involves the use of only three electrodes, which are moved to appropriate positions on the chest. **(Objectives 2 and 3)**
7. Interpretation: Sinus tachycardia

    (a) 170

    (b) Regular

    (c) Narrow, < 0.12

    (d) Positive P waves

    (e) Fixed 1:1 — PR segment 0.16

    (Objectives 4 and 10)

8. **b** Dopamine is indicated to raise the blood pressure in patients with cardiogenic shock. Atropine and epinephrine are not indicated and could extend this patient's infarct or, worse, could cause a life-threatening arrhythmia. Nitroglycerin is not indicated because it could worsen this patient's hypotension.
(Prerequisite Chapter Objective)

9. **d** The change in this patient's ECG is caused by artifact. Artifact can be the result of patient movement, a dry or disconnected electrode, electrical interference, a broken wire, excessive hair, or problems with the amplifier. If this patient were in ventricular fibrillation, she would not be awake. **(Objectives 2 and 15)**

10. Classically, for a 12-lead ECG, electrodes are attached to each wrist, each ankle, and six chest locations. **(Objective 3)**

11. **(a)** Ventricular fibrillation
    (b) Asystole
    (c) Pulseless electrical activity
    (d) Pulseless ventricular tachycardia
    (Objective 15)

12. Premature ventricular contractions (PVCs); PVCs have three characteristics: They occur early; they do not start with a positive P wave; they have an abnormal QRS width. **(Objective 11)**

13. Lidocaine is the drug of choice to suppress premature ventricular contractions when they occur in the context of myocardial ischemia and to prevent the recurrence of ventricular fibrillation. **(Prerequisite Chapter Objective)**

14. Witnessed arrest leading to early access to 9-1-1, early CPR performed by trained professionals, early defibrillation, and quick response time by the paramedics. **(Prerequisite Chapter Objective)**

15. **b (Objective 1)**
16. **d (Objective 1)**
17. **c (Objective 1)**
18. **e (Objective 1)**
19. **f (Objective 1)**
20. **a (Objective 1)**
21. Sinoatrial node; 60–100 **(Objective 7)**
22. Atrium; 40–60 **(Objective 7)**
23. AV node or junction; 40–60 **(Objective 7)**
24. Ventricle; 30–40 **(Objective 7)**
25. **b (Objectives 1 and 2)**
26. **c (Objectives 1 and 2)**
27. **a (Objectives 1 and 2)**
28. **d (Objectives 1 and 2)**
29. **e (Objectives 1 and 2)**
30. 70; count the number of QRS complexes in six seconds and multiply by 10. **(Objective 5)**
31. 68; count the number of small boxes between two R waves and divide into 1500. **(Objective 5)**
32. 150; count the number of large boxes between two R waves and divide into 300. **(Objective 5)**
33. **d (Objectives 6, 8, and 12)**
34. **b (Objectives 6 and 10)**
35. **i (Objectives 6, 8, and 12)**
36. **e (Objectives 6 and 8)**
37. **a (Objective 11)**
38. **g (Objective 13)**
39. **f (Objective 13)**
40. **h (Objective 7)**
41. **b (Objective 1)**
42. **a (Objective 1)**
43. **a (Objective 1)**

44. (Objective 2)

[Figure: Three torso diagrams showing ECG lead placement with negative (−), positive (+), and ground (G) electrode positions.]

45. Atrial fibrillation **(Objective 12)**
46. Sinus tachycardia **(Objective 10)**
47. Sinus arrhythmia **(Objective 11)**
48. Sinus rhythm with isolated premature atrial complex **(Objective 11)**
49. Second-degree variable AV block, or Wenckebach, or Mobitz I **(Objective 13)**
50. Sinus bradycardia **(Objective 10)**

CHAPTER 13 Interpersonal Communication Skills

1. **c** One of the most important aspects of establishing rapport is personalizing the situation: Introduce yourself and find out the patient's name. You should not tell the patient to calm down, nor should you immediately start to evaluate the patient. Sending the wife out of the room could also increase the patient's anxiety. **(Objectives 1 and 4)**

2. Positioning yourself at eye level with the patient, maintaining good eye contact, listening carefully to what the patient says, and holding the patient's hand while you examine/question him are all important techniques for enhancing communication. These methods will also foster the patient's trust and will help to decrease the patient's anxiety and fears. **(Objectives 1, 3, 4, and 6)**

3. **c** Simply telling her to calm down so that you can do your job will only tend to escalate the situation and make it worse. Keeping her informed and reassuring her are the best tactics for gaining her cooperation and decreasing her anxiety. **(Objective 6)**

4. **c** Scene safety is imperative. Before you take any action, make sure that the scene is assessed and secured. **(Prerequisite Chapter Objective)**

5. **b and d** When dealing with hostile patients, one must first try to determine why they are upset. Your "nonverbal" messages are important. Raising your voice or getting too close to the patient too quickly may tend to escalate hostility. **(Objective 5)**

6. **d** Dismissing the friends at the scene may increase the patient's anxiety and may tend to make the crowd even more upset. Keeping them informed, letting them help, and letting one person stay with the patient are much more likely to enhance cooperation. However, confidentiality should be maintained within this process. **(Objective 6)**

7. **a.** 3

   b. 2

   c. 1

   (Objective 2)

8. **(a)** volume, **(b)** pitch, **(c)** rate, **(d)** pronunciation. **(Objective 3)**

9. Good listening is a skill and an art. When good listening is practiced, the patient feels more "free" to talk and rapport is facilitated because the patient senses concern on the part of the provider. Additionally, the provider is likely to obtain a more accurate history. **(Objectives 1 and 3)**

10. Infants

    (a) Support the head when picking up or holding the baby.

    (b) Keep the baby warm and dry, especially if clothes are removed for examination.

    (Objective 5)

11. 9 to 17 months

    (a) Examine the child while he is in the lap of a familiar adult (parent), if possible.

    (b) Remove one section of clothing at a time, and examine toe to head.

    (Objective 5)

12. 18 to 24 months

    (a) Take time to build trust and rapport.

    (b) Use a calm and understanding, yet straightforward, tone of voice (a "sing-song" cadence may be better).

    (Objective 5)

13. 2 to 3 years

    (a) To build trust, allow the child to "play" with a tool (stethoscope, etc.). Allow the parent to handle it to demonstrate that it is safe.

    (b) Speak to the child and not to those around him or her. Children this age can understand much of what is said.

    (Objective 5)

14. 4 to 5 years

    (a) Allow the child to "help," as children this age are very curious.

    (b) Explain what has happened and what the child should expect.

    (Objective 5)

15. 6 to 12 years

    (a) Explain as you go, because these children are somewhat familiar with medical procedures.

    (b) Remain calm and be matter-of-fact. Ask relevant questions.

    (Objective 5)

16. Adolescents

    (a) Remember that privacy is a very important issue at this age, so protect as much as possible.

    (b) "Educate" patients as you examine them. Be matter-of-fact and honest.

    (Objective 5)

17. **e** All of these methods will enhance communication with geriatric patients. **(Objective 5)**
18. Asking questions one at a time, using nonverbal communication skills, and using words that the interpreter will understand are all important techniques to employ. The provider should avoid phrasing questions too quickly because they may be misunderstood or misinterpreted. **(Objective 5)**
19. **c** "Shouting" or talking loudly to a hearing impaired patient should be avoided. This technique only serves to frustrate the patient. **(Objective 5)**
20. Effective communication with colleagues enhances job motivation and performance, which ultimately benefits patient care. Communicating with hospital personnel, medical direction personnel, and bystanders is equally important. **(Objective 7)**

CHAPTER 14: Communication and Documentation

1. Called to a residence; patient is sitting in a chair upon our arrival.
2. Alert, 69-year-old male patient.
3. Chest pain
4. B/P 84/60; pulse 56 and weak; respirations 20.
5. Chest pain, which began 30 minutes ago at rest, is not relieved with nitroglycerin. Pain is described as a "squeezing" sensation in the center of the chest, and the "worst in his life."
6. **S** (Signs/symptoms): chest pain; pale, diaphoretic skin; pulse 56 and weak; BP 84/60

    A (Allergies): none

    M (Medications): Isordil®, Catapres®

    P (Pertinent history): hypertension 15 years, acute myocardial infarction (AMI) 5 years ago

    L (Last meal): not known

    E (Events leading to illness or injury): chest pain, which began 30 minutes ago at rest and has been unrelieved by nitroglycerin. Pain is described as a "squeezing" sensation in the center of the chest, and the "worst in his life."

7. Nauseated, but not short of breath. Pain does not radiate.
8. Skin pale and diaphoretic; ECG shows sinus bradycardia.
9. Oxygen is being administered, and a TKO IV of D5W has been established.
10. The patient describes feeling better as we prepare him for transport.
11. 10 minutes to St. Joseph's Medical Center

    (Questions 1 to 11: Objective 6)

12. Pain does not radiate; there is no shortness of breath. **(Objective 5)**
13. Unit 1 calling OLMD. We are at the residence of a 69-year-old male who is complaining of chest pain. The patient is alert. Initial vital signs were pulse 56 and weak; respirations 20; and B/P 84/60. The patient states his pain began approximately 30 minutes ago while he was reading. The pain is in the center of the chest, does not radiate, and is described as "squeezing" in nature and the "worst pain of his life." He is nauseated, pale, and diaphoretic. He denies any shortness of breath. Medical history includes an AMI 5 years ago and hypertension for 15 years. He takes Isordil®, Catapres®, and nitroglycerin. There are no known allergies. Currently, we have the patient on oxygen and have established an IV, D5W, TKO. The patient states that he is feeling better. Vital signs now are pulse 62; respirations 20; and B/P 94/60. We are preparing to transport the patient to St. Joseph's Medical Center. Our ETA is 10 minutes. **(Objectives 3 and 6)**

14. **S** Chest pain that began 30 minutes ago at rest and has been unrelieved with nitroglycerin. Pain is described as a "squeezing" sensation in the center of the chest, and the "worst pain of his life."

    Nauseated, but not short of breath. Pain does not radiate. Hypertension 15 years, AMI 5 years ago. Allergies, none.

    O B/P 84/60; pulse 56 and weak; respirations 20

    Skin pale and diaphoretic; ECG = sinus bradycardia

    A Possible acute myocardial infarction

    P Oxygen being administered, and a TKO IV of D5W established

    (Objective 4)

15. Visual. Because the individual at the other end of the radio communication cannot see the patient or the situation, verbally "painting the picture" is essential. **(Objective 2)**

16. - Listen to the channel before beginning transmission;
    - Press the transmit button and wait momentarily before speaking;
    - Hold the microphone at a slight angle to the mouth and at a distance of 2 to 3 inches;
    - Minimize background noise;
    - Pronounce each word clearly and speak slowly;
    - Speak calmly;
    - Break the transmission every 30 seconds to recheck the signal;
    - Spell words that medical direction personnel may have difficulty understanding;
    - At the end of the transmission, confirm that the communication was received.

    (Objective 7)

17. Avoid the following:
    - Using proper names when referring to other persons or units in the system (instead, use unit identifiers);
    - Referring to the patient by name;
    - Using slang or profanity;
    - Using words that are difficult to hear.

    (Objective 7)

18. **(a)** Legal
    - to avoid a claim or lawsuit
    - to assist in defense, should there be civil or criminal action taken against the prehospital service or employee
    - to comply with state and/or federal documentation requirements

    (b) System
    - to provide data for medical audits and quality improvement measures
    - to provide data related to response times, placement of ambulances, and patient population data

    (c) Reimbursement
    - to provide the data required for revenue collection

    (Objectives 1 and 8)

19. Treatment Data
    - Basic life support (BLS) provided
    - Advanced life support (ALS) provided
    - Response to therapy
    - Time of drug administration and procedure
    - Transport code
    - Hospital destination
    - Receiving medical personnel signature

    (Objective 9)

20. **b, c, d,** and **e**   **a** is false. The rule of thumb that is applicable to all cases comes from a legal perspective: "If it wasn't written down, it wasn't done." **(Objective 11)**

21. **a, b, c,** and **e**   **d** is false. The PCR should be free of assumptions and judgments. Facts, findings, and observations are most appropriate. Describe *behaviors* of the patient (e.g., "is slurring words," "smells of alcohol," etc.). **(Objectives 10 and 11)**

22. Patients with possible spinal cord injuries; angry, hostile family members or friends; combative or confused patients; restrained patients; possible criminal activity; patients whose conditions deteriorate while they are en route to the hospital; long transport times; breakdown of equipment or the ambulance; deviations from known standards or protocols; and refusals of treatment or transportation. **(Objective 12)**

23. **(a)** vital signs; and **(b)** neurologic assessment.

    Because a patient's condition can change quickly, serial assessments should be conducted and the information recorded; the receiving hospital should be provided with this information, and it can have legal importance for the paramedic. **(Objectives 9 and 12)**

CHAPTER 15: Scene Assessment, Safety, and Control

1. **b** When you are entering a potentially hostile or dangerous situation, the safety of both you and your partner is a priority. If you are injured, you cannot provide assistance to the patient. Although the number of potential patients, the patient's level of consciousness, and other specifics about the location are important, your first priority is to ensure that the scene is safe. **(Objectives 1 and 2)**

2. **b** Again, scene safety is the first priority. **(Objective 2)**

3. **Yes.** Entering an unknown situation warrants careful attention to infectious disease precautions. Identifying risks is the first crucial step. The caller said that there was a lot of bleeding. Protective equipment should be in place before you enter the scene. This includes gloves, masks, and gowns that help to prevent exposure to airborne or blood-borne pathogens. **(Objective 8)**

4. You should stand off to the side, rather than in the front of the door, to lessen the risk of being struck by any objects. **(Objective 2)**

5. Tactfully, but firmly, explain why his condition warrants hospital evaluation. Acknowledge that emotions are high, and that his apparent alcohol consumption may be affecting his judgment. Tell him that you are concerned that his injuries may have serious consequences. You strongly advise him to consent to transport to the hospital. If he still refuses, you could operate under the law of implied consent, given his altered mental status. It is clear that he cannot make a safe and prudent judgment for himself. In some systems, medical direction may be contacted for assistance. Local protocol should be followed. **(Prerequisite Chapter Objective)**

6. Retrospectively, the medical director has provided valuable feedback. Your concern for the patient's welfare and potential injuries was warranted. Additionally, your persistence in transporting the patient was legally correct. Allowing him to refuse (with his altered mental status) could have been considered abandonment, which raises the potential for liability. Postrun review by the medical director, which includes providing feedback to paramedics, is an important aspect of quality assurance and medical accountability. **(Prerequisite Chapter Objective)**

7. Expect the unexpected, and be alert to sudden happenings; be aware of all potentially dangerous neighborhoods and situations; plan the entrance, exit, and escape routes in advance; keep an eye on the surrounding area, not just the patient. It's best to have one person in charge of the scene; be especially careful when you are entering a building; knock, wait, and look before entering a residence; constantly monitor your vehicle and equipment. **(Objectives 1 and 3)**

8. Know the response area; take a few seconds to look around; be aware of an open front door with lights on inside; don't get sidetracked by a "trail of blood"; look through windows of houses and vehicles on approach; stand off to the side when you are knocking on doors. **(Objectives 1 and 2)**

9. **a, b, c,** and **d** These are all appropriate measures to take to gain immediate control of the scene. Removing the hostile bystander yourself is neither appropriate nor necessary because the police are available. It could also be dangerous for you and your partner. **(Objective 6)**

10. Friends, family, and bystanders can be valuable resources at an emergency scene. They must be reassured and informed. However, in certain cases, a conflict may still develop. If bystanders become unruly or agitated, they must be controlled. Sometimes removal is the only solution, but it is best to avoid this, if possible. **(Objective 7)**

11. The environment in which the patient is found; drug paraphernalia, beer cans or liquor bottles, or medication bottles. **(Objective 5)**

12. **c** Narcan® is used to reverse the effects of a suspected narcotic overdose (the patient has pinpoint pupils and needle tracks). The patient's decreased level of consciousness precludes the use of activated charcoal; epinephrine is a cardiac drug, and albuterol is used for treatment of respiratory problems. **(Prerequisite Chapter Objective)**

13. Acknowledge her concern, and explain what you are doing. Reassure her that you are taking good care of her roommate, and that you will take her to the hospital as soon as possible. You may give her a simple task to perform (such as holding up the IV bag or gathering up the patient's personal belongings to take to the hospital) that helps both you and her. **(Prerequisite Chapter Objective and Objective 7)**

14. This can provide "clues" to the situation you are about to encounter. You can prepare for and anticipate potential problems at the scene as well. **(Objective 1)**

15. Family disturbances, bars and taverns, gang territory. **(Objective 1)**

16. **(a)** Consider the potential for hazardous materials exposure on any call to an industrial scene. Don't enter or go near if hazardous material is suspected. Eye, ear, or breathing protection may be required.

    (b) Any setting in which radioactive materials are present poses special threats because radiation is odorless and colorless. Thorough knowledge of what the rescue team may be exposed to is essential. Do not enter the scene until you know what is present.

    (c) Without someone knowledgeable about it to help, large farm machinery can be dangerous. Agricultural chemicals (particularly silo gas) may be present, and confined space rescue may be needed, in some cases. A response area that includes agricultural operations should be surveyed, and preplanning should be done to identify any unusual risks. Rescue/disentanglement procedures should be avoided, unless those present have had special training. **(Objective 4)**

17. **b** Close to the scene or in the middle of the highway may both be unsafe locations. If you arrive before police do, parking between the oncoming traffic and the emergency scene is standard procedure. **(Objectives 1 and 2)**

18. You can eliminate certain distractions at the scene by turning down the stereo/TV, removing pets, and moving small items that are in the room to improve patient access. Additionally, the paramedic should control traffic/access to the area; remove relatives/bystanders who are overly vocal or demanding; and find tasks for concerned relatives/bystanders to do. **(Objective 6)**

CHAPTER 16 Mechanism of Injury

1. Lethal injuries can occur as energy is changed in form. Understanding this "transfer of energy" is an important concept in determination of the mechanism of injury. The most severe form of impact occurs when an outside force meets a moving object straightaway, or "head-on." Thus, the potential for injury in this case is very high. **(Objectives 4, 7, and 8)**

2. The lower region. Compression of the lower torso and significant orthopedic injuries are likely. This often occurs as the "down and under syndrome" in high-speed, head-on collisions. **(Objectives 4, 7, and 8)**

3. **(a)** The car strikes the other car head-on.
   (b) The passenger hits the ground after ejection.
   (c) Internal organs collide during both a and b. **(Objective 5)**

4. **True.** Unrestrained occupants are much more likely than those restrained by seatbelts to suffer serious head trauma and other injuries. Once the occupant is "airborne," the potential for fatal injury increases significantly. **(Objective 7)**

5. **False.** Shear injuries are highly probable with rapid deceleration because the supporting ligaments tear on impact. **(Objective 6)**

6. **True.** The most significant factor in the equation of "kinetic energy" is velocity, or speed. $KE = Mass/2 \times Velocity^2$. This is so because energy changes in form (motion). **(Objective 4)**

7. When trauma produces obvious wounds (whether they are serious or not), prehospital personnel may tend to focus their attention on them. Often the less obvious injuries are more likely to be lethal. Based on the mechanism of injury in this situation, it is important to have a high index of suspicion for potential injuries. This patient has been in a "rollover," and it is likely that he sustained injuries other than the head lacerations. **(Objectives 1 and 7)**

8. Documentation should include a description of the patient's neurologic status to verify the patient's ability to make a conscious, informed decision; there should also be a record of the explanation that you gave to the patient regarding your concerns about his refusal of care and the potential problems that could occur. **(Prerequisite Chapter Objective)**

9. **c**
10. **a**
11. **a**
12. **c**
13. **b**
14. **b**
15. **a**
16. **a**

    (Objective 2)

17. **b** All are factors in enhancing trauma care, but research has shown that the most important factor for improving patient outcome is narrowing the window of time between the incident and definitive care. **(Objective 3)**

18. **c** According to the basic laws of physics and kinetic energy, energy that is "changed in form" can produce more lethal internal injuries. Given the basic equation, increased speed (velocity) has the greatest potential for affecting energy that is changed in form. $KE = Mass/2 \times Velocity^2$ **(Objective 4)**

19. **(a)** Shear is injury that occurs when organs tear at the point of attachment. Shear occurs in organs that are relatively free to move about inside the body, but are held in place at one or two points by a restraining ligament (e.g., aorta, liver, spleen, or kidney). **(Objective 6)**

(b) Compression is direct pressure applied to the heart, lungs, diaphragm, liver, or head and spinal column. Fractures to the skull or spinal column often result in brain or spinal cord injury. **(Objective 6)**

20. • Are there skid marks?
    • Were the victims wearing seatbelts?
    • Is there a "starred" windshield?
    • What was the estimated speed of the vehicles at the time of the collision?
    • Where are the areas of impact of the vehicles? **(Objective 2, 4, and 7)**

21. **(a)** After initial impact, occupants move backward and then may rebound forward. When there are low headrests in a car, the cervical spine can undergo extreme hyperextension, which can result in injury.

    (b) Even if the occupant is wearing a seatbelt, there is a high probability of lateral-medial (sideways) or rotational (twisting) motion of the head and cervical spine. There is little to no protection for the occupants. Unbelted occupants who collide with other occupants may experience internal injuries for which there is little visible evidence.

    (c) Head and cervical spine injuries are very likely to occur. Also, unbelted participants may do serious damage to each other as the vehicle rolls.

    (d) ATVs are one of the most dangerous types of vehicle because of their instability. When the vehicle is moving up an incline and starts to tip over, the operator frequently steps off of it and the vehicle runs over the driver's leg, resulting in ankle and lower leg trauma.

    (e) A side rollover is the most frequent type of tractor rollover. Often the operator either is thrown clear or can crawl clear; thus, he avoids being crushed. Rear rollovers result in fatalities in almost all cases.

    (Objective 8)

22. **b** The lap belt/shoulder harness restrains both the upper torso and pelvis; it also greatly reduces forward motion. Although this type of seatbelt can be very beneficial, injuries still occur even when they are in place. **(Objective 9)**

23. **(a)** The cylinder housing for the air bag is quite hot immediately after deployment, and it may cause minor burns if the victim comes in contact with it soon after the collision.

    (b) The victim may experience respiratory difficulties as a result of inhaling the powder that is placed on the surface of the air bag when it is packed. **(Objective 9)**

24. **c** Even when helmets are worn, they may contribute to head or spinal injury as they bounce on the pavement, potentially compressing the cervical spine. **(Objective 7)**

25. **(a)** Adults tend to turn away from the vehicle to try to avoid the collision. Thus, the point of impact may be on the victim's side. Owing to their higher center of gravity, adults may also go through an "end over end" motion before landing on the ground.

    (b) Children often become transfixed as the vehicle approaches and many times are struck while they are looking directly at the approaching car. If, on impact, the child is thrown, then the relatively large head size of the child increases the chance that she will land on it. **(Objective 10)**

26. **a** Adults who jump from a high distance tend to land on their feet and then fall onto their buttocks or their outstretched hands. This mechanism can produce compression injury to the spine, lower extremity trauma, and fractures of the upper extremities. **(Objective 10)**

27. Shock waves from the blast can cause serious internal injuries; debris can be blown into the victim's body, leading to soft tissue and internal injuries; the victim may become a projectile and be thrown into fixed objects, resulting in almost any type of injury. **(Objective 10)**

28. **c** Increased velocity is associated not only with through and through injuries, but also with an increase in cavitation. It is best to assume that anyone who has been shot with a high-velocity weapon, including many types of rifles, has sustained serious injuries, even if the injuries are not visually apparent. **(Objective 11)**

29. **(a)** Stab wounds:
    1. What type of weapon was used? A sharp weapon sometimes produces bloodless injuries. A dull weapon can rip and tear as it enters, resulting in serious bleeding that is difficult to control.
    2. What type of knife was used? Serrated blades rip rather than cut. Quick entry may transect a vessel and cause little or no bleeding; slow application of a dull knife can produce devastating effects.
    3. Length of the blade, and the number and location of wounds are also important pieces of information.

(b) Gunshot wounds:
1. How large is the projectile, and what are its design characteristics? The larger the bullet, the greater its mass. Bullets such as those with hollow points "mushroom" and flatten out on contact, thereby increasing the amount of surface area that contacts the body. Bullets that are designed to tumble also cause an increase in the size of the injury.
2. Increased speed of the projectile = increased cavitation energy. Distance from gun to target is also an important consideration. **(Objective 11)**

CHAPTER 17 Initial Assessment

1. **c** This information indicates the patient's overall condition, and determination of level of consciousness should precede the evaluation of airway, breathing, and pulses. If the patient is unconscious, a different procedure may be required for checking the airway. **(Objective 2)**
2. Evaluate the airway. For a patient to breathe adequately, the airway must be open and free of any obstruction. **(Objective 2)**
3. Facilitate breathing through comfortable patient positioning; administer a high concentration of oxygen; assist ventilations using a BVM; and closely monitor the patient's respiratory rate. **(Objective 2)**
4. Briefly explain that you are monitoring her husband closely, and that the oxygen should help him immediately. Also, you can tell her that you will be in touch with a physician very soon, and that you will get him to the hospital as soon as possible. **(Prerequisite Chapter Objective)**
5. The medication could be out-of-date, or it may have been exposed to light and rendered ineffective; alternatively, the patient may be having a myocardial infarction. With the occurrence of infarction, nitroglycerin may or may not provide pain relief. **(Prerequisite Chapter Objective)**
6. Speed of capillary refill, the presence of any cyanosis, and pulse oximetry reading, if available. **(Objective 2)**
7. **d** Because there are more P waves than QRS waves, sinus rhythm, first-degree heart block, and wandering atrial pacemaker are ruled out. These rhythms are characterized by 1:1 conduction. In second-degree heart block, there are more P than QRS waves, but there is still a relationship between atrial and ventricular activity. There is no such relationship in this ECG rhythm. **(Prerequisite Chapter Objective)**
8. **e** The therapeutic effect of both of these actions is an increased heart rate. Adenosine is used to decrease the heart rate, and lidocaine suppresses ventricular ectopic activity. Additionally, lidocaine could be harmful and is contraindicated when this rhythm pattern is present. **(Prerequisite Chapter Objective)**
9. Acidotic. The patient's respiratory status and overall condition indicate the presence of hypoperfusion. This is associated with both poor perfusion and the build-up of acids in the blood. Alkalosis is not possible if excess acids are present. **(Prerequisite Chapter Objective)**
10. Talking to him and observing his response; frequently checking his radial pulse (presence, quality, and rate); closely observing his respirations and noting any indication of respiratory distress; and carefully observing the ECG monitor. Also, palpate blood pressure, if it is practical to do so. **(Objective 2)**
11. **c** Obtaining a verbal response should be attempted before eliciting a painful response, such as by pinching or performing a sternal rub. Because the cervical spine could be involved, you should not sit her up until you have determined what happened. **(Objectives 2 and 4)**
12. **d** If the patient can speak, then airway, breathing, and pulse are intact. **(Objectives 2 and 4)**
13. **d** Assessment of the patient's airway, breathing, and circulation status is first priority. The patient's medical history, an ECG, and checking for needle tracks all are part of the focused history and examination, not of the initial assessment. **(Objective 2)**

14. **c** The environmental situation suggests heat exhaustion as the likely cause of this incident. The patient's age is atypical of a heart attack victim, and she allegedly has used no drugs today. Although she has been drinking, she has eaten and thus is not likely to be hypoglycemic. **(Prerequisite Chapter Objective)**

15. **b** Obtaining and correlating the history, as well as performing a physical examination, are part of the focused history and examination, not of the initial assessment. **(Objective 1)**

16. **d** A modified jaw thrust, as opposed to the head tilt/chin lift, should be used to open the airway for a trauma patient if cervical spine injury is suspected. Evaluation of a patient's respiratory status and level of consciousness is performed in the same manner for all patients. Initial assessment is performed on the scene, regardless of whether the injuries are traumatic or medical in origin. **(Objective 5)**

17. **A — alert.** The patient is aware of his or her identity and of the surroundings, and is able to respond appropriately to questions.

    V — verbal. The patient must be stimulated by sound (such as voice) before a response is obtained.

    P — painful. The patient responds only to a painful physical stimulus, such as a sternal rub.

    U — unresponsive. The patient does not respond to any stimulus, whether verbal or painful.

    (Objective 4)

18. Reposition the head. In an unconscious patient who is lying supine, the most frequent cause of obstruction is the tongue. Repositioning usually alleviates this problem. **(Objective 6)**

19. **d** A respiration rate that is lower than 8 or greater than 24 indicates the need to ventilate the patient. Assessing for a tension pneumothorax, checking circulation, and preparing to intubate would occur after the patient has been ventilated. **(Objectives 2 and 6)**

20. **c** Assessments of blood pressure, speed of capillary refill, pulse oximetry, and skin condition augment the circulatory status evaluation, but measurement of pulse is the first priority. **(Objective 2)**

21. **(a)** Carotid artery

    (b) Brachial artery

    (c) Radial artery

    (Objective 2)

22. **b** If ventricular fibrillation is present, the patient should be defibrillated immediately. Currently, a precordial thump is not recommended. Emergency drugs and intubation, when indicated, are secondary in importance to defibrillation. **(Objective 6)**

23. **b, c, d,** and **e** If the patient had experienced a cardiac arrest, there would be no pulse. **(Objective 2)**

24. The paramedic's initial impression of the patient detects an obviously ill appearance, external bleeding, vomiting, sweating, convulsions, and flushed and/or pale skin. Talking and listening to the patient assists in determination of the patient's level of consciousness, breathing status, and degree of pain. The sense of smell can also be helpful in the identification of odors, such as acetone (fruity breath) or alcohol. **(Objective 3)**

CHAPTER 18: The Patient With Airway and Breathing Compromise

1. **Yes.** The history provided indicates airway obstruction by choking. The patient was eating when she became symptomatic. The most common source of obstruction is food. This patient is also elderly. The elderly are the most frequent victims of foreign body airway obstruction. This patient presented clutching her throat, which is the universal sign of distress in a choking patient. The employee described performing the Heimlich maneuver, which is the appropriate treatment for clearing an obstruction in a conscious patient. **(Objective 7)**

2. **No.** Cricothyrotomy is an invasive procedure that may be necessary, but only after the obstruction cannot be relieved by conventional methods. The next appropriate intervention would be to use a laryngoscope to examine this patient's upper airway and Magill forceps to remove or dislodge anything that is found there. **(Objective 7)**

3. One of the most significant problems that can be caused by ventilation is gastric distention. This occurs when the patient is ventilated too quickly and with too great a volume of air. Pharyngeal pressure then exceeds esophageal opening pressures and forces air into the stomach. This air restricts the ability of the diaphragm to contract, thus reducing the available lung volume during ventilations, and making vomiting likely. Respiratory alkalosis also can occur as the result of excessive CO_2 elimination. To minimize the chance of either gastric distention or respiratory alkalosis, ventilations that last 1 1/2 to 2 seconds should be provided. Administer between 12 and 20 ventilations per minute (one breath every 3 to 5 seconds). This allows for adequate inspiration and expiration times. When the bag-valve mask is used, the bag should be squeezed smoothly, not forcefully. **(Objective 7)**

4. Her level of consciousness, heart rate, and skin color should improve, ultimately returning to normal. **(Objectives 4 and 6)**

5. **Yes.** An IV of normal saline or Ringer's lactate should be established at a TKO rate; also, the patient should be placed on a cardiac monitor. **(Objective 7)**

6. In the range of 35 to 45 mm Hg. **(Objective 8)**

7. Based on his ability to speak, you can conclude that he is not experiencing severe breathing problems. **(Objectives 4 and 6)**

8. Inspect the chest for symmetrical movement. Look for the use of accessory muscles and retraction of the intercostal muscles. Note any tenderness, crepitus, or air leakage that may present as subcutaneous emphysema. If possible, auscultate breath sounds with the patient in a seated position. This should be done in a symmetrical pattern; take the time to check all fields. Determine the patient's breathing rate and quality of respirations. Note the location and size of the wound caused by penetration of the knife, as well as the amount of bleeding. Look for more than one entry wound and for other possible injuries. **(Objective 4)**

9. **d** Both the mechanism of injury and the hissing noise coming from the chest indicate a sucking chest wound. **(Objective 3)**

10. This wound should be covered with an occlusive dressing that is taped down on three sides. This technique provides a valvelike action that enables air to escape during expiration, thus preventing tension pneumothorax. It also prevents air from entering the wound during inspiration. **(Objective 7)**

11. **Yes.** This patient requires transport to a Level I trauma center. Rapid recognition of the severity of the patient's actual and potential problems and making an early decision about transport priority are essential. Transport to a hospital that is not a Level I trauma center could delay the delivery of appropriate and definitive care. **(Prerequisite Chapter Objective)**

12. Tension pneumothorax. Open the occlusive dressing to allow air to escape from the pleural space; begin positive pressure ventilation. **(Objective 7)**

13. Although it is a late sign that can be difficult to spot, a deviated trachea is also a good indication of a tension pneumothorax. **(Objectives 4 and 6)**

14. Chest decompression is the definitive treatment for tension pneumothorax. This is performed by inserting large-gauge, 2 1/4-inch needle into the second intercostal space at the midclavicular line. **(Objective 7)**

15. **b** Croup is a viral disease that most often affects children younger than age three. Patients present with stridor, barking cough, and sometimes a low-grade fever. Epiglottitis is a bacterial infection that progresses rapidly and often affects children between the ages of three and seven. They present with significant stridor, drooling, inability to swallow, throat pain, and a high fever. Asthma is caused by bronchial constriction and occurs less frequently in toddler-aged children. Such patients with asthma present with wheezing and respiratory distress. Although pneumonia certainly can occur in a two-year-old, this patient is not symptomatic for pneumonia. **(Objective 3)**

16. **Yes.** The humidity created by the running shower may have decreased the subglottic edema, ultimately improving the child's respiratory efforts. **(Objective 7)**

17. To avoid upsetting the patient; the patient's becoming upset could aggravate her condition. In the field, it is often difficult to distinguish between croup and epiglottitis. If epiglottitis is present, examination of the oropharynx may result in laryngospasm and complete airway obstruction. **(Objective 7)**

18. Stridor, intercostal muscle retractions, and accessory muscle use become more prominent as the obstruction progresses. Severe suprasternal retractions also may develop. **(Objectives 4 and 6)**

19. Nebulized racemic epinephrine. **(Objective 7)**
20. **(a)** right lung; **(b)** bronchioles; **(c)** pulmonary capillaries; **(d)** nasopharynx; **(e)** oropharynx; **(f)** epiglottis; **(g)** larynx; **(h)** trachea; **(i)** bronchus; **(j)** left lung; **(k)** diaphragm; **(l)** alveolus. **(Objective 1)**
21. **b (Objective 1)**
22. **c (Objective 1)**
23. **d (Objective 1)**
24. **a (Objective 1)**
25. Rhonchi **(Objective 5)**
26. Friction rub **(Objective 5)**
27. Rales or crackles **(Objective 5)**
28. Snoring **(Objective 5)**
29. Stridor **(Objective 5)**
30. Wheezes **(Objective 5)**
31. **(a)** 500 mL

    (b) 12 to 20 times per minute

    (c) 95% to 100%

    (Objective 8)

32. When the patient is so large that you cannot reach around his or her waist; and when the patient is noticeably pregnant. **(Objective 7)**
33. The tongue; foreign bodies; swelling of the airways; trauma to the airways. **(Objective 3)**
34. Emphysema; chronic bronchitis; asthma. **(Objective 3)**
35. This patient most likely has a flail chest. Treatment includes spinal immobilization, which is required because of the possibility of spinal injury based on the mechanism of injury; administration of 100% oxygen by positive pressure ventilation, which helps in ensuring an adequate ventilation volume; stabilization of the flail segment with a pillow or towels, which improves the expansion ability of the lungs on the affected side; rapid transport to a trauma center, which minimizes the delay to definitive treatment; and initiation of both an IV line of normal saline or Ringer's lactate delivered at a TKO rate and a cardiac monitor to detect dysrhythmias. **(Objectives 3 and 7)**
36. This patient most likely has sustained a massive hemothorax with hypovolemic shock. Treatment includes administration of 100% oxygen by nonrebreather mask; rapid transport to a trauma center, which minimizes the delay to definitive treatment; initiation of at least one large-bore IV line of normal saline or Ringer's lactate and fluid bolus, which increases circulating volume; and monitoring of cardiac rhythm for possible ectopic secondary to hypoxia. **(Objectives 3 and 7)**
37. This patient most likely is experiencing an acute asthma attack. Treatment includes administration of 100% oxygen by nonrebreather mask; initiation of an IV line of normal saline or Ringer's lactate at the rate ordered by medical direction for possible dehydration; and provision of a beta-adrenergic aerosol such as albuterol to reverse the spasm with little effect on the heart (subcutaneous epinephrine may be indicated if the patient is unable to inhale nebulized aerosol). **(Objectives 3 and 7)**
38. This patient most likely is experiencing pulmonary edema. Treatment includes administration of 100% oxygen by nonrebreather mask; monitoring of cardiac rhythm for ectopic caused by hypoxia, acidosis, and increased workload on the heart; initiation of an IV line of D5W at a TKO rate to prevent increased circulating volume overload; and provision of a diuretic such as Lasix® to decrease the existing circulating volume overload. Morphine and nitroglycerin also may be used as vasodilators to reduce the oxygen demand on the heart. **(Objectives 6 and 7)**
39. **d** Changes in pCO_2, not pO_2, play the most important role in controlling respiration. Muscle movement reduces lung volume during expiration. Chemoreceptors in the medulla, carotid arteries, and aorta monitor pO_2 levels. **(Objective 2)**
40. **d** In complete airway obstruction, no air movement is taking place to enable production of sound. **(Objective 4)**
41. **b** Diminished, absent, or abnormal breath sounds are detected by auscultation of the chest. Distended neck veins are visualized; thus, attempts to detect them are not part of a routine assessment of the chest. **(Objective 4)**

42. **b** If you are unable to visualize the cords during an endotracheal intubation procedure, having another rescuer apply pressure over the cricoid membrane, which is known as the Sellick maneuver, may prove to be helpful. **(Objective 7)**

43. **d** In certain situations, intubation attempts take longer than expected, and the amount of time the patient has been without oxygen is far too long. The pulse oximeter's low saturation limit alarm can alert the paramedic that she should interrupt the intubation attempt to allow the patient to be reoxygenated through the use of appropriate ventilations. A high reading can indicate that the patient is hypoxic, especially in cases of carbon monoxide poisoning and smoke inhalation. Inaccurate readings also may result when there is excessive patient movement, which occurs often during the treatment of infants and children. **(Objective 7)**

CHAPTER 19: The Patient Without a Pulse

1. The amount of time that has passed since the pulseless patient's collapse; whether bystanders have started CPR. **(Objective 7)**

2. The patient in cardiac arrest. With lightning strikes involving several patients, standard triage priorities may be altered somewhat. In this situation, the arrested patient can be saved if the underlying dysrhythmia is corrected quickly. Those who survive a lightning strike are not likely to suffer later cardiac arrest; therefore, they do not need immediate attention. **(Objective 9)**

3. Instruct the coach to stop CPR. Assess the patient's vital signs, including consciousness, airway patency, breathing, and pulse. **(Objective 4)**

4. You should check the cardiac rhythm in at least two leads. **(Objective 7)**

5. Transcutaneous pacing. Although it is recognized as the definitive treatment for bradycardia, transcutaneous pacing rarely changes asystole and does not improve heart rate. Because this lack of success may be due to delays in initiating pacing, it must be started early in conjunction with drug therapy. **(Objective 7)**

6. Epinephrine, atropine, and possibly sodium bicarbonate. **(Objective 8)**

7. The quick response and delivery of CPR and defibrillation help to increase this patient's chance for survival. Effective CPR can prolong ventricular fibrillation until a defibrillator can be applied. Ventricular fibrillation can be corrected with early defibrillation; the outcome of defibrillation is related directly to the timing of its performance. **(Objective 5)**

8. Epinephrine is indicated; it can be administered down the endotracheal tube. Although the optimal dose of epinephrine for endotracheal delivery is unknown, a dose that is at least 2 to 2.5 times the peripheral IV dose (usually 1 mg) may be needed. **(Objective 8)**

9. Lidocaine is the next most appropriate drug and is indicated after the use of epinephrine for the treatment of ventricular fibrillation, per ACLS guidelines. Also, unlike Bretylium®, it can be administered endotracheally. **(Objective 8)**

10. The correct dose of epinephrine for use during cardiac arrest has been studied extensively. Animal studies have demonstrated that high doses cause increased blood flow, but human studies have failed to show improved outcomes. High-dose epinephrine is a class IIb choice under ACLS guidelines, and it could be used in this situation. **(Objective 8)**

11. Atropine may be indicated to increase the patient's heart rate. Dopamine or norepinephrine may be indicated if the patient remains hypotensive. If the heart rate increases, a Lidocaine® drip may be started to prevent the immediate recurrence of ventricular fibrillation after successful defibrillation. **(Objective 8)**

12. **d** This cardiac rhythm is PEA, pulseless electrical activity. PEA includes narrow and wide complex rhythms. There may be no mechanical function of the heart, or cardiac wall motion may be insufficient to generate a pulse. **(Objective 6)**

13. Traumatic arrest is usually the result of massive internal hemorrhage. Restoration of blood volume and control of ongoing bleeding can be accomplished only in the hospital. Patient survival of traumatic cardiac arrest is extremely rare; therefore, this patient should be transported rapidly. **(Objective 9)**

14. Transporting a cardiac arrest patient to the hospital can be an especially difficult task. It requires a coordinated effort among EMS personnel while they are moving the patient and providing care in the back of a moving ambulance. A backboard should be applied before the patient is moved onto the stretcher. Make sure the endotracheal tube is secured. This is also the time to apply an automatic compression and ventilation device, if it will not complicate the transfer of the patient to the ambulance. **(Objective 7)**

15. The endotracheal tube became displaced into the right mainstem bronchus when the patient was moved. You should reposition and rescure the tube, if it will not delay transport. The patient has no other clinical findings of a tension pneumothorax. If breath sounds are heard when the tube is repositioned, you can rule out a simple pneumothorax. **(Prerequisite Chapter Objective)**

16. **Yes.** Resuscitation should begin promptly on all patients who appear to have some potential for survival. The prognosis for cardiac arrest secondary to penetrating chest trauma, as was sustained by this patient, is more favorable than that associated with cardiac arrest secondary to blunt trauma. **(Objective 5)**

17. **a.** 1   **h.** 12
    b. 8   **i.** 10
    c. 5   **j.** 9
    d. 7   **k.** 3
    e. 11   **l.** 2
    f. 4
    g. 6
    (Objective 1)

18. a. **O**
    b. **D**
    c. **O**
    d. **D**
    e. **O**
    f. **D**
    g. **O**
    h. **D**
    i. **D**
    j. **O**
    (Objective 1)

19. 1. **i**
    2. **h**
    3. **g**
    4. **a**
    5. **b**
    6. **e**
    7. **c**
    8. **d**
    9. **j**
    10. **f**
    (Objective 2)

20. Metabolic acidosis; hyperkalemia; tricyclic overdose; prolonged resuscitation. **(Objective 8)**

21. 50 × 100 = 5000 mL or 5 liters. **(Objective 2)**

22. Pulseless electrical activity **(Objectives 6 and 7)**

23. Ventricular fibrillation **(Objectives 6 and 7)**

24. Asystole **(Objectives 6 and 7)**

25. **c (Objective 3)**

26. **c (Objective 2)**

27. **c** Early defibrillation is directly related to the degreee of success in conversion of ventricular fibrillation. **(Objective 5)**

28. **b** The tissue immediately surrounding the site of the infarction is often the source of the dysrhythmias. **(Objective 6)**

29. **c (Objective 6)**

30. **c** Younger patients who have been submerged in cold water have been known to recover fully, even after being submerged for longer than 30 minutes. Usually, they are found in an agonal rhythm, or in asystole. Intubation is extremely important to prevent further airway compromise. Suction should be performed first. **(Objective 9)**

31. **a** and **b** Additional medications, as well as defibrillation, should be withheld if body temperature is lower than 86° F. Initial clinical findings should not cause one to withhold resuscitation efforts. **(Objective 9)**

CHAPTER 20
The Patient With Compromised Circulation

1. Level of consciousness, airway and breathing adequacy, adequacy of pulse, and the presence of severe bleeding can be assessed rapidly in the conscious patient. You can conclude that this patient is conscious, has an open airway, is breathing, and has a pulse, based on her ability to provide appropriate responses to your questions. **(Objective 4)**

2. **No.** Although this patient responds to your questions appropriately and appears to be in no significant distress, it cannot be assumed that her circulation is adequate. She has several physical assessment findings that suggest compromised circulation. She has lightheadedness that could be the result of decreased cerebral perfusion. Also, her skin is pale and cool; this results from capillary constriction, which is part of a compensatory mechanism for redistributing blood to the core when circulation is compromised. **(Objective 3)**

3. A complete medical history; baseline vital signs; rapid head-to-toe physical examination. **(Objective 4)**

4. **Yes.** You should always administer oxygen. Supplemental oxygen helps in meeting the needs of this patient's tissues, which are oxygen-deprived from compromised circulation. An accurate patient history and careful evaluation of the cardiac rhythm help the medical professional to determine whether an electrical conduction abnormality is contributing to compromised circulation. This patient's slow pulse rate, her complaint of lightheadedness, and her pale, cool skin should signal possible cardiac dysrhythmia and inadequate perfusion. **(Objective 7)**

5. Shock, as indicated by this patient's decreasing level of consciousness, pulse, and blood pressure. **(Objectives 2, 3, and 5)**

6. A patient with bradycardia in the presence of compromised circulation requires rapid treatment. The first line of treatment is atropine IV push. Atropine acts by decreasing the effect of the vagus nerve. It does not always work, and when it does, its effect often lasts for only a few minutes. Atropine must be thought of as temporary help. Preparations for transcutaneous pacing should be started immediately. Placing the pads on the patient, while waiting to see if the atropine is effective, decreases the time needed to start the pacing. **(Objectives 2 and 7)**

7. **d** The goal of using the pacemaker is to stimulate cardiac contraction when the electrical conduction of the heart is malfunctioning, especially in complete heart block. Pulses should be palpated at the same rate as the pacer to ensure that there is capture by the heart. **(Objective 7)**

8. Dopamine, epinephrine, and Isuprel® are catecholamines. Catecholamines act on receptors in the heart and small peripheral blood vessels to increase cardiac output and blood pressure. The specific treatment that clinicians should initiate depends on the severity of the clinical situation. The following sequence of interventions recommended by the American Heart Association are in sequence of worsening clinical severity: atropine, trancutaneous pacing, dopamine, epinephrine, and Isuprel. **(Objective 8)**

9. When dispatched for unconsciousness, as well as chest pain, heart attack, and any form of significant trauma, you should think about the patient's condition and possible presentation, and consider what immediate treatment may be needed on your arrival. Determine roles and responsibilities, such as who will gather patient history, handle the patient's airway and breathing problems, and perform other critical procedures. **(Objective 7)**

10. When did the pain begin?

    Does anything make it better or worse?

    What does the pain feel like?

    Does the pain radiate to any other place?

    Rate the severity of the pain on a scale of 1 to 10, with 1 being no pain and 10 being the worst pain you have ever had.

    (Objective 4)

11. Myocardial infarction; abdominal aneurysm. **(Objectives 2 and 6)**

12. **c** This patient presents with signs and symptoms that are characteristic of active gastrointestinal bleeding. These include coffee ground emesis (produced by the mixture of blood with stomach acids), black stools (called *melena*, which is created by the partial digestion of blood as it passes through the gastrointestinal tract), and abdominal pain. This patient is also symptomatic for hypovolemic shock resulting from blood loss. **(Objective 6)**

13. You can assume that his systolic blood pressure is at least 80. In general, an adult's radial pulse cannot be palpated when the systolic blood pressure is lower than 80 mm Hg. **(Objective 5)**

14. **No.** A tilt test is used to determine if a patient has lost a significant volume of blood or body fluid; however, it should not be conducted if the patient, as in this case, is already showing signs of compromised circulation in a supine position. **(Objective 5)**

15. **No.** An IV line of crystalloid solution should be established, preferably with a large-bore IV cannula, while you are en route. Whenever a patient, such as this one, is a candidate for urgent transport because of internal bleeding, you must weigh the value of performing a procedure such as an IV setup at the scene against the transport time that is lost. Whenever possible, it is preferable to establish intravenous lines while you are en route to the hospital. **(Objective 7)**

16. **a, b,** and **d** PASG is indicated for hypovolemic shock when the systolic blood pressure is below 80 to 90 mm Hg with signs of poor perfusion. PASG also has been shown to be beneficial in tamponading certain types of bleeding. Volume replacement with IV fluids eliminates circulation problems that are caused by internal bleeding. The initial infusion is administered at a wide-open rate until the blood pressure is above 90 systolic. Placing the patient in the Trendelenburg position improves perfusion to vital organs by minimizing the amount of blood pooling in the lower part of the body during excessive blood loss.

    Although lidocaine is indicated for ventricular ectopia, the PVCs that this patient is having most likely are caused by hypoxia secondary to blood loss. The more appropriate treatment, in addition to administration of high-concentration oxygen and therapy to improve circulation, is to stop the gastrointestinal bleeding. This can be done effectively only in the hospital setting.
    (Prerequisite Chapter Objective and Objective 7)

17. **Low.** In the average adult, red blood cells account for 40% to 50% of the content of whole blood. The hematocrit is a measurement of the percentage of red blood cells in whole blood. This patient's hematocrit would be low because of his active gastrointestinal bleeding, and because of the hemodilution that results from administration of two liters of IV fluid. **(Prerequisite Chapter Objective)**

18. **Yes.** This patient is in distributive, or low-resistance, shock. This can be determined both by her recent medical history and by the following presenting signs and symptoms, which are consistent with shock: a decreased level of consciousness; a rapid, weak pulse; rapid respirations; cyanotic skin; and decreased blood pressure. **(Objective 6)**

19. Because hypoperfused skin attains the temperature of the environment, hypothermia is a very real threat to the patient in shock. **(Objective 7)**
20. Cyanosis at the lips and mouth is called *central cyanosis*. It indicates that this patient is experiencing hypoxia and hypoperfusion. In general, oxygen-deficient blood must be present in the skin capillaries for cyanosis to be evident. **(Objective 3)**
21. This patient is having a severe anaphylactic reaction with hypoperfusion. She is exhibiting signs and symptoms of uncompensated shock; if these are not reversed quickly, irreversible shock could result. If epinephrine is given subcutaneously in this situation, it may not reach the general circulation in time to be effective. **(Objectives 2, 7, and 8)**
22. In anaphylactic shock, a disruption occurs in the vessels that is caused by loss of tone and vasodilation and by increased permeability. This results in decreased blood return to the heart; ultimately, less blood is available for the general circulation. **(Objectives 1 and 5)**
23. **b** Although increased heart rate is a therapeutic effect of epinephrine, the drug was administered to this patient for its vasoconstricting and bronchodilating actions. Therefore, tachycardia is an adverse reaction in this patient. **(Objective 8)**
24. A functioning heart; an adequate blood volume; an intact vascular system. **(Objective 1)**
25. Conjunctiva; mucous membranes; ear lobes. **(Objectives 3 and 4)**
26. The presence of rales in both lungs, particularly if there is a history of heart failure, makes fluid challenge inappropriate. **(Objective 7)**
27. Because of the possibility that non-demand transcutaneous pacing could discharge during the vulnerable period of the cardiac cycle. **(Objective 7)**
28. **d (Objective 6)**
29. **b (Objective 6)**
30. **e (Objective 6)**
31. **c (Objective 6)**
32. **e (Objective 6)**
33. **a (Objective 6)**
34. **b (Objective 6)**
35. **a (Objective 6)**
36. **b (Objective 7)**
37. **a (Objective 7)**
38. **f (Objective 7)**
39. **g (Objective 7)**
40. **d (Objective 7)**
41. **d** The strength of the radial pulse is a simple indicator of perfusion status. **(Objective 4)**
42. **a** Major fractures, such as pelvic or femoral fractures, can result in a hidden blood loss of 1 to 2 liters, as well as damage to other organs and structures that help maintain adequate circulation. **(Objective 6)**
43. **c** A rigid abdomen and melena for 3 days are strong indicators of gastrointestinal bleeding. Negative orthostatic vital signs indicate that this patient has not had significant bleeding. An appendectomy scar is not related to his current problem. **(Objective 3)**
44. **d** Epinephrine is used to treat distributive shock caused by anaphylaxis. Dopamine often is used to treat hypotension associated with cardiogenic shock. Procainamide is used to treat ventricular dysrhythmias. **(Objective 8)**

Chapter 21: The Critical Trauma Patient

1. **b** Ascertaining the number of victims, evaluating vehicular damage, and setting up flares should not be attempted until the scene is safe. **(Prerequisite Chapter Objective)**

2. Making the scene safe can include summoning additional support; properly positioning the ambulance; placing flares or reflective warning devices; diverting traffic; and stabilizing damaged vehicles. **(Prerequisite Chapter Objective)**

3. Split up and quickly evaluate both patients to determine the severity of the injuries and to decide which patient should be transported first. **(Prerequisite Chapter Objective)**

4. **a** Controlling the hemorrhage takes priority over obtaining a blood pressure reading and instituting any advanced life support measures (IV or PASG). **(Prerequisite Chapter Objective)**

5. **Yes.** Both patients require immediate transport because of life-threatening conditions. Victim #1 has a decreased level of consciousness (LOC) and a tender abdomen. Victim #2 has compromised circulation (signs of shock, hypoperfusion). **(Objective 7)**

6. Obtain baseline vital signs and a brief history; further evaluate the LOC; assess the head and neck for deviated trachea or distended neck veins; observe the patient's chest; palpate the ribs and sternum; auscultate lung and heart sounds; assess the abdomen, pelvis, and extremities for deformities, contusions, abrasions, punctures, burns, tenderness, lacerations, or swelling. **(Objective 5)**

7. **b** In an adult, a closed head injury does not produce enough bleeding to cause signs of hypoperfusion; nor would the forearm fracture cause such signs. There are no clinical indications of a tension pneumothorax. **(Prerequisite Chapter Objective)**

8. Glasgow Coma Score: Eye opening (2), verbal (3), + motor (5) = 10.

    Revised Trauma Score = Glasgow (3), systolic BP (2), + respiratory (4).

    Total Revised Trauma Score = 9.

    Several studies have demonstrated that the paramedic, using this assessment and scoring system, can determine effectively which patients should be transported to a trauma center. **(Objectives 3 and 4)**

9. Because the patient's condition presents a "load and go" situation, the decision is appropriate. Only lifesaving measures such as airway management and bleeding control should be performed at the scene. The patient is critical and requires immediate transport to a trauma center. Any other procedures (e.g., establishing an IV) should be performed while you are en route. **(Objective 7)**

10. Check with dispatch to determine if the police have been dispatched; do not approach the patient until police have secured the scene. **(Prerequisite Chapter Objective)**

11. You should focus the examination on identification and correction of problems such as:
    - Unconsciousness that affects airway patency
    - Any airway or breathing compromise
    - Quick evaluation of the circulation; control of obvious hemorrhage
    - Evaluation of the skin

    (Objective 5)

12. **a** The patient has signs of hypoperfusion with a penetrating chest wound; therefore, a "load and go" situation exists. The setup of ECG and IV and application of PASG (if applicable) can be performed in the ambulance while you are en route to the hospital. **(Objective 7)**

13. **d** Although the other injuries all are possible, the mechanism of injury and the patient's signs and symptoms suggest the strong possibility of tension pneumothorax. **(Prerequisite Chapter Objective)**

14. Needle decompression to relieve the tension pneumothorax. **(Objective 7)**
15. Sinus tachycardia. Yes, this rhythm is expected in times of stress or acute insult to the body. The sympathetic or "fight or flight" response is activated, which increases the heart rate in an attempt to circulate more blood. **(Prerequisite Chapter Objective)**
16. **No.** With all the controversy surrounding the use of PASG, most agree that it should not be used with chest injuries because they may be aggravated further by application of PASG. **(Objectives 5 and 7)**
17. Monitor respiratory status closely, including breath sounds and the work of breathing; check pulses; monitor ECG and palpate BP, if practical. **(Objectives 5 and 6)**
18. **Yes.** The overall goal in trauma care is a 10-minute on-scene time; cases in which a life-threatening procedure must be performed are practical and appropriate exceptions. **(Objective 7)**
19. Ruptured uterus and abruptio placentae. **(Objective 9)**
20. In the fetus, shock and hypoxia could occur, secondary to hypoperfusion of the mother. Fetal survival is greatly influenced by these conditions. Even though you are treating two patients, it is important to remember that the best treatment for the fetus is appropriate assessment and treatment of the mother. This should include oxygenation, control of bleeding, and rapid fluid replacement. **(Objective 9)**
21. high-concentration oxygen and IV Ringer's lactate. Also, you should position the patient on her left side or supine, with the right side of the spine board elevated to about 15 degrees. **(Objective 10)**
22. The golden hour is the time from the initial trauma event until the initiation of definitive care at the hospital. **(Objective 1)**
23. A patient may die within seconds to minutes after a critical injury, usually from major injury to the brain or the cardiovascular system. However, if the patient survives the initial trauma, the next 60 minutes are critical. Paramedics play a key role during this "golden hour" by providing life support measures: maintaining the airway; providing oxygen; limiting hemorrhage; stabilizing fractures; initiating fluid replacement; and delivering patient to the appropriate facility. **(Objective 1)**
24. Rapidly assess the scene and the patient; identify the patient as a high priority; enter the patient into the trauma system; begin transport within 10 minutes of arrival on the scene. **(Objective 2)**
25. **a** Although it is important to obtain the medical history when treating a patient with a sudden illness, it is less likely to be pertinent to a trauma patient's condition than is the mechanism of injury, unless the trauma was the direct result of the medical condition. **(Objective 5)**
26. A patient may appear stable at one moment, then may deteriorate quickly as internal injuries take their toll. The critical trauma victim should be reevaluated every 3 to 5 minutes during transport. **(Objective 6)**
27. **a, b, d,** and **e** A fractured humerus, unless it is associated with obvious signs of shock, is not an automatic load and go situation. **(Objective 7)**
28. **d** Eighty-seven percent of childhood trauma is a result of blunt trauma; 10% results from penetrating trauma and 3% from drowning. Although children do sustain burn injuries, these are not as frequent as injuries sustained in motor vehicle collisions and falls. Because children are smaller than adults, the impact from blunt trauma usually is distributed over a larger portion of the body. Thus, after blunt trauma in children, multiple injuries are more common than isolated injuries.
29. Aggravation of a spinal injury; partial airway obstruction. When the child is placed on a flat surface for spinal immobilization, his proportionately large head size may cause the neck to flex, which may worsen a potential spinal injury. Additionally, this can inadvertently block the airway as the result of tongue position and "kinking" of the trachea. **(Objective 8)**
30. **True.** A child's organs lie close together in a small space and have less protection from injury than do those of an adult. An adult has more tissue and fat in the abdominal cavity, which helps to cushion the organs from injury. **(Objective 8)**
31. **False.** The compensatory mechanisms of healthy children respond more quickly than those of adults. Children tolerate rapid heart rates and increased peripheral vascular resistance better than adults. Thus, they are able to maintain normal blood pressure in the face of hemorrhagic shock. **(Objective 8)**
32. **True.** Children have growth plates at both ends of the long bones. Special caution should be taken by the paramedic to avoid aggravating suspected fractures at or near joints. Any careless movement can damage the growth plate and compromise subsequent bone growth. **(Objective 8)**

Chapter 22: The Critical Pediatric Patient

1. Previous seizures, including febrile seizures, or a diagnosis of epilepsy; medications taken, including compliance with any for known seizure problems; possibility of toxic ingestion or exposure; vomiting and possible aspiration during seizure; recent trauma, particularly head injury; current fever or other signs of illness, especially headache or stiff neck; description of any seizure activity **(Objective 6)**

2. Other procedures that should be included in the examination of this patient include checking his temperature, dehydration status, and blood glucose level; and assessing the patient for any trauma incurred during the seizure. **(Objective 7)**

3. Cooling is performed with tepid rather than cold water to avoid overcooling. Overcooling is a real risk for pediatric patients because they lose heat quickly. A slightly febrile point at which to stop, such as 102° F, is usually ordered because body temperature is likely to continue to drop after active cooling is discontinued. **(Objective 7)**

4. This patient is experiencing status epilepticus because he has had two seizures without a lucid interval between them. Status epilepticus is a true emergency. If left untreated, it could result in severe dehydration, hypoxia, and hypoglycemia. **(Objective 7)**

5. Respiratory depression; hypotension. **(Objective 7)**

6. **Yes.** This patient must be monitored closely; in addition, an IV of lactated Ringer's solution at a TKO rate and dextrose in a 25% solution is indicated because the patient's blood sugar is less than 60 mg/dl. **(Objective 7)**

7. Transport was especially important to ensure a thorough evaluation of a first-time seizure and to make certain that a more rare and major problem, such as meningitis, does not go untreated because it presents subtly. **(Objective 7)**

8. Hypothermia, hypovolemia, and respiratory problems. **(Objective 8)**

9. Drying and heat conservation, which are promoted by covering the infant's head; airway clearing; proper positioning to maintain the airway and encourage fluid drainage; and physical stimulation to promote breathing. **(Objective 9)**

10. **a** Regarding skin color, peripheral cyanosis and sometimes mottling are normal immediately after delivery. Central cyanosis is a more significant sign; it indicates the immediate need for oxygen therapy. After opening and suctioning the airway, you should check the newborn's breathing. Respiratory rate should be rapid, and respirations should be deep enough to cause good chest rise. If the respiratory rate is slow or if depth is shallow, you should attempt a brief period of tactile stimulation and oxygen administration. Assisted ventilation is necessary if these measures do not lead to quick improvement in the patient. Heart rate is the best single sign of oxygenation and perfusion in the neonate. A rate of more than 100 beats per minute is normal. Lower rates call for immediate ventilation. Rates below 60 and those in the 60-to-80 range that do not improve quickly with assisted ventilation require the initiation of chest compressions. **(Objective 8)**

11. Immediate ventilation with oxygen using a bag-valve device. A heart rate less than 100 calls for immediate ventilation. Heart rate is the best single sign of oxygenation and perfusion in the neonate. **(Objective 9)**

12. This reduced compliance can make bagging difficult. Ventilation in the premature newborn may be necessary only with higher pressures than with the full-term newborn. It may be impossible to ventilate with bags that have functional pop-off valves, which generally are not recommended for prehospital pediatric care. When such bags are used, the valve most likely will have to be disabled. **(Objective 9)**

13. It is desirable, when possible, to let the lungs take over. Closely monitor spontaneous respiratory efforts, and try to wean the patient by slowing the rate of ventilation and gradually lowering inspiratory pressure. An increasing heart rate is a good sign that this weaning may work and should be attempted. If the patient is successfully weaned, administer warmed, humidified oxygen. **(Objective 9)**

14. **c** This newborn has an Apgar of 9: 1 for appearance (body pink, but extremities blue); 2 for a pulse over 100; 2 for crying; 2 for active movement; and 2 for respiratory effort. **(Objective 8)**
15. Sinus tachycardia **(Prerequisite Chapter Objective)**
16. Dehydration, which is indicated by a history of vomiting and diarrhea for 3 days; lethargy; cracked lips; sunken eyes; tenting skin; rapid, weak pulse; and rapid respirations. **(Objective 4)**
17. **d** The brachial and saphenous veins generally maintain their diameters better than the more peripheral veins. Although the external jugular vessels are large, they can be a difficult target in the child with a short, fat neck. **(Objective 4)**
18. Administer a rapid fluid bolus of 20 mL/kg of normal saline or lactated Ringer's solution; then, reassess and provide additional infusion, if necessary. **(Objective 5)**
19. Return of central and peripheral perfusion, as evidenced by improved vital signs, skin turgor, and improved mental status. **(Objectives 4 and 5)**
20. **c** Rales and cardiac wheezing are less frequent in children than in adults. Peripheral edema and jugular vein distention are present only rarely in children, even in cases of advanced heart failure. Pink, frothy sputum and rales are most often seen in adults. Pulmonary edema and CHF initially manifest in children as tachypnea and tachycardia. **(Objective 5)**
21. Unexpected death in a previously healthy child that has occurred during the first year of life and in the early morning hours while the child was sleeping; also, the presence of bloody froth around her mouth. **(Objective 4)**
22. **b** Unlike adult patients, for whom convenient standard equipment sizes and doses of medications are available, the size of the child patient determines appropriate equipment needs and medication doses. **(Objective 2)**
23. **a (Objective 4)**
24. Using the heel of one hand, compress the chest at a rate of 100 per minute, while providing a breath after each fifth compression. **(Objective 4)**
25. SIDS is a diagnosis of exclusion. It is applied only when an autopsy and full consideration of the child's history do not produce a clear cause of death. The emotional impact of infant death on the family is so devastating that some EMS systems have protocols that include at least limited resuscitation. One reason to transport is the parents' tremendous need for assistance, which can be met at least initially through hospital social services and contacts with support groups that hospital staff members can provide. **(Objective 4)**
26. The parents need complete support from you and your partner. You must refrain from any speculation or advice that might imply negligence or wrongdoing. Your demeanor should be totally positive and supportive. **(Objective 4)**
27. Infant deaths are among the most stressful of outcomes for many public safety workers who need to look after their own feelings, those of their partners and colleagues, and those of the families involved. Counseling, formal debriefing, and one-on-one venting with close friends all can be helpful. Denial and isolation may be harmful. **(Prerequisite Chapter Objective)**
28. **(a)** Croup, also called laryngotracheobronchitis
    (b) Provide cool, humidified oxygen and a position of comfort (defined as anything that reduces anxiety); also, it may be helpful to use nebulized racemic epinephrine. **(Objective 3)**
29. **(a)** Epiglottitis
    (b) Avoid all anxiety-provoking procedures, including airway visualization, IV initiation, and removal of the patient from parents; these could lead to complete airway obstruction. If complete obstruction does develop, high-pressure, bag-valve mask ventilation may force air around the obstruction. If apnea occurs from complete airway obstruction, intubation with a small-sized tube may be attempted. If intubation is unsuccessful, cricothyrotomy may be required. **(Objective 3)**
30. **(a)** Asthma
    (b) Using a calm, reassuring approach, provide humidified oxygen and nebulized albuterol or terbutaline. You also may need to administer subcutaneous epinephrine if the patient's condition becomes severe; a steroid preparation may be used if transport time is prolonged. **(Objective 3)**
31. **(a)** Foreign body obstruction
    (b) Administer five back blows alternately with five abdominal thrusts. Avoid blind finger sweeps. If repeated attempts fail, visualize the upper airway with a laryngoscope and remove the object with Magill forceps. **(Objective 3)**

32. **(a)** Bronchiolitis

    (b) Provide humidified, high-concentration oxygen by mask, if tolerated; help the patient to achieve a position of comfort; ensure continued parental contact. Nebulized albuterol sometimes is recommended for severe cases. **(Objective 3)**

33. **True.** This procedure requires caution because the trachea in very young children is very compliant, and undue pressure can result in airway compression or even tracheal injury. **(Objective 2)**

34. **True.** Significant gastric distention can cause upward pressure on the diaphragm and may restrict the effectiveness of ventilation. The success of gastric decompression using this method is enhanced by accurate determination of the appropriate tube size for acceptance by the pharynx and the proximal gastrointestinal tract. **(Objective 2)**

35. **False.** This technique is best reserved for patients who are older than eight years of age because the anterior and cephalad position of the glottis in younger children makes blind nasotracheal intubation difficult. **(Objective 2)**

36. **False.** Cuffed endotracheal tubes are not used in children who are younger than eight years of age because the tracheal rings in young children are poorly developed and can be damaged easily. **(Objective 2)**

37. **True.** This is so because in younger children it is difficult to locate landmarks and there is increased risk of severe bleeding. **(Objective 2)**

38. **False.** Direct visualization of the tube as it passes through the cords is the best way to confirm proper placement. **(Objective 2)**

39. When the infant or child is unable to protect the airway; when respiratory efforts are insufficient to support normal oxygenation and ventilation; and when increased intracranial pressure is suspected. **(Objectives 3, 4, 6, and 7)**

40. **d** Preexisting conditions, birth defects, and sudden infant death syndrome (SIDS) account for most deaths that occur during the first twelve months of life. Approximately 80% of nontraumatic cardiopulmonary arrests in children occur during the first year, half of these in the first three months. **(Objective 1)**

41. **c** You should approach all pediatric patients in a nonthreatening manner so that you can avoid worsening the patient's anxiety and aggravating his or her condition. **(Prerequisite Chapter Objective)**

42. **b** Edema, infection, and foreign body injury can constrict air passages and cause stridor. **(Objective 3)**

43. **d** Status asthmaticus is a prolonged, severe attack that is unresponsive to treatment. The child in status asthmaticus is typically exhausted, acidotic, and dehydrated, and has a distended chest caused by trapped air that cannot be exhaled through constricted airways. Carpopedal spasms are associated more often with hyperventilation syndrome. **(Objective 3)**

Chapter 23: Clinical Significance of Vital Signs

1. **b** It is important to give children of this age responsibility for providing the history. However, because of her respiratory distress, this patient may be unable to respond to questioning, and her energy should be reserved for breathing. Therefore, the mother should continue to provide pertinent details. **(Prerequisite Chapter Objective)**

2. **No.** This patient is in obvious respiratory distress and has an abnormal respiratory rate. Although it is important that you measure the respiratory rate accurately in all patients, you should not withhold oxygen while doing so. **(Prerequisite Chapter Objective)**

3. **High.** This patient has multiple reasons for her pulse rate to be elevated. Such an elevation is expected after use of Atrovent; most medications used to treat asthma cause tachycardia. She is also anxious and hypoxic, which results in tachycardia that is caused by stimulation of the sympathetic nervous system. **(Objectives 1, 2, and 3)**

4. The width of the cuff should be 2/3 the diameter of the upper arm. Using a cuff of appropriate size results in an accurate reading. If the cuff is too large, it causes a falsely low reading; if the cuff is too small, the blood pressure reading is falsely elevated. **(Objective 5)**

5. **No.** This patient's irregular pulse is due to sinus arrhythmia. This is a normal phenomenon that is seen often in children. It is caused by the inhibitory vagal effect of respiration on the SA node. **(Prerequisite Chapter Objective)**

6. **(a)** Respirations would decrease because the patient is tiring and is losing the ability to move air; thus, she is retaining CO_2. Initially, the patient would be tachycardic as a result of hypoxia. The heart rate may become bradycardia when there is severe hypoxia and acidosis, and the blood pressure would eventually fall.

   (b) If treatment is effective, respirations should return to a normal range of 18 to 25, and blood pressure to 80 to 110 systolic. A normal pulse rate of 70 to 110 may not occur because of the adverse effects of albuterol administration. **(Prerequisite Chapter Objective and Objectives 1 and 2)**

7. **(a)** Vital signs vary dramatically with age. Elderly patients may not show expected alterations in pulse rate. Systolic blood pressure normally increases with age because of the decreasing elasticity of the arterial walls.

   (b) Beta blockers, such as propranolol, inhibit stimulation of the beta-adrenergic receptors of the heart, thereby preventing the patient from developing a normal tachycardic response. In turn, the blood pressure may also lower because of decreased cardiac output. **(Objective 2)**

8. In dissecting aortic aneurysms, one or more vessels of the aortic arch may be compromised. Disruption through the innominate artery is likely to produce a difference in blood pressure between the two arms. **(Prerequisite Chapter Objective)**

9. **Yes.** Discrepancy between the blood pressure readings in both arms, along with the quality and sudden onset of pain, are highly suggestive of dissecting aortic aneurysm, which is a life-threatening emergency. Serious complications, including death, can develop quickly. Additionally, this patient is already symptomatic of early shock as evidenced by his diaphoretic skin and elevated respiratory rate. **(Objectives 3 and 4)**

10. The pulse pressure, which is the difference between the systolic and diastolic blood pressure readings, has narrowed. This is a classic characteristic of cardiac tamponade. Cardiac tamponade is a complication of dissecting aortic aneurysm that results from aortic rupture into the pericardium. **(Prerequisite Chapter Objective)**

11. **c** This patient's rhythm is pulseless electrical activity. Epinephrine is the initial drug of choice. **(Prerequisite Chapter Objective)**

12. **Yes.** Regardless of his neurologic status, the mechanism of injury is reason enough to immobilize this patient. **(Prerequisite Chapter Objective)**

13. The increased vital sign values could indicate that this patient is in compensated shock. Based on the mechanism of injury and the clinical findings, he could be experiencing bleeding from internal injuries. When a patient presents with tachycardia, the most serious consideration must be given to shock. **(Objectives 3 and 4)**

14. **b** Diaphoretic skin indicates that this patient is vasoconstricted from sympathetic stimulation, which is attempting to compensate for volume loss. Warm, dry skin is associated with both neurogenic and septic shock. Cardiogenic shock usually occurs in the setting of acute chest pain. **(Objective 4)**

15. Urgent. Based on the mechanism of injury and the clinical presentation, this patient needs to be transported without delay to a Level I trauma center. **(Prerequisite Chapter Objective)**

16. **b** Respirations are frequently estimated; thus, they represent one of the most inaccurately assessed vital signs. **(Objective 3)**

17. **a** Hypotension does not occur until a significant amount of blood has been lost. **(Objective 3)**

18. **c** Cardiac output is the amount of blood that is ejected from the heart with each beat. Total peripheral resistance refers to the degree of constriction or dilation of the blood vessels. **(Objective 3)**

19–21. Rapid assessment of the pulse, in conjunction with information on the type of incident sustained and an evaluation of skin characteristics, helps to narrow the possible causes of shock. A patient who has tachycardia and warm, dry skin is manifesting shock from sepsis, anaphylaxis, or spinal trauma. In contrast, if the patient is hypotensive and tachycardic and has pale, cool, moist skin, the condition is most likely either hypovolemic or cardiogenic shock. **(Prerequisite Chapter Objective)**

19. **b (Objective 4)**

20. **a** **(Objective 4)**

21. **b** **(Objective 4)**

22. **b** The cuff is too large. **(Objective 5)**

23. **b** The cuff is too large. **(Objective 5)**

24. **a** The cuff is too small. **(Objective 5)**

25–32. Pulse rate can be affected by many factors. You need to understand what the expected vital signs, including pulse rate, are for patients with specific chief complaints and clinical presentations. When actual vital signs differ significantly from those expected, suspicion about the patient's level of risk should increase quickly. **(Prerequisite Chapter Objective)**

25. **a** This patient has a mechanism of injury and clinical findings that are consistent with hypovolemic shock. Tachycardia is an expected sympathetic compensatory response. **(Objective 2)**

26. **b** This patient has a mechanism of injury and clinical findings that are consistent with neurogenic shock caused by spinal injury. Bradycardia results from lack of sympathetic innervation. **(Objective 2)**

27. **c** Even though this patient has clinical findings that are consistent with an acute myocardial infarction (MI), his ECG indicates normal sinus rhythm. The heart rate associated with this rhythm is 60 to 100 beats per minute. **(Objective 2)**

28. **b** This patient has clinical findings that are consistent with cholinergic poisoning, which results in bradycardia. **(Objective 2)**

29. **b** This patient has a mechanism of injury and clinical findings that are consistent with a head injury and increased intracranial pressure, which can result in bradycardia as part of Cushing's reflex. **(Objective 2)**

30. **a** Amitriptyline is a tricyclic antidepressant. Tricyclic antidepressant toxicity may first manifest as sinus tachycardia. **(Objective 2)**

31. **a** You should expect a gradually increasing pulse when a patient manifests a rising temperature. **(Objective 2)**

32. **b** This patient has a history and clinical findings that are consistent with hypothermia, which can cause a profound bradycardia in which the pulse may not be palpable. The rhythm can be detected only on a cardiac monitor. **(Objective 2)**

33. **b** Atrial fibrillation is the only rhythm that is irregularly irregular with a pulse deficit. **(Objective 2)**

34. **a, b,** and **c** All three cause tachypnea and an increased respiratory rate. Hypothermia may cause a decreased respiratory rate that is so profound that the patient may appear to be not breathing. **(Objective 3)**

35. **a, c,** and **d** A tilt test, which is also known as orthostatic vital signs, is considered positive when there is a pulse increase of more than 20 beats per minute, or a blood pressure drop of more than 20 mm Hg, when the patient is moved from a supine to an upright position. These changes usually occur when 15% to 25% of the normal blood volume is lost.

   a Pulse rate increases by 22 beats per minute.

   c Systolic blood pressure decreases by 22 mm Hg.

   d Systolic blood pressure decreases by 20 mm Hg, and pulse rate increases by 24 beats per minute.

   (Objectives 1 and 2)

36. **a** Cardiac output will be decreased because the blood volume loss decreases venous return. **(Objective 2)**

37. **a** and **b** Third-degree heart block and increased intracranial pressure often result in bradycardia. **(Objective 2)**

CHAPTER 24 — Focused and Continued Assessment

1. **b** Ensuring that the airway is patent is a priority over checking circulation, pulses, or breath sounds, and it must precede steps toward obtaining a SAMPLE history. **(Prerequisite Chapter Objective)**

2. Describe the sensation of difficulty breathing.

   Do you have pain or discomfort anywhere else?

   Do you have any major medical problems?

   Are you taking any medications?

   Have you been outside today; have you been exposed to anything that is potentially harmful?

   Do you have any allergies?

   When was your last menstrual period?

   (Objectives 3, 4, and 6)

3. Possibly, she is having an allergic reaction to the medication. More information would be needed to support this conclusion, but it is a likely possibility. **(Prerequisite Chapter Objective)**

4. **(a)** Blood pressure, skin signs, and capillary refill

   (b) Further respiratory examination, including assessment of breath sounds, the use of accessory muscles, and the work of breathing; it is also important to check the ECG reading.

   A detailed physical examination is important for patients who have a respiratory complaint so that significant findings are not overlooked.

5. **e** Benadryl® is given to prevent any further release of histamine, and epinephrine is given as a bronchodilator and for its alpha effect on the cardiovascular system (peripheral vasoconstriction). Atropine is used to speed up the heart rate in bradycardia, and lidocaine is used for treatment of ventricular ectopy. Neither of these conditions exists in this patient. **(Prerequisite Chapter Objective)**

6. Monitoring her respiratory status, pulse, and blood pressure is most important. It is also important to observe the ECG monitor for any ventricular irritability secondary to the epinephrine and for any improvement in her overall symptoms. **(Objectives 12 and 15)**

7. Benadryl® prevents the release of histamine; it is also a central nervous system (CNS) depressant. This medication may cause symptoms of drowsiness or sleepiness, or other significant signs of an altered level of consciousness, such as confusion, disorientation, or unconsciousness. These signs should be monitored closely. **(Prerequisite Chapter Objective)**

8. The initial assessment should include a quick head-to-toe survey, which ascertains the presence of any life-threatening injuries, such as those that would require critical interventions. Essentially, this examination identifies major injuries that could involve airway compromise or exsanguinating hemorrhage. **(Prerequisite Chapter Objective and Objective 9)**

9. How did it occur?

   Did you feel like you were going to pass out or get dizzy before the fall?

   How did you land?

   Did you lose consciousness after the fall, or at any time?

   (Objectives 4 and 11)

10. Perform a focused history and physical examination. The first part of the assessment focuses on determining what factors are related to the patient's chief complaint. Once these are ascertained, the appropriate physical examination is performed. **(Objectives 1 and 2)**

11. Based on the mechanism of injury, a detailed physcial examination is necessary to rule out potentially serious injuries.

    (a) Vital signs: Assess level of consciousness; pulse rate, strength, and regularity; skin color and temperature; blood pressure.

    (b) Head: Feel for obvious deformities, swelling, or indentations in the skull; check the pupils for size and reactivity to light.

    (c) Neck: Look for any obvious abnormalities, jugular venous distention, or a deviated trachea.

    (d) Chest/Back: Palpate the sternum and ribs; listen to breath sounds and heart sounds; evaluate respiratory rate, depth, and pattern; palpate the back for deformation.

    (e) Abdomen: Check all four quadrants for discoloration, pain tenderness, distention, or rigidity.

    (f) Pelvis: If no pain is obvious, apply gentle compression to the pelvis to verify that it is intact.

    (g) Extremities: Carefully examine the injured ankle; look for appropriate movement, sensation, and circulation; check distal pulses in the ankle.

    (Objectives 11 and 15)

12. **S** — decreased sensation and movement of the lower extremities; signs of an ankle fracture; laceration to the head

    A — none known

    M — Catapres®

    P — high blood pressure

    L — lunch, about an hour ago

    E — slipped and fell; did not have any neurological symptoms or pain prior to the event

    (Objectives 4 and 6)

13. **b** With symptoms that suggest a neck or back injury, this would be the priority (based on the mechanism of injury). This would take priority over obtaining an ECG, stabilizing the ankle fracture, and starting an IV. **(Prerequisite Chapter Objective and Objective 8)**

14. **e** Increasing confusion, agitation, and restlessness may be symptoms of hypoxia, shock, or internal bleeding. These are also signs of increasing intracranial pressure that is consistent with a closed head injury. Based on the mechanism of injury, these complications certainly are plausible. **(Prerequisite Chapter Objective and Objective 8)**

15. **(a)** Gathering the history of the present illness or event (OPQRST)

    (b) Gathering a SAMPLE history

    (c) Obtaining vital signs

    (d) Conducting a rapid physical examination that focuses on the area of the chief complaint

    (Objectives 1 and 2)

16. **O** = onset; when the pain or illness began

    P = provoking or Palliative; when actions or situations bring on the symptoms or relieve the pain

    Q = quality; how the patient perceives the pain

    R = region of radiation or referral; where the pain is located and where it goes

    S = severity; the degree of pain the patient feels

    T = timing; how long and how often this pain has affected the patient

    (Objective 5)

17. **a, b, c, d,** and **e (Objective 15)**

18. **c** Flail chest is accompanied by uneven chest wall movement and signs of fractured ribs. Typically, it does not involve the cardiovascular system, which is associated with jugular venous distention. **(Prerequisite Chapter Objective)**

19. As the paramedic performs the physical examination, the mnemonic (DCAP-BTLS) is useful in facilitating recall of what areas to assess. The conditions in the mnemonic are evaluated as the head-to-toe survey is performed.

    D = deformities
    C = contusions
    A = abrasions
    P = punctures
    B = burns
    T = tenderness
    L = lacerations
    S = swelling

    (Objective 10)

20. **c** **a** involves the focused examination; **b** refers to the initial assessment; **d** is only one part of the continued assessment. **(Objective 12)**

21. Cardiovascular or respiratory complaints usually require that the paramedic perform a detailed physical examination. The areas to be evaluated are:

    Skin..................Check color, temperature, and moisture.

    Head/Face.......Check lips for cyanosis.

    Eyes.................Check pupils for size, equality, and reactivity to light.

    Neck................Note distended neck veins. Also, check in the sitting position. Check the suprasternal area for retractions and for use of accessory muscles.

    Chest...............*Inspection:* Note the presence of barrel chest or rib retractions; note the use of accessory muscles; assess for unequal movement.

    Auscultation: Listen to breath sounds and assess the quality of both sides. Note any rales, rhonchi, or wheezes. Check for irregular heart rhythm.

    Extremities.......*Inspection:* Check for the presence of swelling in the extremities.

    Upper & Lower Palpation: Palpate calves for tenderness and edema. Also, palpate for the presence or absence of pedal pulses; note capillary refill and nail bed cyanosis.

    (Objectives 7, 13, and 14)

22. When the situation is urgent, direct questions can provide information quickly. Open-ended questions elicit a better and more thorough description of what is occurring. *Examples:* Open question — "How does the pain feel to you?" Direct question — "Is this the worst pain you've ever experienced?" **(Objective 3)**

CHAPTER 25: Pediatric Assessment

1. Mentation and level of consciousness are important indicators of general perfusion status. Parental input is sometimes necessary to confirm variations from normal behavior. Signs that should be asked about and observed directly include mood, activity level, attention span, and willingness and ability to cooperate. **(Objective 4)**

2. **c** The examination should be gentle, quick, and limited to the pertinent essentials. Do not separate the child from the mother because anxieties about separation and strangers only make the examination more difficult. Provide concise explanations to both the child and the mother. **(Objective 4)**

3. Your pediatric patient has signs of the early stages of compensated shock, including cool skin, elevated pulse and respiratory rate, slow capillary refill, and mental changes that are different from normal. Based on the mechanism of injury (deceleration, patient unrestrained and ejected) and the anatomic differences characteristic of children (larger internal organs and softer chest wall), this patient could have sustained injury to the spleen and liver. As in adults, expediting transport of critical pediatric patients is essential. **(Objectives 1 and 6)**

4. **No.** Even though it is tempting at times to shade the truth for children and parents, this could compromise patient trust in paramedics and other caregivers. This does not mean that being brutally honest is appropriate, but fair warning should be given to patients about procedures that will hurt or be frightening. **(Objective 4)**

5. To identify developing crisis, which is especially important in this patient because relatively small amounts of bleeding could lead quickly to worsening of his potential shock state. Children lack one important compensatory mechanism for volume loss that adults have—increased cardiac contractility. Because contractility in children is relatively fixed, heart rate and systemic vascular resistance bear a greater burden in maintaining perfusion in the face of volume loss. This, in turn, places greater emphasis on the evaluation of heart rate and skin signs. **(Objectives 1 and 6)**

6. Explain to him that there are several ways in which he can build his confidence. One is to pursue further study of pediatric care. Another way is to increase his contact time with children. Participating in extra training in a pediatric unit, or simply volunteering to help in a day care setting, can prove valuable for developing communication skills and becoming comfortable around children. **(Objective 3)**

7. The mother. Even though the language skills of preschool-aged children may permit them to help with the history, their ability to understand usually exceeds what they can express. This child also may be in too much respiratory distress to effectively answer questions. **(Objective 4)**

8. Rate; mechanics; skin color; breath sounds; arterial oxygen saturation. **(Objective 5)**

9. As with adults, tachypnea is a compensatory response. When fatigue and advancing hypoxia begin to weaken the compensation, breathing slows, and eventually stops. Therefore, a full respiratory reassessment is necessary to detect any change in her condition. **(Objective 5)**

10. **Yes.** People, including children, need to control their bodies, feelings, and decisions. As long as she was able to self-administer the treatment effectively, allowing her to do so was appropriate. **(Objectives 4 and 6)**

11. Parental dignity is part of the pediatric care scenario. Avoid questions and comments that carry a critical or judgmental tone. Parents need to be validated for seeking help (they often feel guilty, even when they have done nothing wrong); they should be included in decision making and explanations and afforded the opportunity to accompany the child during transport. **(Objective 2)**

12. **b** The high activity level of toddlers means that they will become upset about restraint of any kind. **(Objectives 1 and 4)**

13. **a** The infant is likely to be frightened by the sudden appearance of strangers and takes many emotional cues from parents. **(Objective 1)**

14. **c** and **e** Preschoolers have anxiety about blood and mutilation or disfigurement, and body fears are often vivid. Adolescents are acutely aware of possible body disfigurement and other changes in physical image. **(Objective 1)**

15. **d** and **e** School-aged children are very modest and sensitive about exposing their bodies. Among adolescents, peer pressure and a growing awareness of sexual identity add to the need for privacy. **(Objective 1)**

16. Maintaining privacy while exposing the body is essential during the examination. Provide honest communication with an emphasis on positive outcomes; give explanations of procedures and the reasons for them. Ask an occasional question to ensure that she is understanding your explanations. Provide reassurance and praise about her courage and self-control. **(Objective 4)**

17. Talk with the mother first, while providing eye contact with the patient. Leave the patient in his mother's lap and allow him to hold a favorite toy or other possession during the examination. Get as close as possible to his face level, rather than towering over him. Your examination should be gentle, quick, and limited to the pertinent essentials. You may need to be playful to keep his attention focused where it is needed. Keep explanations simple. **(Objective 4)**

18. Treat with adult respect; provide reassurance that is tempered with honest talk about long-term consequences and outcomes. Offer choices whenever possible, and be clear and candid about why information is needed and briefly discuss the possible medical consequences of withholding it. Interviewing the patient privately, before talking with parents, may enhance the history. Take simple precautions to help preserve modesty during the examination. **(Objective 4)**

19. A larger tongue with a sharper angle between the mouth and glottis makes visualizing the cords more difficult. **(Objectives 1 and 4)**
20. The smaller cricoid ring increases the risk that a tube can be inserted that will fit through the glottis but then be stopped by the cricoid just below it. **(Objectives 1 and 4)**
21. Smaller sizes and shorter distances mean that tracheal tubes can be displaced with less movement, leading to bronchial or esophageal intubation. **(Objectives 1 and 4)**
22. **d** Accurate rate determination requires a minimum of 30 seconds of observation; a full minute is preferable in the youngest patients. **(Objective 4)**
23. **d** Tachycardia is a normal compensatory response that bears more of the responsibility for reinforcing perfusion in shock in children than it does in adults. Hypotension, mottling, pallor, and bradycardia are late signs of shock. **(Objective 1)**
24. **b** Like evaluation of color changes, refill measurements may be less reliable if the extremity is cold. The extremity should be held slightly above the level of the heart; if the extremity is lower, the refill may look normal as a result of gravity rather than arterial perfusion. Normal response is 2 seconds or less. Capillary refill is not an absolute sign, but it can be useful in conjunction with other signs during early to moderate shock stages; it is considered more reliable than blood pressure measurements. **(Objectives 1 and 5)**
25. **d** Fontanelles that appear tight or that bulge slightly may be a sign of increased intracranial pressure that is caused by infection (e.g., meningitis), bleeding, or swelling inside the skull that is associated with trauma. **(Objectives 1 and 5)**
26. **d** Soft tissue weakness leads to lowered lung compliance, which makes mechanical ventilation easy in pediatric patients. However, neonates have high lung compliance, especially immediately after birth; thus, more ventilatory effort is required of neonates than of infants. **(Objectives 1 and 4)**
27. **a** Pink membranes inside the eyelids and lips indicate that the central blood supply is well oxygenated. Peripheral color changes more likely are related to circulatory factors. Skin temperature provides information regarding circulatory status. **(Objectives 1 and 5)**
28. **a, c,** and **d** Level of consciousness can be documented objectively using the AVPU scale to describe the best response level to each stimulus. This avoids the inconsistency of using poorly defined adjectives (stuporous, obtunded) to describe unconscious states. **(Objective 5)**
29. **a, b, c,** and **d** **(Objectives 1 and 5)**

CHAPTER 26: Geriatric Assessment

1. Poor lighting, hazardous rugs, bulky clothing. **(Objective 3)**
2. This patient, like many elderly people, may be threatened by the thought of hospitalization and the resulting loss of independence. She also may have fear of being bedridden or institutionalized, and of losing her self-sufficiency. **(Objective 3)**
3. Was there any dizziness or loss of consciousness, or were there other similar warning symptoms before you fell?

    Any altered level of consciousness is pertinent in the history of a patient who has fallen. This could signify a more serious problem, such as a cardiac event, that requires immediate intervention. **(Objective 2)**
4. A thready pulse is usually associated with a rapid heart rate as the body tries to compensate for blood loss. With advancing age, cardiac output drops and the heart rate slows, thus decreasing the body's compensatory ability. The elderly may not have the ability to respond to blood loss because of medications or preexisting cardiovascular disease. Therefore, you should pay special attention to other early signs of shock, such as this patient's clammy skin. With her mentation and blood pressure, you can assume that she is in the early stages of shock. **(Objectives 3 and 4)**

5. **Yes.** Hip injuries are more frequent in the elderly than in any other age group because of the physiological changes of aging. There is a decrease in total skeletal muscle weight and in the density of bones, which makes them more susceptible to fracture, especially that resulting from falls. As a result of slowed reflexes and an impaired sense of equilibrium, the elderly have an increased incidence of falls and injury. **(Objectives 1 and 3)**

6. **Yes.** Spinal injuries, like other bone injuries, can occur with seemingly minor trauma because of chronic bone changes. This patient's mechanism of injury demands special attention to proper spinal immobilization. **(Objectives 1, 3, and 4)**

7. **Yes.** Based on this patient's presentation and your suspicions that she may be in early shock resulting from blood loss, an IV fluid bolus would be appropriate. You should reassess her cardiovascular status and breath sounds to evaluate her response to treatment. **(Objective 4)**

8. Hypoxia secondary to her respiratory condition; alcohol intoxication; excessive medication doses or interactions; depression; neglect. **(Objectives 3, 5, and 6)**

9. With aging, the cough reflex is diminished and the ability to clear secretions is lessened. **(Objectives 1 and 3)**

10. **Yes.** Pneumonia is the leading infectious cause of death in the geriatric age group; it is the fourth leading cause of death overall in patients over 75 years of age. **(Objective 3)**

11. Speak clearly and be positioned in good light and at eye level so that the patient can watch, as well as listen to, the questions. Speak in a normal tone and avoid shouting. Eliminate any distracting noises or sounds that could distract the patient. Writing notes may be necessary. Verify the history with the neighbor if he is knowledgeable about this patient's condition. **(Objective 2)**

12. You should inquire if this patient's condition represents a substantial change from her previous level of function. **(Objective 2)**

13. You should observe the surroundings for indications of inadequate self-care. Look for evidence of drug or alcohol ingestion. Check for a medical identification insignia, "vial of life" programs, or other indicators. Be alert for signs of violence or elder abuse. If possible, identify current versus old medications, including nonprescription drugs. **(Objective 2)**

14. **Yes.** This patient is experiencing an acute mental status change that is sudden in onset and that may be reversible. **(Objective 3)**

15. Remove dentures, if present, to facilitate proper airway management; suction secretions as needed; place her in a stable side position to facilitate drainage of secretions and to avoid aspiration; administer oxygen by nasal cannula; be prepared to assist ventilation as needed. **(Objective 4)**

16. Aging skin may have a thinner outer layer, and capillaries can be fragile and easily bruised. Considering these changes, you should handle this patient gently to avoid additional epidermal bruising and tearing. **(Objectives 1 and 4)**

17. **c** This patient has significant neurologic deficits, which are suggestive of stroke; these include acute onset of mental status change, aphasia, one-sided facial drooping, and decreased reflexes. She also has hypertension, which often accompanies stroke. **(Prerequisite Chapter Objective)**

18. Fewer taste buds may contribute to loss of appetite and poor nutrition; decrease in esophageal activity and gastric motility may cause digestion difficulties and increased risk of aspiration.

19. Dryness of the mucous membranes in the mouth and skin, as well as poor skin elasticity, may cause the false appearance of dehydration; a thinner epidermis and fragile capillaries may lead to easy bruising and tearing.

20. Lung function decreases, which results in decreased oxygen uptake; this may lead to hypoxia. Cough reflex is diminished and the ability to clear secretions is lessened, the combination of which may lead to choking and pneumonia.

21. Cardiac output falls and heart rate slows, thus decreasing compensatory ability. The conduction system degenerates, and the left ventricle thickens and becomes more rigid, which may lead to congestive heart failure.

22. Decline in function and blood flow to the kidneys may contribute to fluid and electrolyte disturbances.

23. Cell loss in certain areas of the brain; decreased blood flow (with increased resistance in the cerebral blood vessels); and reductions in both oxygen consumption and nerve conduction velocity contribute to slowed reflexes; decreased pain perception, sense of equilibrium, and perception of touch and temperature; and an increased incidence of falls and injury.

24. A decrease in total skeletal muscle weight and decreased density of some bones lead to increased frequency of fracture. **(Answers 18–24: Objective 1)**

25. **False.** The elderly are more prone to serious head injury, even with minor trauma. Shrinkage of brain tissue with aging allows more free space inside the skull. The brain can thus move more freely with sudden blows to the head; this leads to increased blood vessel tearing and a greater likelihood of cerebral bleeds such as subdural hematomas. **(Objectives 1 and 3)**

26. **False.** Dryness of the mucous membranes in the mouth and skin may cause you to believe mistakenly that the patient is dehydrated. Also, the skin may have poor elasticity even without dehydration, a fact that can contribute to the misdiagnosis of dehydration. **(Objectives 1 and 3)**

27. **True.** Depression is more common in the elderly than was once believed. **(Objective 3)**

28. **False.** The use of subcutaneous epinephrine is often reserved for younger patients because there is an increased likelihood of adverse cardiac effects with epinephrine, and subcutaneous absorption rates vary. When they are authorized by medical direction, handheld aerosolized bronchodilator agents work more quickly and are effective in relieving bronchial spasms without significant cardiovascular side effects. **(Objectives 4 and 5)**

29. **True.** This is so because of the changes in drug absorption, distribution, metabolism, and excretion that are associated with aging. **(Objective 5)**

30. **d** Assessment of AMI in the elderly presents a considerable challenge to the health care professional because the elderly patient may not present with the classic symptoms. Chest pain is uncommon. The most frequently manifested symptoms of AMI among older patients include shortness of breath, fatigue, and abdominal or epigastric pain. Consider AMI a possibility in any elderly patient who demonstrates an acute change in medical condition or behavior. **(Objective 3)**

31. **a (Objective 3)**

32. **c** Depression is common in the elderly, but it may be difficult to identify because it can accompany other psychiatric or medical illnesses. Alzheimer's disease and delirium are medical conditions. Schizophrenia appears as a less prominent condition than in other age groups. **(Objective 3)**

33. **d** Of the different types of geriatric abuse, physical abuse and physical neglect are encountered most often, but unexplained trauma is the primary finding. **(Objective 6)**

34. **a** and **b** Lung function decreases as aging progresses, resulting in up to a 40% decrease in oxygen uptake. There is no clear evidence of a decline in metabolic activity, but the total number of body cells decreases. **(Objective 1)**

35. **a, b, c,** and **d (Objectives 1 and 2)**

36. **a, b, c,** and **d (Objective 5)**

Chapter 27 Dyspnea

1. Place the patient in a position of comfort to maximize respiratory efficiency; then administer high-concentration humidified oxygen by nonrebreather mask. **(Objectives 7 and 8)**

2. Proventil relieves bronchospasm by relaxing bronchial smooth muscle. **(Objective 9)**

3. Although auscultation difficulty can be associated with lack of experience in auscultating breath sounds, it is likely to be a problem in this patient because there is very little air moving into and out of this patient's lungs because of the severe bronchospasm associated with his asthma attack. **(Objective 6)**

4. **No.** This patient's vital signs are elevated. Mean normal vital signs for a seven-year-old include a systolic blood pressure of 94, a pulse rate of 80, and a respiratory rate of 20. Elevations in blood pressure and pulse may be the result of increased circulating catecholamines such as epinephrine, which is released when the patient experiences breathlessness. His tachycardia and tachypnea may be the result of hypoxia. **(Objective 6)**

5. The patient feels better; respiratory rate and effort decrease; the use of accessory muscles decreases; circumoral cyanosis decreases or disappears; and heart rate and blood pressure may decrease. **(Objective 3)**

6. **No.** It is not indicated in that the patient's condition has markedly improved. Also, Proventil® is contraindicated at this point because it should not be administered in combination with epinephrine. **(Objective 9)**

7. altered mental status, cyanosis, nasal flaring, tracheal tugging, inability to speak, respiratory rate greater than 30 or less than 8, pulse rate greater than 130 or less than 60, intercostal muscle retraction **(Objective 5)**

8. **b** Her medications, as well as her presentation, indicate a chronic respiratory disease. Anaphylaxis, pulmonary embolism, and pneumothorax have an acute onset. **(Objective 5)**

9. It is important to determine her history of medication compliance because this may determine the type and amount of medication you choose to administer to this patient in the prehospital setting. **(Objective 3)**

10. **Yes.** The patient's self-administration of oxygen at 4 liters per minute was not sufficient to relieve her respiratory distress. Therefore, your initial treatment for this patient who is in severe respiratory distress is administration of high-flow oxygen. It is true that some patients with COPD depend on low blood levels of oxygen to stimulate their respiratory drive; however, these patients lose their respiratory stimulus only after receiving oxygen for a duration that exceeds that of the majority of transport times. According to current research, one should never withhold oxygen from a patient with acute decompensation from COPD. The patient should be observed closely to assess whether ventilatory assistance is needed. **(Objective 8)**

11. **Yes.** Cardiac monitoring is especially important for this patient because she is hypoxic, which increases her risk of developing serious, possibly life-threatening, dysrhythmias. Her medications also can cause side effects that include tachydysrhythmias and other rhythm disturbances. Her pulse is irregular as well, which may indicate the presence of ectopia. **(Objectives 6, 7, and 8)**

12. Although both drugs act to reverse bronchospasm, albuterol is preferred because it has fewer cardiac and other side effects. **(Objectives 8 and 9)**

13. Her pCO_2 most likely would be elevated, and her pO_2 decreased. Elevated levels of carbon dioxide and low oxygen levels are expected in COPD patients because of their underlying lung tissue damage, which results in poor gas exchange. **(Objective 3)**

14. Pulse oximetry is a rapid, noninvasive method of determining the oxygen saturation of the blood. This technology is useful not only in helping to determine the severity of the patient's initial condition, but also in monitoring the patient's response to any therapies. **(Objective 8)**

15. **Yes.** Some patients with underlying cardiac disease present with only a complaint of dyspnea and do not report any chest pain or discomfort. This is especially true of the elderly. **(Objective 5)**

16. Orthopnea; pink, frothy sputum. **(Objective 5)**

17. Hypotension. Through its vasodilating action on peripheral vessels, nitroglycerin promotes pooling of the blood in the system's circulation and decreases the resistance against which the heart has to pump. It is useful in treating pulmonary edema, but its use can lead to hypotension. **(Objective 9)**

18. Furosemide and morphine sulfate. These medications are vasodilators, which are effective at reducing venous return (preload). **(Objectives 8 and 9)**

19. An involuntary **(Objective 1)**

20. Carbon dioxide. The accumulation of carbon dioxide in the blood causes the respiratory centers of the brain to increase the rate and depth of ventilation. **(Objective 1)**

21. Increases. Dyspnea is noted when the work of breathing is excessive, or when resistance to air flow increases. **(Objective 2)**

22. Peripheral cyanosis **(Objective 6)**

23. Bradycardia **(Objective 6)**

24. **b** Stridor, which is heard best over the trachea, is a continuous crowing or a musical, high-pitched sound that occurs primarily during inspiration. It usually indicates a partial upper airway obstruction. **(Objective 6)**

25. **d** Rhonchi are low-pitched, harsh sounds that are heard usually on expiration; they are related to mucus or foreign matter in the bronchi, such as occurs with bronchitis or pneumonia. **(Objective 6)**

26. **c** Rales generally are recognized as fine, high-pitched sounds that are heard during inspiration when there is fluid in the alveoli, such as occurs in CHF or pneumonia. **(Objective 6)**

27. **a** Wheezing is a continuous, high-pitched lung sound that is heard best in the lung periphery and is more pronounced during expiration. Wheezing indicates narrowing of the bronchioles, usually by bronchospasm, as is seen in both asthma and COPD. **(Objective 6)**

28. **b** Stridor is heard best over the trachea; it is a continuous crowing or a musical, high-pitched sound that occurs primarily during inspiration. It usually indicates a partial upper airway obstruction. Such an obstruction results from swelling of the oropharynx, as is seen in epiglottitis. **(Objective 6)**

29. **b** Stridor, which is heard best over the trachea, is a continuous crowing or a musical, high-pitched sound associated primarily with inspiration. It usually indicates a partial upper airway obstruction. Such an obstruction is caused by swelling of the oropharynx, as is seen in croup. **(Objective 5)**

30. How long has the dyspnea been present?

    Was the onset gradual or abrupt?

    Does the dyspnea limit your normal activity?

    What were you doing when the dyspnea began?

    Do you have any associated symptoms, such as pain or coughing?

    Does anything make the dyspnea better or worse?

    (Objective 3)

31. Position of comfort, high-concentration oxygen, IV access, ECG monitoring **(Objectives 7 and 8)**

32. Position of comfort, blow-by oxygen, rapid transport **(Objectives 7 and 8)**

33. Position of comfort, high-concentration oxygen, IV access, ECG monitoring, selective beta-2 agonist medications **(Objectives 7 and 8)**

34. Position of comfort, high-concentration oxygen, IV access, ECG monitoring, epinephrine, diphenhydramine **(Objectives 7 and 8)**

35. High-concentration oxygen, spinal immobilization, IV access, ECG monitoring, needle decompression of the right chest **(Objectives 7 and 8)**

36. Coach the patient to slow her respirations; administer high-concentration oxygen as needed. **(Objectives 7 and 8)**

37. **c** **a** is apnea; **b** is hypoventilation; **d** is hypoxemia. **(Objective 2)**

38. **d (Objective 5)**

39. **b** An asthma patient who does not respond to therapies that, when used previously, had resulted in improvement is in jeopardy of respiratory arrest. A previous episode that required intubation or mechanical ventilation is an ominous finding. **(Objective 3)**

40. **a (Objective 5)**

41. **d** A recent history of prolonged immobilization or a surgical procedure may lead to suspicion of deep vein thrombosis with pulmonary embolism. It is likely that such a condition also would be accompanied by hemoptysis. **(Objective 5)**

CHAPTER 28: Nontraumatic Bleeding

1. **c** When the stomach accumulates blood that is partially digested, the emesis may resemble "coffee grounds," which is what this patient has described to you. This not a specific sign of a cerebral vascular accident, a heart attack, or a neurologic condition. **(Objectives 3 and 4)**

2. **e** An elevation in both respiratory and pulse rates indicates the presence of early shock. Because of the initial sympathetic compensation, blood pressure is usually normal, or it may be slightly elevated. Later in shock, as compensatory mechanisms fail, a drop in blood pressure occurs. **(Prerequisite Chapter Objective)**

3. **c** Dark, tarry stool indicates the presence of digested blood from the upper gastrointestinal tract. Initially, this information is most important to obtain because it enables you to approximate the quantity of blood that has been lost. Coughing history, information about medications, and other medical history are also important to obtain, but they are not needed initially. **(Objectives 4 and 5)**

4. **e** Patients with upper gastrointestinal bleeding frequently present with hematemesis, which may be bright red, or "coffee ground" (dark) in appearance. This bleeding comes from the esophagus, the stomach, or the upper part of the small intestine. The gallbladder and spleen are not parts of the gastrointestinal tract. Bleeding from the lower colon or rectum would present from the rectal area, and not through hematemesis. **(Objective 4)**

5. Evaluation of the skin, including the conjunctivae, mucous membranes, and nail beds; abdominal examination; tilt test; and blood sugar determination. **(Objective 5)**

6. Alcohol tends to irritate the lining of the stomach, causing erosion of the capillary beds in the stomach. This condition is known as gastritis. **(Prerequisite Chapter Objective)**

7. Positive. This test is considered positive when, upon sitting, either the blood pressure drops, or the pulse rate increases. This patient experienced both. **(Prerequisite Chapter Objective)**

8. **e** When potential signs of shock are present, oxygen is important because there is an inadequate amount of hemoglobin present; also, fluid must be replaced. Because hypotension is caused by hypovolemia, pressor agents such as dopamine are not indicated. The beta effects of epinephrine would only serve to compound existing tachycardia, which may cause further problems. **(Objective 5)**

9. Even though the patient is conscious, he has significant signs of hypoperfusion and should receive treatment as quickly as possible. **(Prerequisite Chapter Objective)**

10. Pulmonary infection (e.g., bronchitis or pneumonia); tuberculosis or lung abscess; pulmonary embolus, cardiac failure, and valvular heart disease are also possibilities. **(Objectives 3 and 4)**

11. **d** Blood-streaked sputum, productive cough, chest discomfort, fever, and the presence of crackles all suggest the possibility of pneumonia. Gastrointestinal bleeding would present with hematemesis or rectal bleeding. The patient denies any pertinent medical history, which would be associated with chronic obstructive pulmonary disease or congestive heart failure. **(Objectives 3, 4, and 5)**

12. Possibly, although typically, hemoptysis does not cause hypovolemia. Hematemesis is more often the cause. **(Objective 4)**

13. **e** A precautionary IV of normal saline or Ringer's lactate and administration of oxygen are indicated. Even though epinephrine has beta-2 properties, it equally affects beta-1 receptors, thus causing cardiovascular stimulation. Nitroglycerin is used for chest pain, signs of congestive heart failure, or very high blood pressure. **(Objective 4)**

14. Severe respiratory distress can develop in patients with hemoptysis that occurs secondary to obstructed air passages. Even though initial field management involves addressing this problem, the patient may require more aggressive management that can be provided only in the hospital setting. **(Objective 5)**

15. Management considerations for treatment of this patient include these: Ensure a comfortable and upright position to facilitate the patient's breathing; use albuterol (nebulized) to open the patient's air passages. **(Prerequisite Chapter Objective)**

16. **c** Bronchitis and pulmonary embolus would be associated with hemoptysis; gastrointestinal bleeding with hematemesis. Liver disease is associated with ascites, gastrointestinal bleeding, and pulmonary hypertension. **(Objective 4)**

17. **b** An ectopic pregnancy is a serious condition. When rupture occurs, typically it results in intraabdominal bleeding, but it can present with vaginal bleeding. Abruptio placentae and placenta previa occur in the last trimester; hyperemesis gravidarum is excessive vomiting during pregnancy, and preeclampsia is associated with visual disturbances, edema, and high blood pressure. **(Objective 4)**

18. Kidney infection; kidney stones. **(Objective 4)**

19. Hemostasis is the termination of bleeding by mechanical or chemical means through the complex coagulation process of the body. Three factors that affect this are: vasoconstriction, platelet aggregation, and thrombin or fibrin synthesis. The liver is a major organ that affects clotting ability. **(Objective 1)**

20. **b** Rapid respirations and tachycardia are also early signs, but changes in mental status typically occur first. Falling blood pressure is a later sign. **(Objective 5)**

21. Hemophilia; liver disease; leukemia; patients taking medications such as Coumadin®, aspirin, or other blood thinners. **(Objective 2)**

22. **a** Bleeding from the esophagus, stomach, or upper small intestine presents with vomiting of blood, or it is associated with melena if it occurs rectally. Liver disease is associated with upper gastrointestinal bleeding rather than lower gastrointestinal bleeding. **(Objective 4)**

23. Epistaxis may be controlled by pinching the nose after allowing the patient to first blow out all blood and clots. The patient is usually kept in an upright position; suction should be readily available. **(Objective 4)**

24. Airway compromise; pulmonary aspiration; hypovolemia. **(Objective 5)**

25. **True**. Because of the risk of transmission of an airborne infection, respiratory precautions are indicated. The most helpful precaution, when exposed to a patient presenting with hemoptysis, is to wear a mask yourself, and to place one on the patient, if he or she can tolerate it. **(Objective 4)**

26. **True**. Because of the lowered concentration of hemoglobin, all patients should be placed on 100% oxygen at a high flow rate, which maximizes oxygen delivery and minimizes tissue hypoxia. **(Prerequisite Chapter Objective)**

27. **False**. Rapid bleeding from the lungs is indicated by the presence of bright red blood and minimal sputum. Foamy, pink-tinged sputum indicates a small quantity of blood, which has not clotted before being coughed up. **(Objective 4)**

CHAPTER 29: Syncope

1. You should note any signs of obvious distress, which may be evidenced by position of the patient, respiratory rate and effort, use of accessory muscles, facial expression, skin color and temperature, capillary refill, and strength of the pulse.

2. **a** During initial assessment, any patient who is alert but disoriented is not experiencing simple syncope. His condition likely indicates a potentially serious underlying cause. Medical history, 12-lead ECG, and rapid glucose determination are also important to obtain, but none of these is the immediate priority. **(Objectives 4, 5 and 7)**

3. How long have you had these "passing out" spells?

   What were you doing just before the event occurred?

   Did you have any warning symptoms (e.g., sweating, dizziness, visual disturbances)?

   Do you experience palpitations?

   Was anyone else present when you passed out?

   Did you fall, or is there any previous history of trauma?

   Has this ever happened before? How often?

   Do you have any major medical problems? If yes, please describe them.

   Do you take any medications?

   (Objective 4)

4. **d** This rhythm has more Ps than QRSs, with a fixed P-R interval. Sinus bradycardia and first-degree heart block have only one P for each QRS. Second-degree type I and third-degree heart block both have changing P-R intervals. **(Prerequisite Chapter Objectives)**

5. The slow heart rate associated with this dysrhythmia is most likely the cause of the syncopal episode. This can cause a decrease in cardiac output, thereby decreasing cerebral blood flow. **(Objectives 2, 4, 5, and 7)**

6. **a** Epinephrine, dopamine, and transcutaneous pacing also may be indicated; however, the first standard treatment is atropine. **(Objective 8)**

7. **d** The patient is experiencing chest pain. BP is adequate, and he could benefit from nitroglycerin. Dextrose 50% is used for low blood sugar (his is 120), Levophed® for low blood pressure (his is 114/60), and lidocaine for ventricular ectopy (he has none). **(Objective 8)**

8. Emergency department personnel should obtain a 12-lead ECG, gather additional medical history information, and potentially administer thrombolytic therapy.

9. How long have you had these symptoms?

   What were you doing just before the event?

   Did you have any warning symptoms (e.g., sweating, dizziness, visual disturbances)?

   Do you experience any palpitations?

   Was anyone else present when this occurred?

   Did you fall, or is there any previous history of trauma?

   Do you have any major medical problems? If yes, please describe them.

   Do you take any medications?

   Could you be pregnant?

   (Objective 4)

10. **d** Given her age, and the history obtained thus far, it is extremely important to obtain a menstrual history because of the possibility of ectopic pregnancy. The other questions also are important, but they do not relate to a potential threat to life.

11. Positive orthostatic vital signs (tilt test) are a strong indication that the patient has decreased circulating blood volume (hypovolemia). **(Objectives 5 and 6)**

12. **d** Although answers **a, b,** and **c** are possibilities, the patient's clinical presentation (lower left quadrant [LLQ] pain, now resided; syncopal episode; missed period; tender abdomen; and positive tilt test) suggests a ruptured ectopic pregnancy. **(Objectives 6 and 7)**

13. **c** Anaphylactic shock results from an allergic reaction and cardiogenic shock from a heart problem; neurogenic shock involves disruption of the central or peripheral nervous system. **(Prerequisite Chapter Objective)**

14. Oxygen should be administered, and IV (Ringer's lactate) initiated for fluid replacement; it may be necessary to use PASG; the patient must be transported rapidly to an appropriate facility. **(Objective 8)**

15. Ectopic pregnancy — When a fallopian tube bursts secondary to ectopic pregnancy, there is a lot of bleeding because of the increased vasculature of the area. Intraabdominal bleeding occurs, which depletes volume in the intravascular space. This decrease causes a fall in cardiac output, diminished cerebral blood flow, and syncope. **(Objective 8)**

16. **d** Although all the conditions listed here are possible, the patient's history and clinical findings point to orthostatic hypotension as the most likely possibility. The patient has just eaten (ruling out hypoglycemia); further history and physical findings would be needed to support a diagnosis of cerebral vascular accident or hypovolemia. **(Objectives 2 and 3)**

17. Under normal circumstances, when an individual stands, the sympathetic nervous system causes increased peripheral vascular resistance and an increase in heart rate so that cardiac output and blood flow to the brain can be maintained. If these reflex changes do not occur, blood return to the heart decreases because of the pooling of blood in the abdomen and lower extremities. The result is a drop in blood pressure that may be severe enough to cause syncope. **(Objectives 2 and 3)**

18. How long have you had these symptoms?

    What were you doing just before the event?

    Did you have any warning symptoms (e.g., sweating, dizziness, visual disturbances)?

    Do you experience any palpitations?

    Was anyone else present when this occurred?

    Did you fall, or is there any previous history of trauma?

    Do you have any major medical problems? If yes, please describe.

    Do you take any medications?

    (Objective 4)

19. **a** Older individuals are especially susceptible to positional changes in blood pressure, particularly after long periods of inactivity. **(Objective 3)**

20. Definition of syncope: A transient loss of responsiveness (a few seconds to several minutes) after which the patient, when placed in a supine position, regains mentation.

    Pathophysiology of syncope: Syncope occurs most frequently as a result of decreased blood flow to the brain. Normal brain function and maintenance of a responsive state depend on a constant supply of oxygen and glucose. The brain cannot store these nutrients; therefore, an interruption of cerebral blood flow for 5 to 10 seconds results in unresponsiveness. **(Objective 1)**

21. Syncope occurs frequently in otherwise healthy individuals and is usually referred to as simple fainting. However, in response to an unpleasant situation (e.g., feeling afraid, seeing blood, feeling pain), the individual has a temporary sympathetic response that is followed by a reflex vagal reaction that causes decreased heart rate and dilation of the blood vessels. This vasovagal response can cause major, transient decreases in both blood pressure and cerebral blood flow. **(Objective 3)**

22. **a, b,** and **c** A widened pulse pressure is not a related finding in a positive tilt test. Systolic blood pressure falls with a positive tilt test. In widening pulse pressure, the systolic pressure usually is rising. **(Objective 6)**

23. **(a)** Reflex vasovagal response: response to stress (fainting)

    (b) Low blood sugar: inadequate perfusion of glucose to the brain

    (c) Slow or fast heart rate: reduced cardiac output and diminished cerebral blood flow

    (d) Orthostatic hypotension: inadequate adjustment of the peripheral vasculature to constriction upon standing. Blood return to the heart decreases, and cardiac output and blood pressure fall, thus reducing blood flow to the brain.

    (e) Reduced blood volume: Decreased circulating volume causes diminished blood return to the heart and decreased cardiac output, both of which result in decreased cerebral blood flow.

    (Objective 2)

24. Cardiac. Dsyrhythmia or acute myocardial infarction often presents without warning, or while the patient is at rest. Both can be life-threatening; the presence of associated syncope is a valuable clue for the EMS provider. **(Objective 7)**

25. Problems of hypotension and syncope can occur during pregnancy when the enlarged uterus compresses the inferior vena cava and decreases blood return to the heart. **(Objective 3)**

CHAPTER 30: Altered Mental Status

1. **b** Evaluating respiratory status is a priority over checking blood pressure, starting an IV, and taking the patient's temperature. **(Prerequisite Chapter Objective)**

2. Does the patient have a known seizure disorder? Does he take any medications? Has he been seen in the nurse's office for any other medical problems? What was his mental status before your arrival? **(Objective 3)**

3. **Yes.** It is highly likely that it is related. If the brain does not receive adequate amounts of glucose, it becomes irritable (massive discharge of excitable neurons that spread), and seizures may result. **(Objectives 1 and 2)**

4. **Low.** Presentation of a seizure is often associated with hypoglycemia; therefore, this is likely to be the patient's condition. Seizures also can occur in the very late stages of hyperglycemia, but this is not a typical initial presentation. **(Objective 2)**

5. **d** When it has been prepared for IV administration, the consistency of this drug is very thick. It should be administered carefully and slowly. If extravasation occurs, local tissue irritation and possible necrosis can follow. Hypotension, respiratory depression, and tachycardia are not typical side effects of this drug. **(Prerequisite Chapter Objective)**

6. **Yes.** With his known condition and altered mental status, the principle of implied consent would apply. This is the safest and best decision that can be made with the interests of the patient in mind. **(Prerequisite Chapter Objective)**

7. Continued assessment would include monitoring changes in mental status, respiratory status, and pulse, as well as observing for possible seizure. Also, one should closely monitor the IV site and observe for signs of possible tissue infiltration. **(Objective 6)**

8. Glucose is the source of the energy that is needed for most cellular reactions, and the brain is the organ that is most dependent on glucose availability. When it is not available, changes in a patient's personality and/or mental status occur. **(Objectives 1 and 2)**

9. **e** Securing information from the scene and from bystanders about the possible overdose takes priority over checking an ECG and blood pressure. **(Objective 3)**

10. **c** Overdose of opiate-type drugs typically causes the pupils to constrict (pinpoint). Dilated pupils (which result from hypoxia secondary to respiratory depression) may be observed at a later point. **(Prerequisite Chapter Objective)**

11. Heroin and opiate derivatives depress the central nervous system. When this occurs, normal nervous system response is suppressed, which affects the patient's mental status and depresses respirations. **(Prerequisite Chapter Objective)**

12. **c** This medication reverses the effect of narcotic overdose. 50% Dextrose is used for hypoglycemia, and sometimes in coma of unknown etiology. Activated charcoal or syrup of Ipecac would be used in conscious patients who have overdosed. **(Prerequisite Chapter Objective)**

13. Level of consciousness and respiratory status should improve; the patient may become agitated. **(Prerequisite Chapter Objective)**

14. Even if she feels better after the administration of naloxone, she was unresponsive after taking the intravenous drug, and she had never taken it before. It is in her best interest that you evaluate her for possible complications. **(Objective 6)**

15. Level of consciousness (initially, while en route, and on arrival at the hospital, as well as before and after administration of the medication); vital signs and any changes while she was in your care; a description of the conversation and its conclusion regarding transport to the hospital; documentation of all interactions. **(Prerequisite Chapter Objective)**

16. Altered mental status may be reported to EMS as fainting, disorientation, strange behavior, seizure activity, or unresponsiveness. **(Objective 3)**

17. **b** Acute myocardial infarction, hypoglycemia, and status epilepticus could lead to hypoxia. The neurologic signs and symptoms that accompany hypoxia are generalized in nature (e.g., confusion and disorientation). Meningitis also may result in hypoxia, but, more specifically, it may lead to increased intracranial pressure. **(Objective 2)**

18. If the patient cannot provide accurate information, the paramedic is forced to rely on data gathered by observing what the surroundings show and by talking with bystanders on the scene. Initial questions that are important to ask include:

    How quickly did the patient's mental status change?

    Is there evidence of seizure?

    Did the patient injure himself or herself before or during the incident?

    Is there any possibility of substance abuse?

    Is there any pertinent medical history?

    (Objective 3)

19. **d** Focal and Jacksonian episodes are particular types of seizure activity that typically are not associated with loss of consciousness; the postictal state is the period after an episode of generalized seizure activity. **(Objective 2)**

20. **e (Objective 2)**
21. **d (Objective 5)**
22. **c (Objective 5)**
23. **g (Objective 5)**
24. **e (Objective 5)**
25. **f (Objective 5)**

26. **a (Objective 5)**
27. **b (Objective 5)**
28. Very slow and very rapid pulse rates (<40 or >160) can cause generalized hypoperfusion, which reduces cerebral blood flow, causes hypoxia, and alters mental status. **(Objective 2)**
29. (a) Thorough documentation of these findings can be of critical importance. Findings based on the AVPU system are recorded, both initially and subsequently. Careful description of the patient's behavior is most important.
    (b) The overall pattern should be observed. Any abnormal pattern (e.g., Cheyne-Stokes) is observed and recorded.
    (c) Color of the skin and the presence of any perspiration should be noted. Hot, dry skin could indicate fever resulting from infection or exposure; generalized rash may indicate an allergic reaction; bruising could indicate a clotting or bleeding problem.
    (d) Check both eyes for reaction to light; note any abnormal movement.
    (e) Muscle strength is evaluated according to the patient's level of responsiveness. If the patient is unresponsive, any signs of abnormal posturing upon stimulation should be noted. If the patient is responsive, muscle strength is assessed by instructing him or her to squeeze both of the examiner's hands, and to push against the examiner's hands with his/her hands or feet. **(Objective 4)**
30. **a, b, d,** and **e** Hypoperfusion causes altered mental status that results from the generalized effects of hypoxia. It is not related specifically to intracranial pressure. **(Objective 2)**
31. The management approach depends on the specific findings in each particular patient; however, attention to the basics of airway, breathing, and circulation should be applied with all patients. Administration of high-concentration oxygen, use of cardiac monitoring, and establishment of IV access also are important for all patients. **(Objective 6)**

CHAPTER 31 Chest Pain

1. **Yes.** Initial assessment reveals anxiety, pale, sweaty skin, and labored respirations. All could be indications of shock, particularly when they occur in the presence of chest pain. **(Prerequisite Chapter Objective)**
2. **a** Obtaining a 12-lead ECG, requesting morphine sulfate, and starting a TKO IV all are important, but none of these is the first priority. **(Objective 5)**
3. **c** There is only one P wave for each QRS; thus, a higher degree of block is not present. **(Prerequisite Chapter Objective)**
4. A slow heart rate usually indicates the presence of a dysrhythmia. This occurs when the heart muscle is deprived of oxygen. Vagal stimulation also can slow the heart rate. **(Objective 4)**
5. **Yes.** In the presence of hypotension, this is most likely a treatable bradycardia in most EMS systems; however, local protocol should be followed. **(Prerequisite Chapter Objective)**
6. **a** Dopamine is a second-line drug that is used to treat slow heart rate, and it is first-line for the treatment of hypotension. Epinephrine is used primarily in cases of cardiac arrest and in certain cases of breathing difficulty. Lidocaine is used for ventricular irritability. **(Prerequisite Chapter Objective)**
7. Field management should comprise close cardiac monitoring, including a 12-lead ECG, if available; establishment of IV access; and rapid transport. The benefits of morphine, used alone or in conjunction with nitroglycerin, should be considered if the patient's hypotension is improved. These drugs help to alleviate chest pain, and they reduce the workload on the heart. These agents can be very useful in the prehospital setting. **(Objectives 3 and 5)**

8. **Yes.** Thrombolytic agents dissolve blood clots that obstruct coronary blood flow. The sooner they are administered, the sooner blood flow is restored to the myocardium, thus reducing the amount of muscle damage and necrosis. Later complications of myocardial infarction also are directly related to the speed with which thrombolytics are administered. Thus, minimizing "door to drug" time is essential. Recent studies have shown no improvement in patient outcome associated with the prehospital administration of thrombolytics. However, obtaining 12-lead ECGs in the field may be effective in reducing the time to thrombolytic administration. Time is the key factor. **(Objective 5)**

9. **d** A chest radiograph and fluid challenge may be important for this patient, but the first priority is to administer thrombolytics, if they are indicated; then, the patient must be admitted to the coronary care unit for close monitoring. **(Objective 5)**

10. **c** The most important element of the history is an accurate characterization of the type of pain that the patient is experiencing because this information determines the approach to patient management. Allergies, radiation of the pain, and medical history also are relevant, but none is the first priority when gathering historical information. **(Objective 2)**

11. **c** Information about associated symptoms and additional patient history are important, as is starting a precautionary IV. However, given the patient's chief complaint, these do not take precedence over quick application of the ECG monitor. **(Objectives 3 and 5)**

12. **c** Atrial fibrillation would exhibit neither a constant P wave, nor any regularity in the R to R pattern. Sinus arrhythmia is characterized by a slight variation in the pattern, secondary to respirations. The premature beats do not have wide QRS complexes; therefore, they cannot be PVCs. **(Prerequisite Chapter Objective)**

13. Myocardial ischemia, esophageal spasm, pulmonary embolus, or gallbladder disease. Any of these conditions may be considered initially, given her chief complaint and presenting symptoms. **(Objectives 1 and 4)**

14. Explain that you believe it is in her best interest to go to the hospital, even though she is feeling better. Although the precipitating event may not be cardiac in origin, one cannot be sure of this without further evaluation at the hospital. **(Prerequisite Chapter Objective)**

15. Pain that originates in the esophagus may be virtually indistinguishable from pain of cardiac etiology, possibly because both structures share a common nerve supply. Esophageal pain usually arises in the presence of acid (either ingested or from the stomach), or it may be caused by severe spasms of the esophageal muscles. The patient may describe characteristics that are similar to those of cardiac pain, such as retrosternal pressure with radiation that is not necessarily relieved by antacids. To further complicate the issue, nitroglycerin, which is taken for cardiac ischemic pain, often relieves esophageal symptoms. All of these patients should be treated as if they have cardiac disease because historical features do not separate esophageal from cardiac processes. **(Objectives 1 and 4)**

16. **a, b, d,** and **e** Increased intracranial pressure is associated with ischemia to the cerebral circulation. **(Objective 4)**

17. **e** Cardiac ischemia and the resulting pain can be described by patients in various ways. Knowledge of these various descriptions is important because each could indicate an acute cardiac event. **(Objectives 1 and 2)**

18. Dysrhythmias are the most common specific cause of sudden death caused by heart disease. Careful monitoring is essential in cardiac patients because rapid recognition and treatment of dysrhythmia could be lifesaving. **(Objectives 4 and 5)**

19. **Yes.** Activity is not necessary for the development of cardiac ischemia. Some patients have chest pain at rest or after eating a large meal. The pain may be dismissed as "indigestion." **(Objectives 2 and 4)**

20. **e** Abnormal pulse findings can be significant without the presence of hypotension. Because dysrhythmia frequently occurs in association with a cardiac event, it always should be considered life-threatening. **(Objective 4)**

21. **d** Digoxin, epinephrine and Inderal® are not indicated for the presence of chest pain alone. **(Prerequisite Chapter Objective)**

22. **a** The other conditions listed here do not typically describe "tearing" and back pain; this is specific as a chief complaint for an aneurysm, which can result in acute aortic dissection. **(Objectives 1 and 4)**

23. **c** Cardiac and gastrointestinal conditions typically are not associated with deep respiratory inspiration or coughing. **(Objective 4)**

24. The most important element of assessment is the history. Questions to be asked include:

    What is the character of the pain? Where it is located?

    Does the pain go anywhere else?

    Are there any associated symptoms?

    What is your medical history?

    What medications are you taking currently?

    (Objectives 2 and 3)

25. Morphine sulfate is effective in relieving acute cardiac chest pain and in reducing anxiety. Anxiety may lead to agitation and increased catecholamine release, which contributes to stress on the injured heart muscle. Morphine usually is considered in conjunction with, or after failure of, nitroglycerin. **(Objective 5)**

26. Patients with significant coronary artery disease frequently experience cardiac chest pain when cardiac muscle demands more oxygen than can be supplied by the blood flow through the coronary arteries. Short-lasting episodes (duration less than 5 to 10 minutes) of chest pain that resolve with rest and reveal no signs of permanent muscle damage are called *angina attacks*. If the pain lasts longer than 5 to 10 minutes and cardiac muscle damage is revealed later by ECG reading or blood testing, the episode is called an *acute myocardial infarction* or, more commonly, a heart attack. **(Objective 4)**

CHAPTER 32: Palpitations and Dysrhythmias

1. **c** Checking her pulse and breathing provides a quick evaluation of her overall cardiovascular and respiratory status. When there is associated chest pain, this is particularly important. Obtaining a 12-lead ECG reading, assessing blood pressure, and checking for distended neck veins are also important to her care, but they are secondary steps. **(Prerequisite Chapter Objective)**

2. History: Does the pain go anywhere else?

    Is there anything that makes it better or worse?

    Are there any visual disturbances?

    Has this ever happened before?

    What is your medical history?

    Physical examination. Check for distended neck veins, peripheral edema, and the presence and quality of peripheral pulses.

    (Prerequisite Chapter Objective and Objectives 2, 4, and 5)

3. **a** A short-lasting episode (duration less than 5 to 10 minutes) of chest pain that resolves with rest and reveals no signs of permanent muscle damage is called angina pectoris. Congestive heart failure is evidenced by associated signs of fluid retention; transient ischemic attacks also are associated with temporary reduced blood flow (i.e., cerebral circulation); Wolff-Parkinson-White syndrome is a specific dysrhythmia that is not necessarily associated with chest pain. **(Prerequisite Chapter Objective and Objective 2)**

4. Many dysrhythmias (including bradycardia) reduce cardiac output and produce symptoms related to decreased blood flow and perfusion (e.g., falling blood pressure). Additionally, if the patient is having an infarct, the damaged area of the heart may pump ineffectively, thereby causing decreased cardiac output. **(Objective 6)**

5. **e** This is the treatment of choice for symptomatic bradycardia. Adenosine is used to treat tachydysrhythmias; lidocaine is used for ventricular irritability. **(Objective 6)**

6. The rule of thumb is to treat the patient, not the dysrhythmia. Signs of adequate perfusion would indicate that the patient did not require emergent treatment in the field. However, this patient is demonstrating signs of hypoperfusion, evidenced by her pale skin and falling blood pressure. This rule of thumb is particularly appropriate in the presence of chest pain with suspected myocardial infarction and an associated bradycardia. Increasing the heart rate with atropine subsequently increases myocardial oxygen demand; thus, the benefit of this treatment should be weighed carefully against this disadvantage. **(Prerequisite Chapter Objective and Objectives 5 and 6)**

7. Treatment with nitroglycerin is not recommended in the presence of her hypotension because it may compound this problem. If her heart rate stabilizes and blood pressure improves, its value for pain relief could be considered. **(Prerequisite Chapter Objective)**

8. Mobitz II and third-degree heart blocks represent potentially dangerous situations for the patient. Mobitz II can progress to complete heart block, which is associated with a high mortality rate. Atropine may increase the atrial rate and worsen the AV block. Paradoxically, its use can also cause the ventricular rate to fall, which further diminishes the hemodynamic status. If atropine is used in this setting, transcutaneous pacing must be made available immediately. **(Objective 6)**

9. **e** This is a wide complex tachycardia without any P waves. Atrial flutter is characterized by the presence of flutter waves in the baseline (referred to as a "sawtooth pattern"). This is not present. PSVT and sinus tachycardia both have P waves. Torsades de pointes is a wide complex tachycardia, but QRSs are constantly changing. These QRSs are consistently the same. **(Prerequisite Chapter Objective)**

10. Unstable. The patient is showing significant indications of hypoperfusion: shortness of breath; diaphoresis; a rapid, weak pulse; and hypotension. **(Objectives 2, 4, and 6)**

11. **d** Adenosine is used to treat narrow complex tachycardia. Defibrillation is used for ventricular fibrillation. Magnesium sulfate may be administered for this dysrhythmia, but not initially if, as in this case, the patient's condition is unstable. **(Prerequisite Chapter Objective and Objective 6)**

12. **e** This rhythm indicates marked ventricular instability; it is likely to progress to ventricular fibrillation and requires rapid intervention. This rhythm may be seen mostly in elderly patients, and it is always considered an urgent situation. Occasionally, patients with this rhythm may present in a stable condition; however, instability is more common. (When a patient's condition is unstable, cardioversion is the first-line treatment before the use of medications.) **(Prerequisite Chapter Objective and Objective 6)**

13. Sinus rhythm with couplet PVCs. **(Prerequisite Chapter Objective)**

14. Lidocaine is used to treat ventricular irritability. Although the rhythm has converted, the bolus and maintenance drip may help to prevent a recurrence of this life-threatening dysrhythmia. **(Prerequisite Chapter Objective and Objectives 5 and 6)**

15. Dopamine IV piggyback drip to treat and maintain his blood pressure. Cardiogenic shock frequently is associated with this dysrhythmia, and dopamine may be required if the rhythm does not convert, and/or if blood pressure remains low after conversion. **(Prerequisite Chapter Objective and Objectives 5 and 6)**

16. Palpitations are an awareness of forceful heart beating, usually at an increased rate. This sensation may occur normally during or after strenuous exercise; however, when it is associated with mild exertion, it suggests underlying poor physical conditioning, dysrhythmia, heart failure, or anemia. Other possible triggering mechanisms include smoking, stress, fatigue, alcohol ingestion, and the use of caffeine or stimulant-type drugs. **(Objectives 1 and 2)**

17. **a, b, c,** and **e**   Stimulant drugs are associated more often with tachydysrhythmias. **(Objective 6)**

18. **d, e**

19. **b, e, f**

20. **a, b**

21. **b, c, e**

22. **b, e, f**

   (Answers 18 to 22: Prerequisite Chapter Objective and Objective 3)

23. Is the patient stable or unstable?

    Is the heart rate fast or slow?

    Are the QRS complexes wide or narrow?

    Is the rhythm regular or irregular?

    Are the P waves associated with QRS complexes?

    (Objectives 2, 4, and 5)

24. **a** Sometimes hypoperfusing bradycardia leads to PVCs that are caused by hypoxia or that occur as escape beats. After administration of oxygen, the rate should be treated (atropine, TCP); then, if necessary, the PVCs should be addressed (lidocaine, magnesium sulfate). Improving the rate hopefully will result in improved perfusion and oxygenation of the myocardium, thus eliminating the PVCs. Dopamine could be used to treat the rate, but only after administration of atropine and TCP. It can also be used to improve hypotension, but only after the rate is treated. **(Objective 6)**

25. Common causes of tachycardia include exercise and anxiety; it can also occur as compensation for certain medical problems, such as blood loss, fever, and hypoxia. It can be an expected physiologic response, particularly when the rate is lower than 160. **(Objectives 2 and 6)**

26. **a** Rapid ventricular rates that occur in response to atrial fibrillation can be problematic for older patients and for those with heart disease. The lack of coordinated atrial contraction compromises the efficiency of ventricular filling and decreases cardiac output. Over time, microemboli (tiny blood clots) can be caused by sluggish blood in the atria; these can lead to cerebral vascular accidents. **(Objective 6)**

27. **True**. Premature ventricular contractions caused by hypoxia usually indicate irritability of the cardiac muscle. The first treatment for any PVC activity is to administer high-concentration oxygen. **(Objective 6)**

28. **False**. Because atrial fibrillation can be very difficult to cardiovert, this treatment is not used routinely. Medication is the standard treatment; medication usually is administered in the hospital as opposed to the prehospital setting. One exception is diltiazem, which is currently used more frequently in the prehospital than the hospital setting. **(Objective 6)**

29. **True**. With its short half-life, adenosine is used most often and should be considered when there are long transport times, or when patients are awake with no signs of hypoperfusion. Verapamil is also effective, but because it often causes significant hypotension, adenosine is the first choice for field use. **(Prerequisite Chapter Objective and Objective 6)**

30. **True**. PVC activity may warn of impending ventricular tachycardia or ventricular fibrillation. Certain types of PVCs are of particular concern and could indicate the possibility of impending ventricular tachycardia or ventricular fibrillation. These include the occurrence of more than 6 PVCs per minute, R on T phenomenon, multifocal PVCs, bigeminy, and couplets. **(Prerequisite Chapter Objective and Objective 6)**

31. **True**. Even though the cause of the disturbance is often benign, most patients consider palpitations to be serious and are concerned that the symptom signals heart disease. **(Objective 1)**

32. **True**. The body compensates for the effects of dysrhythmias and always attempts to perfuse the heart and brain. When symptoms are significant, hypoperfusion to these areas is indicated. **(Objectives 2, 5, and 6)**

33. **True** These drugs in particular have associated dysrhythmias in the presence of toxicity. **(Prerequisite Chapter Objective and Objective 6)**

34. **False**. Ventricular tachycardia (wide complex) is much more likely than narrow complex tachycardia to produce a rapid fall in cardiac output. **(Objectives 5 and 6)**

Chapter 33: Headache

1. When did the headache start, and how severe is it?

   Where is the pain located?

   Are there any associated symptoms?

   Has there been a toxic exposure?

   What is the patient's medical history?

   Does the patient have a history of either bleeding abnormalities or use of blood thinners?

   Is the patient pregnant?

   (Objective 2)

2. Women who are in the latter half of pregnancy, in labor, or in the early post-partum period who complain of headache and have blood pressure elevation should be considered to have preeclampsia. This is a potentially life-threatening condition for both mother and infant. **(Objective 2)**

3. Fever, neck stiffness, history of bleeding abnormalities, severe hypertension, pregnancy, exposure to fumes, and abnormal neurologic examination. **(Objective 2)**

4. The headache is related to stress; the location of the pain is bilateral and involves the occipital and frontal areas; the patient has had similar previous headaches. **(Objective 4)**

5. Even though most headaches do not result in findings of neurologic abnormality, you should regard the headache patient as having a potentially serious condition. In general, patients with a chief complaint of headache that is severe enough to call 9-1-1 should be transported for physician evaluation. **(Objective 6)**

6. This patient's presentation was more suggestive of tension headache than of meningitis. She was afebrile and had none of the other findings that are frequently associated with meningitis. In addition to headache, fever, and neck stiffness, patients with meningitis may complain of photophobia, nausea, vomiting, and chills. This patient's neck pain may be the result of a spasm of muscles, which in turn can cause tension headache. **(Objective 4)**

7. **Yes.** Your neurologic examination should be limited at this time to include only a determination of the patient's mental status according to the AVPU scale. In other words, you should determine the following: Is the patient alert? Does he respond to verbal stimuli? Does he respond to pain, or is he unresponsive? **(Objective 3)**

8. **Yes.** Headache that begins suddenly (within seconds) rather than gradually (over minutes to hours) usually indicates a more serious problem. **(Objective 2)**

9. Aggressive airway control with hyperventilation, and recognition of the need for transport. The patient presenting with headache who displays any neurologic abnormality should be considered to have a potentially life-threatening condition and must be transported immediately. **(Objective 6)**

10. Posturing is a grave sign of increased intracranial pressure; it demonstrates the severity of this patient's condition. **(Objective 3)**

11. **Yes.** IV access is indicated when any potentially life-threatening condition is recognized, but it should not delay transport. **(Objective 6)**

12. **Yes.** Coumadin® is a blood thinner. Patients presenting with headache who are taking blood thinners can bleed into their brains, either spontaneously or after seemingly minor injury. **(Objective 2)**

13. **No.** This additional history, although it is important, should not alter your treatment approach for this patient. Increased intracranial pressure should be treated the same way in all cases, regardless of the cause. However, it is important to convey this historical information to hospital personnel. **(Objective 6)**

14. Patients with suspected intracranial hemorrhage should be transported to a hospital with neurosurgical capabilities. By definition, a level I trauma center provides these services. **(Objective 6)**
15. **e (Objective 5)**
16. **c** This patient is experiencing pulseless ventricular tachycardia. Immediate defibrillation is critical to this patient's outcome. **(Prerequisite Chapter Objective)**
17. Exposure to carbon monoxide. In the late fall or early winter, faulty heaters can emit carbon monoxide and can cause carbon monoxide poisoning. Carbon monoxide is the most likely inhaled substance to cause headache. **(Objective 4)**
18. **Yes.** After the patients have been removed from the source of carbon monoxide, treatment includes ensuring a patent airway, providing adequate ventilation, and administering high-concentration oxygen. **(Objective 6)**
19. A patient with high carbon monoxide levels may have a bright red skin appearance, but more often, the patient has normal or pale skin and lip coloration. Usually, cyanosis does not appear in these patients because arterial oxygen tension is normal. **(Objective 2)**
20. **No.** The pulse oximeter is unreliable for determining effective patient oxygenation in cases of carbon monoxide poisoning. False readings can occur because hemoglobin may be saturated with carbon monoxide. **(Prerequisite Chapter Objective)**
21. A hyperbaric chamber **(Objective 6)**
22. Meningitis and subarachnoid hemorrhage **(Objective 4)**
23. **g (Objective 4)**
24. **e (Objective 4)**
25. **f (Objective 4)**
26. **d (Objective 4)**
27. **c (Objective 4)**
28. **c** An effective antihypertensive medication that is used often in the prehospital setting is nitroglycerin; it is given either sublingually or orally in spray form. Naloxone is a specific antidote for narcotic agents; it is used to reverse the effects of narcotics. Lidocaine is an antiarrhythmic and anesthetic that is used both to suppress ventricular ectopic activity and as a local anesthetic. Lasix® is a potent diuretic that is used in conditions of fluid overload to rid the body of excess fluid. **(Objective 6)**
29. **b** Glaucoma is a condition of the eyes. Although it is not life-threatening, glaucoma can cause permanent blindness; it is important that glaucoma patients with severe headache receive prompt evaluation by an ophthalmologist. **(Objective 5)**
30. **d** When you are describing a patient's level of consciousness, avoid using words like *stuporous, lethargic, obtunded*, and the like. Such terms are not very informative because people seldom agree on what they mean. Instead, you should describe the patient's state of consciousness in terms of reactions to specific stimuli or responses to specific inquiries. **(Objective 3)**
31. **a** Your interview questions should be phrased in such a way that you avoid putting words into the patient's mouth. In particular, you should refrain from asking questions that can be answered with *yes* or *no*. **(Objective 2)**
32. **c** Tension may cause spasm in scalp and neck muscles, which can result in tension headache. Should an intracranial mass or bleeding be present, sensory fibers are activated to send impulses that are interpreted as pain. **(Objective 1)**

Chapter 34: Weak, Dizzy, and Malaise

1. Conditions affecting the brain (stroke or a specific nerve), electrolyte disturbances, infection and fever, hypoperfusion, hypoglycemia, toxicologic conditions, and cardiac ischemia. **(Objective 1)**

2. **c** It is essential to find out this information first. It will assist you in determining the potential cause of the patient's problem. The other questions listed here are also relevant, but their value is enhanced by obtaining this information first. **(Objective 3)**

3. A respiratory examination, a neurologic examination, a blood glucose determination, and an ECG reading. **(Objective 3)**

4. **c** Anemia is accompanied by a history of bleeding; cerebral vascular accident and specific nerve aliments are associated with one-sided weakness; an inner ear disorder is manifested by dizziness. **(Objective 1)**

5. Sinus tachycardia with peaked T waves. **(Prerequisite Chapter Objective)**

6. **c** Peaked T waves, loss of P waves, and a widening QRS are specific changes associated with potassium abnormalities; these are not characteristic of calcium, magnesium, or sodium disorders. **(Objective 1)**

7. **e** Dopamine is used to treat low blood pressure in patients who are in cardiogenic shock; epinephrine is administered as a cardiovascular system stimulant or as a bronchodilator. **(Objective 5)**

8. ECG changes, respiratory compromise, and any indication of hypoperfusion. **(Objectives 4 and 5)**

9. Describe what your dizziness feels like.

    How long have you been experiencing it?

    Do you have any major medical illnesses?

    Do you take any medications?

    (Objective 3)

10. **d** Anemia is a condition characterized by a low hemoglobin level in the blood, decreased red blood cell production, and increased red cell destruction or blood loss. Hypoperfusion is described as a symptom similar to lightheadedness, and malaise is a more generalized weakness. **(Objective 1)**

11. Inner ear disorders or central nervous system disorders, particularly tumor, hemorrhage, or an ischemic condition that affects the cerebellum. **(Objective 1)**

12. Patients who have vertigo may exhibit ataxia (incoordination) or an unsteady gait. These signs, when present, support a diagnosis of this condition. **(Objectives 1 and 3)**

13. **Yes.** Because this is a vague complaint, the suspected condition and other potentially life-threatening conditions should be considered and evaluated immediately by a physician. **(Objectives 4 and 5)**

14. **No.** As stated above, the patient's condition could have been life-threatening. Therefore, it was appropriate to provide immediate access to physician attention (with or without admission to the hospital). **(Objectives 4 and 5)**

15. **c** When only the brain or a specific nerve is involved, symptoms are manifested in one side, or part, of the body. **(Objective 1)**

16. **(a)** Anemia is defined as a deficiency of hemoglobin in the blood. Because hemoglobin carries oxygen to the tissues, low hemoglobin levels result in the delivery of less oxygen. Consequently, the anemic patient feels weak, tired, and sometimes short of breath. The most common causes of anemia are related to chronic blood loss.

    (b) Whether bacterial, viral, or fungal, infection frequently causes malaise or weakness. The more systemic an infection has become, the more probable it is that a patient will show signs of malaise.

    (c) In elderly or diabetic patients, cardiac ischemia may present without the typical complaints; it may be demonstrated by lethargy or weakness alone. **(Objective 1)**

17. Alteration of mental status and decreased cerebral blood flow. **(Objective 1)**

18. Any cause of decreased cardiac output, such as hypovolemia or dysrhythmia, can lead to lightheadedness. Also, the central nervous system can be affected by hypoxia, medications (sedatives and antihistamines), and psychogenic causes (such as hyperventilation syndrome), all of which produce this symptom. **(Objective 1)**

19. **b** Hypoperfusion typically presents as syncope, or lightheadedness; inner ear infection manifests with vertigo; cerebral vascular accident is associated with one-sided, as opposed to generalized, weakness. **(Objective 1)**

20. **f (Objective 2)**

21. **a** When evaluating the patient who complains of weakness, dizziness, or malaise, the paramedic must attempt to define the complaint(s) further. Patients who complain of weakness, dizziness, and malaise present a challenge to even the most experienced EMS provider. Historical data concerning the patient's symptoms (vertigo, lightheadedness, generalized weakness, localized weakness) are the most useful for directing management. Twelve-lead ECG, rapid blood glucose determination, and medical history all are relevant to the assessment, but none of these is the most important aspect. **(Objective 3)**

22. **(a)** Rapid blood glucose determination **(b)** cardiac monitoring **(Objective 5)**

CHAPTER 35 Diabetic Emergencies

1. Large vessels in the brain develop atherosclerotic plaque formation more often in diabetics than in nondiabetics; thus, cerebral vascular disease is a major contributor to the decreased life expectancy of diabetics. **(Objective 4)**

2. Type II, non–insulin dependent diabetes mellitus. This patient is taking the oral hypoglycemic agent Tolinase®, which is prescribed for treatment of Type II diabetes. Also, Type II diabetes usually appears after age 40. **(Objective 3)**

3. Signs and symptoms of dehydration include orthostatic hypotension, tachycardia, skin tenting, and blood sugar greater than 350. This condition is more common among patients older than 60 years of age and in institutionalized individuals. Alternatively, in a patient presenting with stroke, blood pressure is usually elevated and pulse rate is slow. **(Objective 8)**

4. **Yes.** This patient's assessment findings strongly suggest dehydration, which requires isotonic fluids (normal saline or lactated Ringer's solution) for volume replacement. Fluid replacement is the mainstay of therapy for patients with nonketotic hyperosmolar coma. **(Objective 7)**

5. Basilar breath sounds should have been assessed before any fluid bolus was administered to this geriatric patient. Because many geriatric patients exhibit some degree of congestive heart failure, chronic basilar crackles are not an uncommon finding. Therefore, information on baseline basilar breath sounds is essential. **(Prerequisite Chapter Objective)**

6. Blood pressure should increase, pulse should decrease, and dizziness and neurologic deficits may completely resolve. **(Objectives 7 and 8)**

7. Mortality may be as high as 50% in patients with nonketotic hyperosmolar coma. Ultimately, this patient will need insulin (which you cannot administer in the prehospital setting) and volume replacement for successful treatment. **(Objectives 6 and 7)**

8. In the unconscious adult, consent for life-saving treatment measures is said to be implied. In the case of children, if the parent or legal guardian is unavailable, emergency treatment to sustain life also may be undertaken under the principle of implied consent. **(Prerequisite Chapter Objective)**

9. Low. All of your assessment findings are consistent with a low blood glucose measurement. Eating a special diet and taking medication by injection both suggest that the patient has insulin-dependent diabetes. Her cur-

rent episode had an acute onset; signs and symptoms of central nervous system dysfunction were described by her friends as "acting drunk" before losing consciousness. Tachycardia and slow or normal respiratory rates are seen often in hypoglycemic patients, as is diaphoresis that results from an increased sympathetic response. **(Objectives 5 and 8)**

10. The signs and symptoms of hypoglycemia are rapidly and easily reversible. Its quick diagnosis and management are essential in preventing irreversible brain damage. **(Objective 6)**

11. **No.** This patient's level of consciousness is too low to allow safe administration of oral glucose solution. This form of glucose administration is appropriate only if the patient is competent to administer the liquid without assistance, which clearly this patient is unable to do. **(Objective 7)**

12. So that with this blood sample, a more precise blood sugar evaluation can be done at the hospital. **(Objective 7)**

13. D50 is extremely irritating to the veins; it should be administered slowly over 3 to 5 minutes, with a maintenance IV continuing to run open. **(Objective 7)**

14. **e** Providing your patient with immediate reassurance and privacy will minimize the fear and embarrassment that she will experience as she becomes more alert. Informing her of what happened also will help to calm her. The duration of the interval between her last meal and the administration of insulin most likely will reveal the cause of her hypoglycemic episode. **(Objective 7)**

15. Recommend that the patient take complex carbohydrates. Explain that a quick boost of simple sugar without a more prolonged carbohydrate load leads to repeated episodes of hypoglycemia. **(Objective 7)**

16. In addition to documenting the patient's response to treatment, it is standard practice to require the patient's legal guardian to sign a refusal of treatment and/or transport form after the potential risks of refusing treatment have been explained. **(Prerequisite Chapter Objective)**

17. Diabetic ketoacidosis. This patient exhibits all of the characteristics of diabetic ketoacidosis, including polydipsia, polyphagia, polyuria, nausea, Kussmaul respirations, and fruity-smelling breath. **(Objective 8)**

18. **Yes.** Decreased potassium levels resulting from dehydration can lead to serious dysrhythmias. **(Objectives 7 and 8)**

19. **c** Fluid and electrolyte replacement via isotonic IV solution administration is the only appropriate and safe prehospital treatment for a patient with diabetic ketoacidosis. **(Objective 7)**

20. Adults can be given boluses of 500 mL, which may be repeated as needed to a total volume of 2 liters. **(Objective 7)**

21. Foot problems are common in diabetic patients. Ulcers form and do not heal well because of poor blood supply, impaired wound healing, and decreased nerve function. **(Objective 4)**

22.

	Type I (IDDM)	Type II (NIDDM)
Pathology	No insulin production	Decreased insulin production
Age of onset	Childhood Peak age: 10–14	Adulthood older than age 40
Required treatment	Insulin	Diet control, oral agents, insulin
Tendency for ketoacidosis	Strong	Weak

(Objective 1)

23. **(a)** Insulin is released into the bloodstream in response to elevations in blood sugar. It assists glucose uptake by the cells, allows excess glucose to be stored in the liver and muscle, and is used in fat synthesis.

    (b) Glucagon is released into the bloodstream to elevate blood sugar when glucose is not getting into cells, either because of inadequate food intake or lack of insulin, thus causing the body to perceive a fasting state. It causes the breakdown of stored sugars in the liver, and then breaks down stored body fat. **(Objective 1)**

24. Heart disease and cerebral vascular disease. Large vessels of the heart, brain, and lower extremities develop atherosclerotic plaque formation more often in diabetic than nondiabetic patients. As a result, heart disease and cerebral vascular disease are major contributors to the decreased life expectancy of diabetics. **(Objective 4)**

25. Oral hypoglycemic agents work by causing the release of insulin from the pancreas. **(Objective 9)**

26. It should be diluted to D25; D50 is too hypertonic to be administered to pediatric patients. **(Objective 7)**

27. Unrecognized hypoglycemia results in death. The cells of the body, especially those of the brain, depend on glucose to function. Without glucose, the cells may find other sources of energy, but their breakdown products are toxic and eventually lethal if the hypoglycemic process is not reversed. Permanent brain damage may occur in patients who survive hypoglycemic events; this is so because the cells of the brain, similar to other body cells, lack the ability to store or to use other sources of energy. **(Objective 6)**

28. **b (Objective 8)**
29. **a (Objective 8)**
30. **a (Objective 8)**
31. **b (Objective 8)**
32. **a (Objective 8)**
33. **b (Objective 8)**
34. **d (Objective 8)**
35. **d** It is likely that all blood vessels in diabetics are abnormal. Small vessel disease is caused by thickening of the lining of the vessels. Large vessels develop atherosclerotic plaque formation. **(Objective 4)**
36. **b** Without adequate insulin to assist glucose uptake by the cells, the circulating blood level will increase. **(Objective 8)**
37. **d** When glucose is not getting into the cells, because of either inadequate food intake or lack of insulin, the body perceives a fasting state and releases glucagon to elevate blood sugar. Glucagon causes the breakdown of stored sugars in the liver, and then of stored fat. Fat metabolism results in ketone production as a breakdown product. Ketones are acidic. It is this process that leads to diabetic ketoacidosis. **(Objective 8)**
38. **b (Objective 2)**
39. **c** Alcoholics generally have depleted most of their stored thiamine, and some evidence suggests that Wernicke's encephalopathy can be precipitated by a large load of glucose that rapidly exhausts the small remaining reserve. **(Objective 7)**
40. **c** Propranolol is a beta blocker that is commonly prescribed for angina, hypertension, and tachydysrhythmia. **(Objective 9)**

CHAPTER 36: Abdominal, Genitourinary, and Back Pain

1. **b** Your initial assessment, including determination of pulse and breathing status, takes priority over the medical history, BP, and ECG. **(Prerequisite Chapter Objective)**
2. **d** Acid-neutralizing and antiinflammatory agents also may be used for gastrointestinal problems, but they do not specifically reduce acid secretion. ACE inhibitors are used for the treatment of cardiac conditions. **(Prerequisite Chapter Objective)**
3. **c** Atypical pain is defined as "not typical"; this pain is typical. Referred pain is experienced at a site that is distant from the affected site; visceral pain is localized poorly and is usually intermittent. **(Objective 1)**
4. **Yes.** The patient demonstrates signs of shock, which include an altered level of consciousness, a weak and rapid pulse, pale and sweaty skin, and rapid respirations. **(Prerequisite Chapter Objective)**
5. **Yes.** The reduction in cardiac output that results from intraabdominal bleeding and shock can cause airway, breathing, and circulatory compromise. **(Objectives 4 and 5)**
6. **d** Other types of cardiac medications exert effects to dilate coronary arteries (coronary vasodilators), improve conduction through the AV junction (digoxin), and lower heart rate (beta blockers). **(Prerequisite Chapter Objective)**
7. **d** Pain associated with acute appendicitis occurs initially in the periumbilical region, then is focused in the right lower quadrant; pain from cholecystitis is in the right upper quadrant; kidney stone pain is focused in the back and flank areas; however, typically, it is not accompanied by signs of shock or decreased femoral and peripheral pulses. **(Objective 7)**
8. Ringer's lactate or normal saline; at a fast rate   The patient is exhibiting signs of shock; there is possibly internal bleeding. **(Prerequisite Chapter Objective)**

9. Typically, no. Although this is a controversial issue, the prehospital use of narcotic analgesics for patients with abdominal pain is not recommended. Administration of narcotics can mask ongoing symptoms and can impair evaluation of the patient's condition by the emergency department physician or surgeon. **(Objective 8)**

10. Abdominal aortic aneurysm is one of the most rapidly lethal conditions that can present with acute abdominal pain. It is caused by localized weakening and dilation of the wall of the aorta; it usually results from atherosclerosis. An estimated 2% to 7% of the adult population experiences this condition; there is an 11% incidence in men older than 65 years of age. Mortality that results from ruptured abdominal aortic aneurysm is nearly 80% in such patients who present in shock. **(Objectives 4, 5, and 7)**

11. When did the pain begin?

    Where is the pain?

    Describe the pain.

    Do you feel pain anywhere else?

    Do you have any other symptoms associated with the pain?

    Is there anything that makes it better or worse?

    Rate your pain on a scale of 1 to 10 (with 1 being least severe).

    (Objective 3)

12. Placement of the patient in a comfortable position; performance of a tilt test; inspection and palpation of the abdomen. **(Objective 6)**

13. History and physical findings suggest the following possibilities: appendicitis; intestinal obstruction; aortic aneurysm; gastroenteritis; possible diverticulitis; kidney stone (although this is not as likely). **(Objective 7)**

14. Given the time constraints and noisy environment of the prehospital setting, auscultation of the abdomen has limited value in the prehospital evaluation of patients with abdominal pain. Even when it is performed, auscultation does not alter patient management decisions. **(Objective 6)**

15. Acknowledge that you are glad that he feels better. Explain that his symptoms could indicate a nonurgent problem (e.g., gastroenteritis) but that they are also consistent with more serious conditions that require further evaluation in the hospital and could require immediate surgery. Tell him that you strongly recommend that he pursue this possibility and agree to transport. **(Objective 7)**

16. Change in the level of consciousness; change in vital signs; any indication or signs of hypovolemia. **(Objectives 7 and 8)**

17. Reassure her that you are there to help her; quickly evaluate her overall appearance, looking for signs of any immediate distress (e.g., respiratory or circulatory compromise). **(Prerequisite Chapter Objective)**

18. Ruptured ectopic pregnancy is the leading cause of death occurring during the first trimester of pregnancy; mortality results primarily from acute hemorrhage. If the ectopic pregnancy ruptures, the patient usually experiences sudden, severe abdominal pain that originates on one side of the lower abdomen. All women of childbearing age with acute lower abdominal pain must be considered for this potential problem. Determination of menstrual history is related directly to this situation. **(Objectives 4 and 7)**

19. Do you have any other symptoms associated with the pain?

    Is there anything that makes the pain better or worse?

    Do you have any blood in your urine? Do you experience discomfort while urinating? **(Objective 3)**

20. **c** The patient's age, history, and symptoms are not suggestive of acute myocardial infarction; her menstrual period history is normal; there is no evidence of gastrointestinal bleeding, which would be present with a bleeding ulcer. **(Objective 7)**

21. **Yes.** Patients with suspected kidney stones require further diagnostic testing to either confirm the diagnosis or determine another cause for the problem. **(Objective 7)**

22. **(a)** Visceral pain fibers are located in the walls of hollow organs and in the capsules of solid organs. This pain is often the earliest sign of an acute intra-abdominal process; it is usually intermittent, it worsens with time, and it may be described as dull, cramping, or even gaseous. Visceral pain is poorly localized and ill defined; usually, it is felt in the midline of the abdomen. **(Objective 1)**

    (b) Referred pain is experienced at a location distant from the affected site. Pain that originates in the abdomen can occur also at an extra-abdominal location; it is usually intense, and it most often occurs in association with an inflammatory condition. **(Objective 1)**

23. **b** Cardiac pain could be described this way, but typically it is not aggravated by coughing. Visceral pain is intermittent, may be described as dull or crampy, and is poorly localized. Referred pain is the pain that occurs in another area of the body, which is not the primary source of the pain. **(Objective 1)**

24. Somatic. It may be caused by bacterial or chemical inflammation of the peritoneum, and it occurs after the onset of visceral pain in many disease processes. Once parietal peritoneal irritation occurs, the abdominal examination reveals localized tenderness that corresponds to the specific inflamed area. **(Objectives 1 and 2)**

25. Referred pain is experienced at a location distant from the affected site because overlapping nerve segments provide sensation to both areas. **(Objective 1)**

26. **(a)** To characterize the pain episode

    (b) To identify factors suggestive of a potentially life-threatening condition

    (Objective 3)

27. Sudden, severe abdominal pain suggests an intra-abdominal catastrophe. Abdominal pain precedes the onset of associated symptoms such as nausea and vomiting in most cases of acute abdominal pain that require surgery. Pain that awakens the patient from sleep usually indicates significant disease. Acute, severe abdominal pain that occurs in a previously healthy patient and lasts longer than six hours usually requires surgical intervention. **(Objective 4)**

28. **d** If peritoneal involvement is extensive, as may occur with leakage of blood, gastric juice, or intestinal contents into the intraabdominal cavity, somatic pain progresses from a well-localized to a generalized pain that involves the entire abdomen. This produces the "boardlike" muscle rigidity that characterizes an acute abdomen. **(Objectives 2 and 4)**

29. **b, c,** and **d** All structures of the gastrointestinal tract may bleed when disease is present. The appendix is outside the gastrointestinal tract; if it is inflamed or if it ruptures, typically there is no significant gastrointestinal bleeding. **(Objective 5)**

30. Melena indicates "old" blood; it originates in an upper gastrointestinal tract (e.g., stomach or small intestine). Melena is indicated by the presence of "dark tarry stools," as described by the patient. **(Objective 5)**

31. **b** Gastroenteritis is commonly known as "stomach flu." It can be accompanied by fluid losses and possible dehydration, but it is typically not life-threatening. Sepsis, hypovolemia, and/or hemorrhage are potential and frequent complications of the other conditions listed here. **(Objectives 4 and 7)**

32. To determine the extent and location of the underlying problem, while taking care to avoid causing unnecessary discomfort for the patient. Establishing rapport and providing explanations during assessment promote the patient's understanding and cooperation; such an approach also greatly enhances the yield of information. **(Objective 6)**

33. **False**. Doing so unnecessarily increases the patient's pain and serves to make the patient more guarded and less cooperative for the next examiner. It does not provide any information that will alter the prehospital patient management approach. **(Objective 6)**

34. **True**. Once the aneurysm ruptures, bleeding is very rapid and is associated with a very high mortality rate. **(Objective 7)**

35. **True**. Bleeding vessels, organ rupture, and fluid losses can accompany acute abdominal conditions; these can lead to hypoperfusion and dehydration. **(Objective 7)**

36. **True**. Sepsis is a potential cause of hypoperfusion and hemodynamic compromise in patients with acute abdominal pain. Serious intra-abdominal infection can lead to bacterial invasion of the bloodstream, particularly among elderly patients and those with impaired immune function due to cancer, malignancy, diabetes mellitus, or human immunodeficiency virus (HIV) infection. **(Objective 7)**

37. **True**. As more of the peritoneum becomes involved, local abdominal tenderness is accompanied by guarding (an increase in abdominal wall muscle tone when palpated) and muscle rigidity over the involved structure. **(Objective 2)**

38. **False**. Any pain of this description should be considered a true emergency that carries the potential for a serious intra-abdominal problem. **(Objective 4)**

39. **True**. Some patients with acute cardiac disorders complain primarily of acute abdominal pain. Patients with acute myocardial infarction (AMI) may present with abdominal pain that is not associated with chest pain as the only manifestation of decreased blood flow to the heart muscle. This atypical presentation of AMI is most common among elderly patients, diabetic patients, and those with myocardial infarction that involves the posterior or inferior wall of the heart. **(Objective 7)**

CHAPTER 37 Pregnancy and Child Birth

1. **d** It is very difficult to hear fetal heart tones in the field setting without specialized equipment (Doppler). Asking her if this is her first baby is important, but you can check contractions while obtaining this and other relevant information. Obtaining a blood pressure is important, but it is not the initial priority. **(Objective 7)**

2. How far along is the pregnancy?

   Do you have abdominal pain?

   Has there been any vaginal bleeding?

   Has the bag of waters ruptured?

   Are you having contractions? **(Objective 7)**

3. You should ask her if she has experienced any visual disturbances, headaches, or other discomforts; check her hands, face, and extremities for swelling. Also, evaluate her medical history for conditions such as diabetes, hypertension, and kidney disease. **(Objectives 4, 6, and 7)**

4. **c** High blood pressure, associated with edema of the face and hands, indicates preeclampsia. Blood pressure normally drops somewhat during pregnancy, so this reading (140/94) could be significant. It is also her first pregnancy, which places her at a higher level of risk. Placenta previa most likely would be associated with vaginal bleeding. Abruptio placenta would present with some signs of abdominal rigidity and/or shock. **(Objectives 4 and 6)**

5. You should take your partner aside and tell him that you think the patient should go to the hospital because she could be preeclamptic. To the patient, acknowledge that what your partner said about early labor is true; however, explain that because of her blood pressure reading, you must suggest that she consent to being transported to the hospital. **(Objective 4)**

6. Seizures. If the patient is preeclamptic and is in labor, the risk of seizures should be strongly considered. When a pregnant patient has a seizure, the mother's life is in danger, as is that of the fetus, because of the hypoxia that is associated with seizure activity. **(Objectives 2 and 4)**

7. **Yes.** This condition is seen most frequently in very young and older primigravidas (first-time pregnancies). Also, it often occurs in women who have had multiple pregnancies, or who have a history of hypertension, diabetes, or another chronic illness. **(Objective 4)**

8. **a, b, c, and d** Also, the patient in labor should be placed on her left side whenever possible to promote blood return to the heart and oxygenation to the fetus. This is particularly important if, for any reason, you suspect that the fetus has been deprived of oxygen. **(Objectives 4 and 6)**

9. Magnesium sulfate, or possibly diazepam. If available, magnesium sulfate is typically the drug of choice for treatment of eclamptic seizures. Diazepam must be used with caution because it can cause respiratory depression while controlling seizure activity. **(Objective 9)**

10. Paramedics may not always agree on the assessment findings of a patient. The important thing is that the best patient care be provided. If it requires you to "overrule" your partner at the time, do so as tactfully as you can, and discuss the reasons why later. Another option in this situation (particularly if it cannot be resolved) is to contact medical direction for advice. Explain your reasons after the call, and reassure your partner that your actions were not meant to belittle him or her in any way, but that you observed a finding that required you to intervene. **(Prerequisite Chapter Objective)**

11. Because you know that any bleeding during the last trimester of pregnancy is considered an abnormality, this is an immediate concern. Most such situations require prompt attention and possibly an emergency cesarean section. You need to perform a rapid assessment and quickly transport her to the hospital. **(Objectives 3, 4, and 7)**

12. **d** Abruptio placenta typically is associated with pain; this patient denies pain. Ectopic pregnancy occurs during the first trimester; hyperemesis gravidarum is a condition that is associated with some pain. Toxemia of pregnancy occurs during the second or third trimester; it is characterized by high blood pressure, excessive swelling, and CNS alteration. Bleeding is not associated with toxemia of pregnancy. **(Objectives 4 and 7)**

13. Place the patient on 100% oxygen; this provides the best environment for circulation of oxygen to the fetus. An IV (Ringer's lactate or normal saline) should be established and titrated to the patient's blood pressure. Place the patient on her left side. If signs or symptoms of shock worsen, a second IV line should be established. **(Objective 4)**

14. **Yes.** When shock occurs, blood flow is maintained to the most essential organs. The fetus is the first to have blood shunted away; this precedes even diversion of blood from the skin. If the mother has decreased cardiac output, such as occurs in trauma or shock, fetal circulation is affected immediately. It is possible for the mother to withstand a great deal of blood loss without showing evidence of shock, while the fetus may be dying of hypoxia. Signs of shock or hypoperfusion in the mother should signal the potential for immediate danger to the fetus (fetal distress); urgent transport to an appropriate facility is essential. **(Prerequisite Chapter Objective and Objective 3)**

15. Acknowledge that her bleeding is a cause for concern; reassure her that you are taking immediate steps to provide the best treatment for both her and the baby. Explain that immediate treatment provided by you and emergency department personnel can result in the best possible outcome. **(Prerequisite Chapter Objective and Objective 4)**

16. Check the perineal area to determine if she is crowning, or if there is a presenting part. **(Objectives 7, 8, and 10)**

17. **d** The situation is now critical. Breech extremity presentation requires a cesarean section, which cannot be performed in the prehospital environment. Therefore, immediate transport to the hospital is the only appropriate action. **(Objectives 5 and 10)**

18. Breech extremity presentation tends to prolong labor. Prolonged labor can lead to hypoxia in the infant, which is associated with a high mortality rate. Delivery should never be attempted in the field setting. **(Objectives 3 and 5)**

19. **f**
20. **e**
21. **b**
22. **g**
23. **c**
24. **h**
25. **a**

    (Answers 19 to 25: Objective 1)

26. **(a)** Increased blood volume, heart rate, cardiac output, and total body water; decreased blood pressure.

    (b) Increased oxygen consumption, tidal volume, and depth of respirations; enhanced perception of dyspnea.

    (c) Increased size of kidneys and improved blood flow to them; increased frequency and urgency of urination; increased urine production, especially at night.

    (d) Gums may bleed; heartburn; nausea and vomiting during the first trimester; constipation and hemorrhoids.

    (e) Stretch marks on breasts, lower abdomen, and thighs; increased perspiration; skin pigmentation (mask of pregnancy is a darkening of the skin that is seen particularly on the face, forehead, cheeks, and nose); increased nail and hair growth.

    (f) Increased backache, pelvic discomfort, and muscle cramping, especially during the third trimester and at night. **(Objective 2)**

27. **b** With significant stress, the fetal heart rate drops below its normal rate of 120 to 160. Monitoring must be done with a Doppler or Fetascope, both of which are rarely available in the field. The mother's blood pressure and heart rate are not good indicators of fetal status, nor is pulse oximetry that checks the abdomen (uterus). **(Objective 3)**

28. Spontaneous abortion: the uterine muscles contract to expel the contents, causing crampy abdominal pain. Vaginal bleeding usually occurs.

    Threatened abortion: the occurrence of vaginal bleeding during the first half of pregnancy, possibly associated with abdominal cramping; however, the fetus remains viable. Twenty percent of threatened abortions progress to fetal demise and abortion, and more than one half of those fetuses exhibit chromosomal abnormalities that are not compatible with life. **(Objective 4)**

29. **b, c, d,** and **e**   Age is not a specific risk factor for ectopic pregnancy. **(Objective 4)**

30. **b**   All the others listed here are problems that contribute to infant morbidity and mortality, but none does so as universally as premature or preterm labor. **(Objectives 3 and 4)**

31. Abruptio placenta is the premature separation of the placenta from the uterus; it occurs most often in the third trimester. It is always accompanied by bleeding, which may or may not be visible, depending on the point of separation. In any case, the bleeding is significant, and both mother and baby are in a life-threatening situation. **(Objective 4)**

32. **a**   Meconium-stained amniotic fluid is not associated with bleeding; it does not indicate imminent delivery and has no association with the incidence of placenta previa. Fetal asphyxia can occur if the thick meconium is aspirated because it can block the airway. **(Objective 5)**

33. **(a)** Place your hand into the vagina, and push up on the fetal head to decrease cord compression until management can be assumed by a physician in the emergency department.

    (b) Rapid transport to the hospital is indicated for any breech presentation or other condition that causes prolonged labor. If you must deliver a frank breech, allow the fetus to deliver spontaneously to the level of the umbilicus. If the head does not deliver spontaneously, insert a gloved hand and support the infant's maxilla while exerting mild downward traction.

    (Objective 5)

34. **c**

35. **a**

36. **b (Answers 34 to 36: Objective 8)**

37. The patient is straining as if to have a bowel movement; the vagina is bulging; the fetal head is visible at the vaginal opening. **(Objective 10)**

38. Establish a sterile field: support the head; encourage the mother not to push as the head emerges. Once the head is delivered, suction the nose and mouth; deliver one shoulder at a time (usually the upper first); clamp the cord; warm and stimulate the infant. **(Objective 11)**

39. Uterine massage; encouraging the infant to breastfeed. **(Objective 5)**

40. Maintaining body temperature is a primary concern. Dry the infant as soon as possible, using an infant warmer, if one is available. If not, use warm towels. Covering the head is also important for maintaining warmth; this can be accomplished easily using a blanket. **(Objective 12)**

CHAPTER 38 Fever

1. When did the fever begin, and how high is it?

   What is the pattern of the fever?

   Are there any associated symptoms?

   (Objective 7)

2. Explain that this is a routine precaution that is taken during examination of any patient, especially one who presents with a fever. Explain that gloves are worn to protect the baby from exposure to possible germs or infection, as well as for the protection of others from the spread of an unknown illness that the baby may have. **(Prerequisite Chapter Objective)**

3. **Yes.** The temperature should be measured rectally with any patient who exhibits an altered level of consciousness or confusion, is younger than 5 years of age, or has a history of seizures. A rectal temperature reading is the most accurate reflection of core body temperature. Techniques such as temperature strips or audiothermy when used to measure temperature may not be as accurate as using a thermometer. **(Objective 10)**

4. The possibility of meningitis should be considered in any child with a fever. A sustained fever, as well as a higher body temperature, is most commonly found with a more serious illness such as meningitis. Associated complaints and findings of tiredness, poor feeding, skin rash, and bulging fontanelles are also highly suggestive of meningitis. **(Objective 8)**

5. Lethargy, anorexia, purpura. **(Prerequisite Chapter Objective)**

6. Neck stiffness is a significant sign of meningitis, but it is especially difficult to evaluate this in young children. **(Objective 8)**

7. **No.** The normal pulse rate range for a 2-month-old is 100 to 160. The pulse can be expected to increase at a rate of 10 beats per minute for each 1.3-degree F (0.6-degree C) rise in temperature. **(Prerequisite Chapter Objective and Objective 8)**

8. The risk for a child of developing a serious infection, such as meningitis, is greater than that for an adult because children lack a fully developed immune system. **(Objective 9)**

9. Acetaminophen is effective in lowering temperature elevation by blocking the production of prostaglandins. Aspirin is no longer considered appropriate for use in children with a fever because it is now known to provoke Reye's syndrome. **(Objectives 11 and 12)**

10. Ice and cold baths should be avoided because they can cause overcooling through shivering and constriction of skin blood vessels, which increases the core temperature. Alcohol baths are also discouraged because the alcohol can be absorbed through the skin. **(Objectives 11 and 12)**

11. The physician might recommend prophylactic treatment for both of you because you were exposed to a potential case of meningitis. **(Prerequisite Chapter Objective)**

12. Treatment, including administration of high-concentration oxygen and preparation to assist ventilations, should begin immediately. Based on this patient's presentation, his change in level of consciousness and signs of respiratory distress could indicate oxygen insufficiency. If this is not corrected, it could pose an immediate life threat. Airway management is always a high priority of the initial assessment procedure. **(Prerequisite Chapter Objective)**

13. Further assessment of this patient's respiratory and cardiovascular status, including evaluation of breath sounds, measurement of vital signs, and use of the cardiac monitor, is the next assessment priority. These areas are important because they pose the most imminent life threats. **(Prerequisite Chapter Objective)**

14. Cardiac monitoring is especially important for this patient because he is at high risk for the development of dysrhythmia owing to his age and his past and current conditions. **(Prerequisite Chapter Objective)**

15. **Yes.** In the elderly, temperature regulation by the hypothalamus is often compromised. Because baseline temperature is usually lower than normal, a life-threatening infection can occur without a significant temperature elevation. **(Objectives 2 and 9)**

16. Advanced age and diabetes. Both of these factors are associated with impaired immunity. **(Objective 9)**

17. A decreasing level of consciousness; pale, cool, moist skin; hypotension. **(Objective 8)**

18. Field management of this patient in septic shock would include blood pressure support provided by the administration of fluids; vasopressors such as dopamine may be used if the blood pressure does not respond to volume replacement. Immediate transport to the emergency department is necessary so that the patient may be started on a course of antibiotics. **(Objective 11)**

19. Airway control and assisted ventilations are the highest priority because of this patient's decreased level of consciousness and slow respiratory rate. **(Prerequisite Chapter Objective)**

20. Sympathetic stimulants such as cocaine and amphetamines can produce a hyperactive, hypermetabolic state that is associated with the development of fever. **(Objectives 4 and 5)**

21. Remove her clothing, and place cold compresses to her groin and axilla. **(Objective 11)**

22. Diazepam is used to treat seizures that are associated with cocaine toxicity. **(Objective 11)**

23. Body temperature can be estimated clinically and quickly by noting the appearance of the skin, which may be flushed and warm to the touch. The skin is usually dry; however, in this patient, it may be diaphoretic because of the seizure activity. **(Objective 10)**

24. Loss; production. **(Objective 1)**

25. Hypothalamus **(Objective 2)**

26. Shivering; vasoconstriction. **(Objective 5)**
27. 96.6° ; 99.6° **(Objective 3)**
28. Radiation; evaporation; convection; conduction. **(Objective 1)**
29. **b (Objective 3)**
30. **c (Objective 3)**
31. **a (Objective 3)**
32. Fever is an elevation in body temperature. **(Objective 3)**
33. Infection **(Objective 4)**
34. Bacteria and viruses reproduce more slowly at temperatures that are higher than the normal core temperature. **(Objective 5)**
35. **(a)** This patient may be experiencing an acute myocardial infarction, which can result in the release of pyrogens when tissue is destroyed. These pyrogens cause an increased production of prostaglandins, which raise the thermostatic "set point" of the hypothalamus to a higher level.
    (b) This patient may be experiencing heat exhaustion because high humidity decreases the ability of the body to dissipate the heat produced by evaporation that is associated with increased exercise.
    (c) This patient may be experiencing a stroke, which can cause structural damage that directly affects the hypothalamus.
    (d) This patient may be experiencing a urinary tract infection, which results in pyrogen release that is caused by infectious agents in the urinary system.
    (Objectives 4, 5, and 6)
36. **c (Objective 7)**
37. **b (Objective 8)**
38. **c (Objective 6)**
39. **b (Objective 8)**
40. **d (Objective 11)**
41. **True. (Objective 10)**
42. **False.** Axillary temperatures are somewhat unreliable, and it takes 5 to 7 minutes to obtain a reading; therefore, this method is not recommended for use in the prehospital setting. Oral temperatures are taken in most situations. **(Objective 10)**
43. **False.** Rectal temperature readings are measured in patients with a history of seizures because this method is safer. **(Objective 10)**

CHAPTER 39: Eye, Ear, Nose, and Throat Complaints—Medical

1. **Yes.** A chief complaint of eye pain could indicate a serious and emergent condition, such as acute glaucoma or retinal artery occlusion. If it is accompanied by vision loss, this complaint is more significant. Further assessment in the emergency department is warranted. **(Objective 3)**
2. Ask questions that elicit a specific description of the pain and its severity. You should also ask questions such as:
    Are you having any visual disturbances?
    Is there any history of trauma or eye surgery?
    Has this ever happened before?
    (Objective 10)

3. Acute glaucoma. This condition occurs most frequently in the elderly. It begins with unilateral eye pain that causes nausea and vomiting. The patient often appears quite ill and complains of decreased vision and "seeing halos" around lights. There are no signs of infection, although retinal artery occlusion and cerebral vascular accident (CVA) are also possibilities, considering the patient's age and medical history. **(Objective 4)**

4. If medications to decrease intraocular pressure are not initiated promptly in the emergency department, the patient can become blind within hours. **(Objective 4)**

5. **b** Airway problems can occur with a significant nosebleed. Ensuring airway potency takes priority over steps to control bleeding, evaluate circulatory status, or start an IV. **(Objective 8)**

6. The irritating effect of swallowed blood (from a nosebleed) on the gastrointestinal tract can produce nausea and vomiting. If bleeding is severe, rapid, or prolonged, signs and symptoms of hypovolemia can develop. **(Objective 8)**

7. **c** Obtaining information related to the patient's medical history is significant at this point in the assessment to determine if there have been previous episodes, how they were managed, and what the potential causes were. This information takes precedence over an ECG reading and checking for allergies. Examination of the nose is limited to what can be accomplished by inspection; probing for foreign bodies is not appropriate. **(Objective 10)**

8. Upright on the stretcher. Because this patient has been swallowing blood and is nauseated, she should be positioned so that she is leaning forward; this permits blood flow from the nostrils rather than the throat. Suction should be readily available. **(Objective 8)**

9. **c (Objective 1)**

10. **e (Objectives 1 and 2)**

11. **b (Objectives 1 and 2)**

12. **g (Objective 2)**

13. **d (Objective 7)**

14. **a (Objective 7)**

15. **f (Objective 7)**

16. It converts sound waves into nerve impulses, which allow us to hear; it provides information to the brain to maintain balance. **(Objective 6)**

17. **a, b, d,** and **e** Conjunctivitis is a localized infection and an irritation of the anterior surface of the eye. Although the condition requires treatment, it typically does not cause vision loss, blindness, or other serious complications. **(Objectives 4 and 5)**

18. When a light is shined into the eye, the normal response is for the pupil to constrict. If the pupil does not react, something in this pathway is not working properly. A fixed and dilated pupil may indicate trauma (local or intracranial) or glaucoma. The presence of an artificial eye also should be considered. **(Objective 10)**

19. **a** Peritonsillar abscesses can penetrate deeply to form abscesses in the deep spaces of the neck, thereby threatening airway patency. Pharyngitis, strep throat, and tonsillitis typically do not cause acute problems related to the airway. **(Objective 9)**

20. A red, painful eye; a patient with sudden onset of decreased vision. **(Objective 3)**

21. **d** The patient has the classic symptoms of a dystonic reaction, such as sitting forward, drooling, and stating that she feels like she is going to swallow her tongue. Other signs and symptoms typically would accompany an allergic reaction (e.g., hives, itching, skin reddness, or localized swelling). Also, the physical symptoms indicate that the condition is not simply anxiety, or a conversion reaction. **(Objective 9)**

22. **False.** The patient who wears contact lenses usually is quite adept at removing them and should be allowed to do so if the eyes are painful. **(Objective 2)**

23. **True.** Normal saline typically is more easily tolerated by the patient and thus is preferable to cold water. **(Objective 2)**

24. **True.** Topical anesthetics may be used for pain control in the presence of a suspected foreign body. They should be administered only after a patient has consented to be transported; this approach prevents an inappropriate refusal of care after pain relief is attained. **(Objective 2)**

25. **True.** If bleeding is significant, the collection of blood in the back of the throat and the choking sensation that results can cause airway patency problems. Adequate suction and airway adjuncts should be readily accessible. **(Objective 8)**

26. The most common causes of epistaxis are local trauma, low atmospheric humidity, upper respiratory infection, and allergy. The overuse of nasal spray and the use of cocaine and medications that increase bleeding (aspirin and Coumadin®) also increase the risk of anterior nosebleeds. Hemophilia is an uncommon cause, but it should be considered. A patient who has hypertension has a more difficult time controlling a nosebleed, if it occurs. **(Objective 8)**

27. A patient with a partial airway obstruction should be transported in a position of comfort; oxygen should be administered. Intubation should be considered only as a last resort because this procedure may further aggravate closure of the airway. **(Objective 9)**

CHAPTER 40 Nontraumatic Extremity Complaints

1. Information on the onset and intensity of the pain is important initially. Before you obtain further information or perform the physical examination, it is essential to ask the patient if there has been any recent trauma to the leg, if he or she has been bedridden for any reason, and if he or she has undergone any surgery recently. **(Objective 4)**

2. **a** Checking pulses is the first priority. Absence of a pulse indicates that there is no blood circulation to the extremity. If this is discovered to be the case, the potential for the patient to lose the extremity is increased. Range of motion, sensation, and Homans' sign all are evaluated in the course of the assessment, but these are not the initial priority. **(Objective 4)**

3. **d** Coumadin® is a blood thinner that is used to minimize blood clot formation in susceptible patients. It does not have antidysrhythmic properties, it does not function as a diuretic, nor does it directly affect blood pressure. This patient is at high risk for blood clot formation. Thus, the use of Coumadin® is medically appropriate for his care. **(Prerequisite Chapter Objective)**

4. **b** The patient's history of recent surgery and bed rest indicates that he is a likely candidate for the development of deep vein thrombosis. The presence of a pulse essentially rules out an arterial occlusion. There is no known history of arthritis or a bleeding disorder, which would be associated with septic arthritis or hemarthrosis, respectively. **(Objective 2)**

5. The affected area is extremely painful to the touch; it is also swollen and red, and the patient has a positive Homans' sign. These signs and symptoms are indicative of deep vein thrombosis. **(Objective 2)**

6. Appropriate management of this patient would consist of the administration of 100% oxygen; the initiation of an IV line at a TKO rate; transport of the patient in a position of comfort; and monitoring of the neurologic and vascular status of the extremity while en route. **(Objective 2)**

7. **c** If a portion of a deep vein thrombosis (DVT) breaks loose (embolus), passes through the vascular system, and becomes a pulmonary embolus, this can be life-threatening. Circulatory and respiratory compromise may ensue quickly. Heart attack and aortic aneurysm both involve blockage or other arterial circulation problems. A DVT typically does not affect the heart valves. **(Objectives 1, 2, and 3)**

8. Deep vein thrombosis; arterial occlusion; arthritis; compartment syndrome; hemarthrosis; sickle cell crisis. **(Objective 2)**

9. Describe the pain in terms of character, intensity, and specific location.

   When did the pain start?

   Does the pain radiate anywhere else?

   (Objective 4)

10. **Yes.** The patient's medical history of sickle cell disease combined with her current condition indicates that most likely she is experiencing sickle cell crisis. Because defective red blood cells cannot carry oxygen effectively, the patient can suffer from tissue hypoxia. She requires oxygen, emergency drugs, monitoring, and evaluation at an appropriate medical facility. **(Objectives 1 and 3)**

11. **b** In terms of hydration and oxygenation, IV fluids are important in the management of sickle cell crisis. A TKO IV of D5W or normal saline would be insufficient for her metabolic needs. **(Objective 2)**

12. In sickle cell crisis, abnormal red blood cells (sickle cells) block small blood vessels and prevent blood flow. Blockage and hypoxia occur, resulting in severe aching pain that is located most often in the abdomen, chest, back, and extremities. **(Objective 2)**

13. **c (Objective 2)**

14. **d (Objective 2)**

15. **b (Objective 2)**

16. **e (Objective 2)**

17. **a** Any patient who has single-extremity pain with evidence of decreased warmth, color, or pulse could have an arterial occlusion. Rapid identification is crucial if the extremity is to be saved. If the clot is not removed within six hours of its origin, the extremity could require amputation. **(Objectives 1, 2, and 3)**

18. A thrombus is a stationary blood clot that forms on the wall of a blood vessel or organ. An embolus occurs when a portion of that blood clot (thrombus) breaks loose and travels through the vascular system. An embolus also may consist of air or fat. **(Objective 2)**

19. **d** Arterial emboli usually originate from the heart, but they can originate from the other areas listed here. They may be in the left ventricle (post AMI), or they can occur in the atrium as a result of valvular stenosis or atrial fibrillation. **(Objective 2)**

20. Character, intensity, location, onset, and radiation. **(Objective 4)**

21. Immobilization of the extremity; confinement to bed for long periods; obesity; recent surgery; use of some types of birth control pills; trauma to the extremity; taking a long trip with limited time to stretch. **(Objective 2)**

22. **True.** Weakness or paralysis of one side of the body (both arm and leg) is a classic sign of a cerebral vascular accident. **(Prerequisite Chapter Objective)**

23. **True.** Circulatory compromise to an extremity is detected best by evaluation of the presence and quality of both distal pulse and capillary refill. **(Objective 4)**

24. **False.** This description indicates blockage of an artery, not a vein. **(Objectives 2 and 4)**

25. **True.** Symptoms in the arms that are caused by stress or activity that does not involve the affected extremity and that are not relieved by rest could indicate cardiac ischemia. **(Prerequisite Chapter Objective)**

26. **False.** If a patient has an acute arterial occlusion that is associated with significant circulatory compromise, a vascular surgeon may be needed immediately. In this case, the patient should be transported to a hospital that has this capability. **(Objectives 1 and 3)**

27. The five Ps are *p*ain, *p*aresthesia, *p*allor, *p*ulselessness, and *p*aralysis. **(Objective 2)**

CHAPTER 41 Poisoning and Overdose

1. Because clinical signs of serious poisoning may be delayed for many hours, rapid identification of the toxic agent is important so that therapy can be planned and possible deterioration anticipated. An antidote may be available for a specific substance. **(Objective 3)**

2. Knowing the time of ingestion is critical for effective antidote administration and gastric emptying. **(Objective 3)**

3. **Yes.** Taking 20 pills is not an accident. All patients with intentionally abusive ingestions must be transported, and a psychiatric evaluation of suicidal intent is mandatory. Tylenol® is involved frequently in suicidal poisonings. Initially, there may be only mild nausea, or no symptoms at all. However, over several days, vomiting, abdominal pain, and jaundice can occur because there is potentially fatal injury to the liver. Prompt treatment is needed to avoid complications. **(Objective 3)**

4. Although Tylenol® is well bound by activated charcoal, Ipecac® is safe for very early ingestions. **(Objective 4)**

5. 8 ounces of water **(Objectives 4 and 5)**

6. N-acetyl cysteine; it must be administered within eight hours of the ingestion. **(Objective 4)**

7. **Yes.** You should always bring the pill bottles or the container of suspected poison to the hospital with the patient. You also should bring any other medications that you find in the home. This helps to narrow the possibilities when there is an unknown ingestion, and it may offer evidence of a mixed overdose. **(Objective 3)**

8. You should inspect it for any pills or pill fragments and report any findings to emergency department personnel. You should also note and report any blood in the vomitus. Gastrointestinal hemorrhage can occur with uncontrolled vomiting, as a complication of Ipecac®. **(Objective 3)**

9. **c** Large amounts of iron-containing vitamins can be toxic to small children. **(Objective 3)**

10. **a** Assessment of toddlers is usually difficult. They do not want to be touched, especially by a stranger; therefore, you must do what you have to do as quickly as possible. Separating the mother from the patient probably would make the examination more difficult. **(Prerequisite Chapter Objective)**

11. Be calm, patient, gentle, and honest. Explain what you are going to do before you do it. **(Prerequisite Chapter Objective)**

12. Large amounts of iron-containing vitamins can be very toxic; vomitus may provide a clue as to whether the swallowed vitamins contained iron. Iron is very irritating to the stomach, and early vomiting after iron ingestion occurs often. Vomiting also provides evidence when there has been a more significant ingestion than was suspected initially. **(Objective 4)**

13. Iron is not bound to activated charcoal. If the amount ingested is thought to be small, Ipecac® should not be given because the development of spontaneous vomiting provides a clue that there has been a more significant ingestion than was initially suspected. **(Objectives 4 and 5)**

14. **Yes.** Rapid development of unresponsiveness occurs with serious overdoses of amitriptyline. **(Objective 2)**

15. **Yes.** Intubation is appropriate because of both her reduced level of consciousness and the need to protect her airway. **(Objective 3)**

16. Start an IV and attach ECG monitor leads. The rapid development of hypotension and of wide complex tachycardia is common with this type of overdose. **(Objective 4)**

17. Check the label on the bottle for the number of pills included, the date they were prescribed, and the directions to the patient. Determine the number of pills that she should have taken already per her prescription; then, check to see how many are left in the bottle. Subtract this number from the original number of pills prescribed. **(Objective 3)**

18. Her pupils would be dilated and her skin flushed and dry. **(Objective 3)**

19. Sodium bicarbonate. Wide complex tachycardia responds to the administration of sodium bicarbonate. **(Objective 4)**

20. | Complication | Treatment |
    | --- | --- |
    | Seizures | Administer IV benzodiazepines. |
    | Hypotension | Treat with IV fluids, then with norepinephrine, if it is needed. |

    (Objectives 3 and 4)

21. Ingestion; inhalation; injection; skin contact. **(Objective 1)**

22. It coats the stomach and prevents absorption; it makes the toxin inert; it opposes the action of the poison. **(Objective 5)**

23. Anticholinergic **(Objective 2)**

24. Opioid **(Objective 2)**

25. Adrenergic **(Objective 2)**

26. **No.** Administering Ipecac® is contraindicated if the patient is already vomiting. **(Objective 5)**

27. **Yes.** Ipecac® is indicated for the ingestion of large amounts of aspirin. **(Objective 5)**

28. **No.** Ipecac® is contraindicated in patients who have already seized and who have a mental state depression that would increase the possibility of aspiration. **(Objective 5)**

29. **No.** Ipecac® is contraindicated in patients who have ingested a caustic substance. **(Objective 5)**

30. **No.** Ipecac® is contraindicated in patients who have mental state depression that would increase the possibility of aspiration. **(Objective 5)**

31. Signs and symptoms: headache, nausea, confusion, seizures, unresponsiveness, and hypoperfusion **(Objective 3)**

    Management: administer high-concentration oxygen; transport to a facility with a hyperbaric chamber, if possible. **(Objective 4)**

32. Signs and symptoms: pinpoint pupils, decreased respirations, hypotension, bradycardia, hypothermia, and sedation **(Objective 3)**

    Management: administer high-concentration oxygen; assist ventilations, if needed; start an IV; administer Narcan®; monitor respirations; and transport. **(Objectives 4 and 5)**

33. Signs and symptoms: pinpoint pupils, sweating, hypothermia, bradycardia, vomiting, diarrhea, and increased salivation and bronchial secretions **(Objective 3)**

    Management: wear personal protective clothing when handling the patient; manage the airway; administer high-concentration oxygen; wash skin with soap and water; start an IV; administer intramuscular (IM) and IV atropine; and transport. **(Objectives 4 and 5)**

34. Signs and symptoms: feeling panicky and short of breath at first, followed by unresponsiveness, seizures, bradycardia, and respiratory arrest **(Objective 3)**

    Management: use personal protection from the toxin; manage the airway; assist ventilations, if needed; administer high-concentration oxygen; start an IV line; administer sodium nitrite and sodium thiosulfate; and transport. **(Objectives 4 and 5)**

35. Signs and symptoms: difficulty swallowing, difficulty breathing, and severe pain **(Objective 3)**

    Management: give water or milk to drink; intubate early if there is stridor or respiratory distress; and transport. **(Objective 4)**

36. Signs and symptoms: rapid heart rate, tremor, diaphoresis, vomiting, and seizures **(Objective 3)**

    Management: manage the airway; apply the cardiac monitor; administer activated charcoal if the patient is alert; and transport. **(Objectives 4 and 5)**

37. Signs and symptoms: agitated behavior, hyperthermia, hypertension, tachycardia, seizures, heart attack, stroke **(Objective 3)**

    Management: vomiting is not likely because cocaine entered the body through inhalation rather than ingestion; treatment is symptomatic. **(Objective 4)**

38. **d (Objective 5)**
39. **a (Objective 5)**
40. **a (Objective 3)**
41. **c (Objective 3)**
42. **d (Objective 3)**

CHAPTER 42 Drugs of Abuse

1. Cocaine; amphetamines; alcohol; PCP; LSD **(Objective 8)**
2. Because of the patient's paranoia, you need to avoid any sudden movement or other actions that the patient may find threatening. **(Objective 8)**
3. **Yes.** Myocardial infarct has been associated with the abuse of drugs, especially cocaine. Additionally, the increase in both heart rate and blood pressure that is caused by drug use places excessive demands on the heart. **(Objective 3)**
4. Cocaine use causes stimulation of the sympathetic nervous system. **(Objective 2)**

5. **Yes.** In cases of severe cocaine overdose, hyperthermia often occurs. **(Objective 3)**

6. Benzodiazepines **(Objective 8)**

7. The primary life threat is respiratory depression. Patient management includes assisting ventilation with a BVM (bag-valve mask) and a high concentration of oxygen. **(Objective 1)**

8. Pinpoint pupils **(Objective 8)**

9. You should be especially cautious because IV drug abusers have a high incidence of communicable diseases such as hepatitis B and HIV. **(Prerequisite Chapter Objective)**

10. Narcan® (naloxone hydrochloride); 0.4 to 2.0 mg IV is the usual dose, but higher doses are recommended for a patient who is experiencing respiratory compromise. Dose administration may vary according to the system's protocols. **(Objective 8)**

11. Needle track marks **(Objective 8)**

12. Withdrawal can be precipitated by Narcan® (naloxone hydrochloride), which makes the patient more difficult to manage and transport. Therefore, smaller doses should be administered to protect the respiratory drive without waking the patient. **(Objective 8)**

13. Repeat administration of Narcan up to a maximum of 10 mg **(Objective 8)**

14. Protecting him from injury during the seizure (e.g., not restraining the patient or forcing an airway into his mouth, if the teeth are clenched; moving any furniture or potentially dangerous objects away from the patient); administering oxygen, if possible; keeping the patient turned on his side; having suction available **(Objective 1)**

15. **a** In a person who has chronically abused alcohol, seizures can occur when alcohol intake is stopped or decreased. They usually occur approximately one day after the last drink is taken and are of the generalized tonic-clonic type. **(Objective 5)**

16. Thiamine and D50. Thiamine should be given before, with, or within a short period of time after dextrose is administered. **(Objective 6)**

17. **b** Delirium is a change of consciousness or orientation; tremens refers to an excessive output of the sympathetic nervous system that causes dilated pupils; diaphoresis; elevated BP, pulse, and temperature; and shakiness. **(Objective 6)**

18. Benzodiazepines such as diazepam (Valium®) or chlordiazepam (Librium®). **(Objective 6)**

19. **(a)** snow, flake, blow, coke

    (b) adam, eve, ecstasy, ice, crank

    (c) pot, mary jane, weed, grass

    (d) LSD, PCP

    (e) heroin

    (Objective 7)

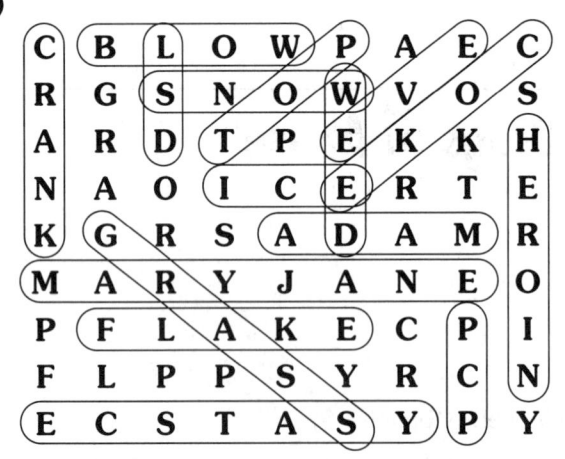

```
C B L O W P A E C
R G S N O W V O S
A R D T P E K K H
N A O I C E R T E
K G R S A D A M R
M A R Y J A N E O
P F L A K E C P I
F L P P S Y R C N
E C S T A S Y P Y
```

20. **(a)** Narcotic

    (b) Lysergic acid diethylamide (LSD)

    (c) Inhalants

    (d) Barbiturates

    (e) Alcohol

    (Objective 8)

21. Activated charcoal **(Objective 8)**
22. Narcan® **(Objective 8)**
23. Nitroglycerin **(Objective 8)**
24. **d (Objective 4)**
25. **d (Objective 7)**
26. **d (Objective 5)**
27. **c (Objective 7)**

CHAPTER 43 Environmental Emergencies

1. A better description of the snake that is consistent with that of a poisonous type; puncture wounds corresponding to the location of the snake's fangs; surrounding swelling and erythema with bloody drainage from the wound. **(Objective 1)**

2. **Yes** and **No.** Keeping the extremity immobilized at the level of the heart helps to minimize venom absorption. Ice should not be used because it can cause local tissue destruction. Tourniquets are no longer recommended; however, if one has been applied by a bystander, it should be left in place until intravenous access is established. Then, it should be removed slowly. **(Objective 1)**

3. Keep the patient calm; remove any rings, watches, or other bands that can cause vascular compromise, if swelling occurs; establish an IV before slowly removing the tourniquet that was applied before your arrival; monitor the patient's status closely; evaluate for swelling—mark the edge of the swelling with a pen and note the time; transport the patient in a position of comfort to a facility that is capable of providing antivenin. **(Objective 1)**

4. **Yes.** The initial appearance of the bite does not reflect the severity or likelihood of envenomation. Symptoms and signs of toxicity can develop over time. **(Objective 1)**

5. Evidence of stridor; increased secretions; swelling of the tongue or oropharynx; the use of accessory muscles of respiration. **(Objective 1)**

6. **No.** Clinical findings of tachycardia, tachypnea, respiratory distress, and wheezing indicate a severe allergic reaction that demands an aggressive approach with rapid institution of therapy. **(Objective 1)**

7. Administer high-concentration oxygen; give epinephrine 1:1000 SQ promptly; establish an IV line with normal saline or Ringer's lactate; administer diphenhydramine intravenously; apply the cardiac monitor; remove the stinger with forceps or by scraping the skin with a straight-edge blade; apply ice locally to decrease pain; transport the patient in a position of comfort. **(Objective 1)**

8. A bee sting kit containing autoinjectable epinephrine and an oral antihistamine might be helpful. With previous exposure, there is increased risk for a more severe response. Symptoms that manifest soon after the sting occurs and that progress rapidly are indicative of a severe response that requires prompt and aggressive management. A bee sting kit would be especially helpful for this patient because of the language barrier, which causes him difficulty in communicating his problem. **(Objective 1)**

9. Classical heat stroke is caused by damage to the hypothalamus and heat regulatory center that results from prolonged exposure to heat. **(Objective 4)**

10. Altered mental status; a rectal temperature of 105° F or higher. **(Objective 4)**

11. Hot, dry skin; abnormal vital signs; hypotension; a weak, rapid pulse; rapid, shallow respirations; advanced age; chronic cardiovascular disease; wearing excessive clothing in a hot, humid environment. **(Objectives 3 and 4)**

12. Rapid cooling **(Objective 4)**

13. **(a)** The airway should be intubated because the patient is unresponsive.

(b) An IV line of normal saline or Ringer's lactate should be administered cautiously to avoid overload and pulmonary edema (administer a 250- to 500-mL bolus, if cooling does not restore blood pressure.

(c) Cooling is achieved by the use of cold packs placed on the neck, axilla, groin, and chest over the large vessels. Air conditioning or a fan can enhance cooling by convection and evaporation. Monitor rectal temperature, and stop cooling measures when it reaches 102° F.

(Objective 4)

14. Shivering, seizures, and dysrhythmias. **(Objective 4)**

15. Frostbite. The history of prolonged exposure to cold temperatures, the complaint of numbness, and the appearance of the skin are consistent with severe frostbite. The possibility of alcohol consumption by the patient may be a contributing factor because it clouds thought processes. It can also lead to decreased perception and appreciation of environmental risk. Alcohol use is associated with almost all cases of urban frostbite; it directly contributes in 50% of all cases. **(Objective 6)**

16. **No.** In general, patients have the right to refuse any medical care that may be offered, but they must understand the ramifications of their decision. This patient cannot be assumed to understand all the ramifications of his refusal because his mental state has been altered by alcohol consumption. **(Prerequisite Chapter Objective)**

17. **d** Ideally, the affected extremity is transported best in a supported, elevated position. Frostbitten skin can be covered with dry, sterile dressings. Care should be taken to keep any blisters or bullae intact. Rubbing frostbitten skin increases the potential for tissue damage. Rapid rewarming is the definitive care for frostbite, but this is best performed in the emergency department. If a frostbitten area is allowed to thaw and refreeze, greater tissue destruction results than if the tissue remains frozen until the patient arrives at the hospital. **(Objective 6)**

18. Establish a TKO IV with normal saline or Ringer's lactate; administer diphenhydramine intravenously; remove the stinger, if it is present; apply ice locally at the site to decrease pain; and transport the patient in a position of comfort. **(Objective 1)**

19. Move the patient to a cool place; replace fluid and salt losses with an IV of normal saline or Ringer's lactate, if he is unable to tolerate oral fluids because of his nausea; do not massage his legs; and transport the patient in a position of comfort. **(Objective 4)**

20. Establish a TKO IV of normal saline or Ringer's lactate; administer diazepam or morphine sulfate for pain relief; apply ice for a short time to reduce pain; provide local wound care in the form of elevation, irrigation with sterile saline, and application of sterile dressings; and transport the patient in a position of comfort. **(Objective 1)**

21. Provide local wound care with elevation and irrigation using sterile saline; cover with sterile dressings; immobilize to reduce bleeding and further damage; and transport the patient in a position of comfort. **(Objective 1)**

22. Establish a TKO IV of normal saline or Ringer's lactate before descent; and transport the patient in a position of comfort to an emergency department at an appropriate altitude for further evaluation and observation, and for possible admission. **(Objective 7)**

23. Provide full spinal immobilization; establish a TKO IV of normal saline or Ringer's lactate; and transport the patient to an appropriate trauma center. **(Objective 5)**

24. Radiation; convection; conduction; evaporation. **(Objective 2)**

25. Shivering—augments heat production metabolically;

    vasoconstriction—reduces heat loss by shunting blood to the core.

    (Objective 2)

26. Remove the patient from the cold environment and protect him or her from further cooling; if possible, move the patient promptly to a warm environment such as a heated ambulance, and replace any wet clothing with warm blankets; administer warm, humidified, high-concentration oxygen using a nonrebreather mask or bag-valve mask, if necessary; monitor cardiac rhythm; establish an IV access using a large-bore catheter with normal saline or Ringer's lactate, warmed if possible; perform rapid glucose determination; avoid rough handling; and transport the patient to a definitive care center that is capable of providing controlled, active rewarming. **(Objective 6)**

27. **E (Objective 4)**
28. **S (Objective 4)**
29. **S (Objective 4)**
30. **E (Objective 4)**

31. **E (Objective 4)**
32. **E (Objective 4)**
33. **c** The J wave (Osborn wave, hypothermic hump) is frequently seen in Lead II; it is described as a "hump" or elevation of the ST segment at the junction of the QRS complex and the ST segment. Its size increases as core body temperature drops. **(Objective 6)**
34. **c** Measurement of core temperature is important in the evaluation of patients with heat-related illness. Core temperatures are taken most reliably using rectal thermometers. **(Objective 4)**
35. **d** In the United States, the factor predisposing an individual to hypothermia that is seen most frequently is the use of alcohol. Alcohol counteracts many of the normal physiologic responses to cold by promoting vasodilation and impairing the heat-generating mechanism of shivering. By clouding the thought processes, it can also lead to a decreased perception and appreciation of environmental risk. **(Objective 3)**
36. **b** The venom from a brown recluse spider has a high concentration of enzymes that can produce extensive local tissue destruction. **(Objective 1)**
37. **c** If infection occurs after an animal bite, the patient may complain of pain and localized swelling or rash. Systemically, there may be fever, chills, aches in muscles and joints, weakness, or malaise. **(Objective 1)**
38. **c** Lithium interferes with sweat production, which impairs dissipation of heat. **(Objective 3)**
39. **d** Because individuals with respirations and a pulse typically survive, those in cardiac or respiratory arrest as a result of a lightning strike are the first priority. **(Objective 5)**
40. **c** In severe hypothermia, ACLS drugs and electrical therapy should be used rarely, if at all, because these therapeutic measures are generally ineffective and may cause harm to the patient. **(Objective 6)**

CHAPTER 44 Aquatic Emergencies

1. Alcohol ingestion was an important predisposing factor in this case of immersion syndrome. Intoxicants impair judgment and lead to inappropriate and dangerous actions. They also predispose the individual to unconsciousness, exhaustion, hypothermia, and hypoglycemia, all of which make aspiration and drowning more likely. **(Objective 2)**
2. She probably experienced immersion syndrome in which sudden death occurs as a result of contact with water, usually cold water. This poorly defined syndrome is probably the result of severe bradycardia or cardiac arrest with subsequent loss of consciousness and aspiration. **(Objective 7)**
3. Airway management should be done in conjunction with precautions to protect the cervical spine. In situations in which the mechanism of injury clearly suggests the potential for head and spine injury, it is important to manage the airway and spine appropriately. Endotracheal intubation is indicated if the victim is apneic or unresponsive, or if respirations are inadequate. All submersion victims should receive 100% oxygen. Always assume that hypoxic brain injury has occurred in the unresponsive submersion victim, and hyperventilate with 100% oxygen. Suction may aid ventilation. Use pulse oximetry, if available, to monitor oxygenation. **(Objective 5)**
4. A submersion victim who is hypothermic and in cardiac arrest should be transported rapidly to the nearest appropriate facility, preferably one with advanced rewarming capabilities such as cardiopulmonary bypass. Dysrhythmias are treated according to Advanced Life Support guidelines, with the exception that only one course of ACLS drugs should be administered until the patient is warmed to 92° F. If the patient is hypothermic, defibrillation and other ACLS strategies are likely to be unsuccessful until the patient is rewarmed. Prolonged CPR may be needed. **(Objective 5)**

5. This patient had several factors that are associated with a poor outcome, including fixed and dilated pupils, Glasgow Coma Score under 5, and asystole upon arrival at the hospital. Still, submersion victims with all these findings have completely recovered, particularly if they were hypothermic. Hypothermia greatly reduces cerebral oxygen requirements and thus increases the time the brain can withstand anoxia. Hypothermic near-drowning victims, particularly children, have sustained submersion times longer than 40 minutes with complete neurologic recovery. **(Objective 4)**

6. **b** Air embolism typically manifests within seconds after a diver surfaces. Common symptoms are altered mental status, seizures, weakness, visual disturbances, difficulty speaking, dizziness, headache, dyspnea, and hemoptysis. Although neurologic findings of an air embolism resemble those associated with a stroke, stroke is unlikely based on this patient's age. Most patients with decompression sickness notice symptoms within 4 hours of surfacing, and some may be asymptomatic for 12 hours or more. Subcutaneous emphysema causes a crackling sensation on palpation of the skin. **(Objective 7)**

7. The type of equipment used, the number and depth of all dives in the past 48 hours, how much in-water decompression took place if any, and the approximate water temperature. **(Objective 6)**

8. Most patients with decompression sickness (DCS) notice symptoms within 4 hours of surfacing, but some may be asymptomatic for 12 hours or longer. DCS is usually not a risk unless one has been exposed to depths of at least 33 feet. Unlike decompression sickness, air embolism can occur after ascent from a dive as shallow as 4 feet. **(Objective 6)**

9. Air embolism occurs when the diver either surfaces too quickly or breath-holds during ascent. **(Objective 2)**

10. 8 Does not open eyes = 1, pulls hand away when pinched = 5, makes garbled sounds that the examiner cannot understand = 2. **(Prerequisite Chapter Objective)**

11. As soon as air embolism is suspected, the patient should be placed in Trendelenburg's position on his left side. This position keeps air bubbles away from the brain and coronary arteries. **(Objective 6)**

12. Hyperbaric facility. Recompression is the mainstay for patients with DCS and air embolism. Because recompression is provided in a hyperbaric oxygen chamber, all patients with suspected DCS or air embolism should be transported as quickly as possible to the closest hyperbaric facility. **(Objective 6)**

13. Patients with submersion times shorter than 5 minutes who regain spontaneous circulation with less than 10 minutes of resuscitative effort generally have good outcomes. **(Objective 4)**

14. **c** Because there appear to be no life-threatening conditions, it is appropriate to use all of these techniques except examining him in private. A child of this developmental age gets very distressed by separation from his or her mother; therefore, such separations should be kept to a minimum or avoided altogether, if possible. **(Prerequisite Chapter Objective)**

15. All submersion victims should be transported to the hospital for evaluation and observation because of the possibility of postsubmersion syndrome, or secondary drowning. This syndrome usually occurs within 12 hours of rescue, but it can be delayed for as long as 72 hours. Its existence emphasizes the importance of hospital evaluation after any submersion accident. **(Objective 5)**

16. **Yes.** Bathtub drowning should alert the EMS provider to the possibility of child abuse. **(Objective 2)**

17. Drowning is defined as death by submersion in a liquid, usually water. Near-drowning involves a submersion accident in which the patient survives for at least 24 hours after submersion. **(Objective 1)**

18. **(a)** Wet—occurs when water or other liquid is aspirated into the lungs, usually after the victim has lost protective airway reflexes and is unable to suppress respirations.

    (b) Dry—occurs when laryngospasm during the initial struggle prevents water from entering the lungs, leading to death by airway occlusion and asphyxiation rather than aspiration.

    (c) Postimmersion (secondary)—occurs when respiratory distress develops after an initial period of recovery.

    (d) Immersion—occurs when there is sudden death after contact with water, usually cold water; it is probably the result of bradycardia or cardiac arrest with subsequent loss of consciousness and aspiration.

    (Objective 3)

19. **(a)** Ears—pain, diminished hearing, tinnitus, dizziness

    (b) Sinuses—headache, cheek pain, upper tooth pain, or nosebleed

    (Objective 6)

20. Resuscitation efforts should be attempted in the water only when circumstances prevent removal, such as with entrapment in a partially submerged vehicle. Even then, CPR cannot be performed effectively in the water. **(Objectives 5 and 6)**

21. **No.** Mouth-to-mouth breathing is difficult to perform without significant practice, requires the use of techniques that are inconsistent with BSI precautions, and requires many sets of free hands working in the water. **(Objectives 5 and 6)**

22. **d** Most patients with decompression sickness notice symptoms within 4 hours of surfacing, but some may be asymptomatic for 12 hours or longer. **(Objective 6)**

23. **d** Aspiration of polluted water can result in bacterial contamination, infection, or chemical inflammation of the lungs, depending on the pollutants. Patients with submersion times shorter than 5 minutes who regain spontaneous circulation with less than 10 minutes of resuscitative effort generally have good outcomes. Prolonged submersion is associated with poor outcome. Hypothermic near-drowning victims, particularly children, have sustained submersion times longer than 40 minutes with complete neurologic recovery. **(Objective 4)**

24. **c** Salt water is more concentrated than plasma; its aspiration results in fluid from the circulation passing into the lungs, having been drawn there by osmosis. **(Objective 3)**

25. **c** All forms of drowning lead to poor ventilation and severe hypoxia. **(Objective 5)**

26. **c** When fresh water is aspirated, it is absorbed quickly through the alveoli into the circulation by osmosis. **(Objective 3)**

27. **c** The jaw thrust maneuver moves the tongue off the back of the oropharynx without manipulating the cervical spine. **(Objective 5)**

CHAPTER 45 Behavioral Emergencies

1. Plan a team approach to continue monitoring scene safety and to gather as much information as possible in a reasonable time frame. Ask two or three open-ended questions, and listen actively for the patient's responses so that you can sort out details and make sense of the situation. An understanding, calm, and nonjudgmental approach sets the tone and enables you to establish a rapport with the patient. **(Objective 3)**

2. **a** Agreeing with his delusions can serve to further his psychotic behavior. To discontinue talking with him or to tell him that he is bizarre would likely produce heightened paranoia and agitation.

   (Objectives 1 and 3)

3. **Yes.** Patients with obvious psychiatric illnesses usually are oriented in the face of significant hallucinations and delusions. So, this patient's behavior would be an expected finding. **(Objective 1)**

4. **d** Haldol® is a major tranquilizer that is used to treat patients with psychotic disorders. Anxiety may or may not require medication; depression is treated with antidepressant drugs (such as tricyclics); and bipolar illness usually is treated with lithium. **(Prerequisite Chapter Objective)**

5. **Yes.** Situational crises that are experienced in life can cause various behavioral reactions. In the case of this patient's underlying illness, certainly a situational crisis could exacerbate his symptoms. **(Objective 1)**

6. First, you should seek the patient's cooperation by providing him with a brief explanation of why he should remain dressed. If he does not respond to this, you should tell him firmly that he must wear clothes outside of his home and to the hospital. **(Objectives 1 and 3)**

7. Consult with local law enforcement if a mental health "hold" is needed to transport against the patient's will. Usually, the legal requirement is that a patient must be a danger to himself or others, or be gravely disabled and unable to function independently. Local protocol dictates how care in such situations is to be provided. You must not leave a patient who may harm himself or others. **(Prerequisite Chapter Objective and Objective 9)**

8. If the patient is holding a gun, her intent is serious and should be considered as such. In acute situations that involve potential suicide, it is important that you listen intently to the patient and try to gain trust. You should be considering techniques for establishing trust. **(Objectives 3 and 5)**

9. Many systems have a crisis emergency team and/or a mental health expert who can be dispatched to the scene. If such a system is in place, it should be activated. **(Objective 1)**

10. Try to build trust. Move slowly, and avoid any attempts to hold the patient or to use physical restraint. It is important that you ask her direct questions about suicidal thinking and planning, so that she understands that you are taking the risk seriously. Keep her focused on the immediate situation. Validate her feelings by explaining that having suicidal thoughts is common, but acting on those thoughts is unacceptable. Help the patient to understand that there are alternatives. **(Objectives 3 and 5)**

11. **Yes.** Several aspects put her at high risk, according to the scale:

    a (age) = 1, d (depression) = 2, e (excessive alcohol or drug use) = 1,

    s (separated, divorced, or widowed) = 1, o (organized suicidal plan) = 2,

    n (no social support) = 1, for a total of 8 points. **(Objective 5)**

12. **c** Given the potential danger of the situation, options a and d, which involve leaving her, are unacceptable. Additionally, this could be considered a case for abandonment. Restraining a suicidal patient also is undesirable and in fact may accelerate the situation. **(Objectives 3, 5, and 9)**

13. Tell the patient that you understand that he has not asked for help, but his wife is concerned, so you just want to check him over to make sure he is alright. Establishing rapport with the patient and exhibiting a supportive and caring attitude are essential to effective patient communication. **(Objectives 1, 3, and 6)**

14. **No.** Even though the patient appears to be alert and oriented, it would not be appropriate to leave without performing further assessment. Many EMS calls for behavioral emergencies present as patients who need some emotional support in a crisis situation. **(Objectives 1 and 9)**

15. Acknowledge that he is in pain and is experiencing a difficult time. A compassionate approach and the sense of touch help to demonstrate your concern. Ask if there is someone whom you could call (e.g., a close friend or a member of the clergy) to come and be with him. Reassure him that you are there to help and not to cause further distress. **(Objectives 1, 3, and 6)**

16. Reinforce to the patient that emotional upsets can affect one's general health, and that it is advisable for him to seek a medical opinion. The finding of elevated blood pressure could be a sign that he needs medical care. You cannot force him to go to the hospital, but you can strongly encourage him to seek assistance on his own; share this recommendation with his wife. **(Objectives 6 and 8)**

17. Depending on the area of service, there may be community resources available to assist them in this situation. If such are available, provide appropriate information to the patient and his wife. Ask again about other resources, such as children, siblings, neighbors, or church members. Sometimes, providing these suggestions facilitates action, and the patient will seek support. **(Objective 1)**

18. **f**

19. **a**

20. **b**

21. **c**

22. **g**

23. **d**

24. **e**

    (Answers 18–24: Objectives 1 and 2)

25. Situational crisis; maturational crisis. **(Objectives 1 and 2)**

26. Determine if there is a risk to the patient or to others. Rapid intervention to lessen the danger to all involved is crucial. Some examples of a behavioral emergency include suicidal thoughts, severe psychosis, violent behavior, severe depression, and mental derangement so extreme that a person is incapable of self-care. **(Objective 1)**

27. Observations on approach; speech characteristics; mood; thought processes; and orientation. **(Objective 4)**

28. **(a)** Reduce outside stimulus. This can be achieved by isolating the patient from the people or events that are causing additional agitation. It is also helpful to reduce noise, movement, and bright lighting, and to control environmental factors such as heat and cold.

    (b) Delegate specific small tasks to family members, friends, and others. The presence of a loved one or a respected clergy member can help in calming the situation.

    (c) Keep the patient well informed about what steps are going to be taken to manage the situation.

    The emergency team needs to balance support for the person's emotions with efforts to contain and resolve the problem. Establishing eye contact and touching the patient help in gaining rapport. **(Objectives 6 and 8)**

29. Violence. Move and talk in a slow and deliberate manner—lowering environmental stimuli can help the patient to focus on your instructions. Avoid making moral judgments about the patient's lifestyle or behavior. Try to anticipate the patient's needs before they become issues that disrupt the scene. **(Objective 7)**

30. Illness and injury are not only physical experiences; they also have a psychological component. In fact, the psychological aspects of pain, sickness, incapacitation, and disfigurement can have a remarkably negative impact on physical illness and injury. Treatment of the whole person entails a number of important elements. For the health care professional, the ability to communicate effectively with people is one of the most important skills; it is manifested by the demonstration of genuine concern, kindness, and sensitivity to the needs of others.

    Sick and injured people need guidance, direct contact, warmth, and understanding. Adding psychological awareness to technical skills humanizes both the patient and the paramedic, and both are better for the combination. **(Objective 6)**

CHAPTER 46 Truncal Trauma

1. **b** Patient #2 has potentially life-threatening injuries and her treatment takes priority over that of Patient #1. Calling for a second unit will free you up to take care of the more seriously injured patient. **(Prerequisite Chapter Objective)**

2. **c** Increasing dyspnea, narrowing pulse pressure, and distended neck veins indicate possible pericardial tamponade. Most cases of cardiac tamponade occur with penetrating trauma. Although other injuries are possible, signs and symptoms support this conclusion. **(Objective 9)**

3. **a** Studies have shown that patients with thoracic injury have a greater chance of dying before they reach the hospital if PASG is applied. **(Objectives 4, 5, 8, and 9)**

4. Gloves should be worn while you are performing the patient examination and treatment procedures. **(Prerequisite Chapter Objective)**

5. Although its incidence is low (2%), in penetrating trauma, cardiac tamponade occurs more frequently with stab wounds than with gunshot wounds. Classical findings include: penetrating trauma, distended neck veins, decreased arterial pressure, and muffled heart sounds. This patient displayed the classic symptoms. **(Objectives 2, 3, and 9)**

6. **a** Before you can take care of the patient, assurance of scene safety is the priority. Gasoline spills and highway traffic are considerations. **(Prerequisite Chapter Objective)**

7. Rib fractures; flail chest; myocardial contusion; and spleen, liver, and kidney injuries. **(Objectives 1 and 2)**

8. **a, b,** and **d** Auscultation of the abdomen provides little information. Bowel sounds are absent in 65% to 93% of patients with internal organ injuries, but they are an unreliable indicator in the separation of patients with and without injury. Also, properly listening for bowel sounds requires a quiet environment, which is not practical in the prehospital setting. **(Objectives 4 and 9)**

9. **d** The patient is disoriented and has sustained a serious injury. She is developing signs of shock, and alcohol ingestion is suspected. Therefore, she probably is not capable of making a treatment decision. It is in her best interest, and yours, to treat and transport her. **(Prerequisite Chapter Objective)**

10. You should administer high-concentration oxygen, assess the chest, continue with the overall assessment, start an IV of Ringer's lactate, splint her leg, and monitor vital signs. **(Objective 9)**

11. Ruptured spleen; fractured ribs; possible injury to the diaphragm, stomach, left kidney, and/or pancreas; possible C-spine or back injury; injury to the left arm. **(Objectives 1, 2, and 3)**

12. **e** All of these indicate a possible intra-abdominal injury. **(Objectives 5 and 7)**

13. The patient should be asked questions that will assist in the determination of whether there is an underlying medical or cardiac problem that may have precipitated the fall. Examples of such questions are listed below:

    What happened?

    How did you feel before the fall?

    Did you slip and fall *or* get dizzy?

    Did you pass out before the fall occurred?

    Do you have any major medical problems? **(Objective 5)**

14. **a, b, c,** and **e** These are all appropriate assessment and treatment measures for use en route to the hospital. Dopamine is used for shock of cardiogenic origin, not for hypovolemic shock. The treatment for hypovolemic shock is to replace lost volume (e.g., start a second IV if BP drops). **(Objectives 5, 8, and 9)**

15. **b**

16. **g**

17. **d**

18. **c**

19. **e (Answers 15–19: Objective 10)**

20. **(a)** Heart, esophagus, trachea, mainstem bronchi, and large blood vessels.

    (b) Pleural spaces that contain the lungs. **(Objective 1)**

21. **b** Mechanism of injury is one of the most important factors in the determination of risk and type of injury in truncal trauma. It is extremely important to reevaluate the available data and to communicate the information to the receiving facility. **(Objective 3)**

22. **c** Time saved in the field is a key factor in attainment of an early diagnosis in the emergency department, as well as in reduction of the interval between occurrence of the injury and patient arrival in the operating room. Both of these factors have shown to *decrease* overall mortality. Applying PASG is controversial; knowing exact injuries is less important; and IVs should be started while en route. **(Objective 4)**

23. **c** Impaled objects are best removed in the operating room, not in the field. If they are removed prematurely, massive bleeding can result. Only when the object prevents extrication and resuscitation efforts should field removal be performed (in very rare cases, if at all) with careful medical direction. **(Objective 9)**

24. **(a)** Apply an occlusive dressing.

    (b) Primary treatment is to ensure adequate oxygenation. Traditional external stabilization may not offer any benefit, but it is not harmful. (Position the patient injured side down.)

    (c) Eviscerated contents should be covered with moist saline gauze to prevent further contamination and drying. Do *not* attempt to push organs back into the peritoneal cavity. This increases the likelihood of infection and complicates surgical evaluation of the injury.

    (d) Listen for breath sounds, treat for shock, and transport rapidly.

    (e) Provide careful observation (and suspicion for the injury) and adequate oxygenation; protect the airway.

    (Objective 9)

25. **c** With blunt trauma, the spleen is the most frequently injured organ, followed by the liver. **(Objectives 1 and 2)**

26. Pneumothorax. The pleura normally allows the lungs to expand throughout the entire chest cavity and yet slide on the inner chest wall. The parietal and visceral sheaths of the pleura are held together by negative pressure, similar to that exhibited by two panes of wet glass that are stuck together. If this space is torn and becomes exposed to air (e.g., by a broken rib, a bullet, or a knife), air rushes into this space and causes the lungs to "collapse" in the chest cavity. **(Objectives 5 and 9)**

27. **e (Objective 9)**

28. After the skin at the selected site is appropriately prepped, a large-bore (14-gauge) needle is inserted through the chest wall into the pleural space. (*Note:* The second intercostal space at the midclavicular line is a common site for needle decompression of the chest. However, insertion through the pectoralis major can be difficult, and the risk of injury to the internal mammary artery suggests that the fourth or fifth intercostal space is a better site.) **(Objective 6)**

29. Tension pneumothorax; air embolism. **(Objective 7)**
30. **(a)** Cardiac tamponade **(b)** myocardial contusion **(Objective 7)**
31. Penetrating **(Objective 2)**
32. According to recent studies:
    - Application of PASG does not increase the total length of prehospital time.
    - Application does increase the blood pressure.
    - Application does not decrease the length of time that the patient spends in the emergency department, operating room, or hospital.
    - When PASG is applied, an overall increased mortality is seen for all patients.
    - Patients with a prehospital time longer than 30 minutes and PASG application do not have a better survival rate.
    - Patients with thoracic injury have a greater chance of dying before they arrive at the hospital, if PASG is applied.
    - Patients with major abdominal injury do not have an overall better survival rate, nor do they have a better chance of seeing a trauma surgeon, when PASG is applied.

    (Objective 8)

CHAPTER 47: Head, Eyes, Ears, Nose, Mouth, and Throat Trauma

1. **Yes.** Assessment of airway, breathing, and circulation takes the usual precedence in treatment of the head-injured patient. Because most head-injured patients have a mechanism of injury that indicates a possible spine injury, spinal immobilization also should be performed. After the ABCs have been assessed and all of the necessary interventions are under way, the degree of disability, or neurologic impairment, should be assessed. **(Objective 8)**

2. Opens eyes when pinched = 2, pulls hand away when pinched = 5, makes no sounds = 1; Total Score = 8. **(Objective 4)**

3. A changing level of consciousness, increasing blood pressure, and slowing heart rate all result from increasing intracranial pressure that is caused by brain swelling or intracranial bleeding. An unreactive dilated pupil, in the setting of depressed mental status, is an ominous sign that indicates critically elevated intracranial pressure. **(Objective 5)**

4. Hyperventilation using a bag-valve mask at a rate of no more than 20 to 22 times per minute could have been initiated; controlled hyperventilation lowers the blood carbon dioxide level, which in turn causes constriction of the cerebral arteries. This constriction of blood vessels provides extra room for expansion caused by swelling or bleeding. Too much hyperventilation may constrict blood vessels too much and decrease cerebral blood flow to below needed levels, thus causing ischemic injury. **(Objective 6)**

5. Vomiting and seizures are common complications among head-injured patients. Intubation prevents aspiration from vomiting and hypoxia, which can lead to seizures. **(Objective 8)**

6. The patient's level of consciousness and how it changed over time should be reported. Changes, for better or for worse, serve as feedback about ongoing treatments and provide guidelines for future interventions. **(Objective 3)**

7. The initial management is essentially the same for all head-injured patients; these procedures should be followed in all patients with significant head injury and an impaired level of consciousness. The paramedic usually cannot distinguish between the various types of head injuries, and there is no need to do so. **(Objective 8)**

8. **b** A nosebleed that is caused by injury usually arises from the anterior part of the nose; it is best controlled by simply pinching the nostrils. Such nosebleeds are usually self-limited; thus, there is rarely a need for inserting a pack because compression accomplishes the same purpose. Leaning forward would have little or no effect on the bleeding. The use of a trumpet should be avoided with any distorted normal anatomy. **(Objective 8)**

9. **e** Any stressor to the body, including emotional upset and blood loss, stimulates the sympathetic nervous system to release the catecholamines epinephrine and norepinephrine. These catecholamines increase heart rate and other actions of the sympathetic nervous system. **(Prerequisite Chapter Objective)**

10. Transport the tooth in saline or milk for possible reimplantation. **(Objective 8)**

11. Swelling, bruising, tenderness, crepitus at the fracture site, and misalignment of the upper and lower teeth. **(Objective 3)**

12. **No.** Endotracheal tubes placed nasally usually are not recommended in patients with severe facial trauma who have unstable fractures or distorted normal anatomy; this is true particularly in the treatment of those with midface fractures because tubes can be accidentally placed into the cranial vault with disastrous results. **(Objective 8)**

13. **(a)** frontal lobe, **(b)** zygoma, **(c)** maxilla, **(d)** mandible, **(e)** parietal lobe, **(f)** temporal lobe, **(g)** occipital lobe **(Objective 1)**

14. **(a)** auricle, **(b)** external auditory canal, **(c)** tympanic membrane, **(d)** stapes, **(e)** incus, **(f)** malleus, **(g)** internal auditory canal **(Objective 1)**

15. **(a)** conjunctiva, **(b)** sclera, **(c)** cornea, **(d)** anterior chamber, **(e)** iris, **(f)** lens, **(g)** posterior chamber, **(h)** retina **(Objective 1)**

16. Using jaw thrust, or by placement of a nasopharyngeal or oropharyngeal airway. However, nsopharyngeal airways usually are not recommended in severe facial trauma with unstable fracture or distorted normal anatomy, particularly midface fracture. You cannot be sure that this patient does not have a nasal or facial fracture. **(Objective 8)**

17. Removal improves access and prevents breakage and possible aspiration of the dentures. **(Objective 8)**

18. Alert, Verbal, Pain, Unresponsive; the last three refer to the patient's response to stimulus and provide a gross estimate of awareness of the environment. **(Objective 4)**

19. **(a)** eye opening, **(b)** best motor response, **(c)** verbal response **(Objective 4)**

20. **(a)** cerebrospinal fluid leakage from the ear, **(b)** Battle's sign, **(c)** raccoon eyes **(Objective 3)**

21. **(a)** naloxone, **(b)** glucose **(Objective 8)**

22. **(a)** late, **(b)** late, **(c)** early, **(d)** late, **(e)** early, **(f)** late **(Objective 5)**

23. **(a)** Cover with sterile gauze and keep free from gross contamination. Avoid using direct pressure to prevent further displacement of the fracture.

    (b) Leave the object in place. It will be removed and treated in the hospital.

    (c) Allow to drain.

    (d) Avoid applying pressure, place a hard shield over the ruptured eye, cover the other eye, and transport the patient in a supine position.

    (Objective 8)

24. **c** The Glasgow Coma Scale judges verbal, ocular, and motor responses. The best responses by the patient are totalled into a number score that ranges from 3 to 15. A patient with a score of 8 or less is considered to be in a coma. **(Objective 4)**

25. **c** It may also be the result of a direct blow to the orbit or of any mechanism that increases pressure inside the chest, such as trauma to the chest or abdomen, or that associated with hanging. **(Objective 2)**

26. **d** Cushing's reflex is manifested by increasing blood pressure and slowing heart rate, which result from increasing intracranial pressure. **(Objective 5)**

27. **d** Controlled hyperventilation at no more than 20 to 22 breaths per minute lowers the blood carbon dioxide level, which, in turn, causes constriction of the cerebral arteries. This limitation of blood flow to the brain creates more intracranial space for expansion caused by swelling or bleeding. **(Objective 6)**

28. **c** Patients often become sleepy or lethargic, although in some cases, they become agitated. As the pressure increases, they become more difficult to wake. Eventually, they become comatose. **(Objective 5)**

29. **d (Objective 7)**

30. **b** The middle meningeal artery runs directly under the thin temporal portion of the skull. Because this portion of the skull is thin, it is a common fracture site. Such a fracture can tear the middle meningeal artery and cause intracranial hemorrhage. **(Objective 2)**

CHAPTER 48 Orthopedic Injuries

1. A priority of care is spinal immobilization because management of possible spinal injuries begins the moment you arrive at the scene. **(Objective 2)**
2. For injuries to the upper extremities, check for grasp or light touch sensation. For injuries to the lower extremities, check sensation to pinprick and light touch, having the patient resist against pressure to flex or extend the toes and flex or extend the knees against resistance without actual movement. **(Objective 3)**
3. Tenderness of the bone or injury site upon palpation; swelling over the injury site, ecchymosis (bruising) over the injury site; obvious deformity; bony crepitus; shortening of the extremity; abnormal rotation of the extremity; decrease or complete loss in function because of pain. **(Objective 1)**
4. You should apply manual traction to the extremity that is distal to the fracture site in an attempt to bring the bone fragments back into alignment so that blood flow can be restored. **(Objective 6)**.
5. Traction splint. Sager and Hare traction splints are the most frequently used. **(Objective 4)**
6. **Yes.** The patient is showing signs and symptoms of shock, which is a complication of this type of fracture. **(Objective 1)**
7. c **(Prerequisite Chapter Objective)**
8. d **(Objective 2)**
9. The patient's skin should be evaluated by pinprick and light touch. **(Objective 3)**
10. *Air splint*

    Advantages: Stabilizes the fracture in alignment and can be used as a pressure dressing for lacerations or open fractures; most are constructed of clear plastic material that allows the wound to be viewed, which decreases the likelihood that the emergency physician will overlook any lacerations or open fractures; it can remain in place during the radiographic process because it is radiolucent.

    Disadvantages: Is expensive; it can compromise circulation to the distal extremity, and application may require excessive manipulation.

    (Objective 4)

    Ladder splint

    Advantages: Can be bent to conform with the shape of the extremity; it is strong, light-weight, and impervious to wind and water; cost is low, and it is easy to store.

    Disadvantages: Shows up on radiograph and may cover fractures that are splinted; it does not immobilize as well as the air splint; it may be bent or reshaped, which causes the fracture to be resplinted in an undesirable position; it must be applied by wrapping the splint to the extremity, which conceals any open fractures or lacerations from view. **(Objective 4)**

    Box splint

    Advantages: Same as those listed for the ladder splint.

    Disadvantages: Is weakened when wet; it may hide wounds; it may be reshaped, which causes the fracture to be resplinted in an undesirable position.

    (Objective 4)

    Vacuum splint

    Advantages: Is versatile, reusable, and nonconstrictive.

    Disadvantages: Is expensive.

    (Objective 4)

11. Motor function; sensory function; circulatory function. **(Objective 2)**
12. Because the hospital was only 5 minutes away, it was inappropriate to remain on the scene for 20 minutes. Based on the mechanism of injury, this patient could be experiencing multiple trauma. Therefore, splinting of the arm should have been done while en route. **(Prerequisite Chapter Objective)**
13. To prevent additional complications such as nerve, spinal cord, or vascular damage. **(Objective 2)**
14. Pelvis; femur. **(Objective 1)**
15. **d (Objective 2)**
16. **c (Objective 4)**
17. **b (Objective 5)**
18. In-line immobilization in a neutral position without actual traction. **(Objectives 2 and 5)**
19. Compress the pelvis both anteriorly over the symphysis pubis and laterally over the iliac crest; the pelvis will feel unstable, and the patient will localize pain during the compression; treat shock, if present; little can be done in the field to directly stabilize a pelvic fracture. **(Objectives 1 and 2)**
20. Manually stabilize the head and neck to prevent self-inflicted spinal cord injury. **(Objective 2)**

CHAPTER 49 Burn Injuries

1. Close enough to the location of the patient(s) to allow rapid access, yet far enough away to be safe from explosion, water runoff, and airborne chemical contamination. **(Objective 5)**
2. **a (Objective 7)**
3. To protect the patient's privacy, prevent hypothermia, and reduce the risk of contamination to her burned skin. **(Objectives 3 and 7)**
4. Facial burns, singed nasal hair, soot around her mouth. **(Objective 6)**
5. You should consider intubation if the patient develops signs of respiratory distress, such as dyspnea, wheezing, or a decreased level of consciousness. It would be extremely difficult to intubate the patient at this time because she is still conscious. However, local protocols may allow for nasal intubation or sedation or paralysis before oral intubation. **(Objective 7)**
6. Shoulders or back **(Objective 7)**
7. **No.** Because of the patient's potential for airway compromise secondary to possible inhalation burns, she should be transported immediately. When transport time is less than 60 minutes, IV placement may be delayed until the time of arrival at the receiving hospital. **(Objective 7)**
8. **c (Prerequisite Chapter Objective)**
9. **b (Objective 5)**
10. Cardiac dysrhythmia **(Objective 6)**
11. **Yes.** Deep tissues, such as muscle, nerves, blood vessels, and bone, can be destroyed as electrical current flows through the body, even though the skin appears normal. **(Objective 6 and 7)**
12. The hospital with the specialized burn unit. This is necessary because of the classification of this patient's burn. According to the American Burn Association, this is a major burn injury because it is an electrical burn and it is an injury to the hand. All major burns require rapid transfer to the nearest trauma center or regional burn center. **(Objectives 4 and 7)**
13. (1) **c** (2) **a** (3) **b** (4) **b** (5) **b** **(Objective 2)**
14. Flame; flash; scald; contact. **(Objective 1)**
15. Smoke inhalation; carbon monoxide poisoning. **(Objective 3)**

16. Hands; feet; face; perineum. **(Objective 4)**
17. Destination decisions **(Objective 4)**
18. Associated trauma **(Objective 3)**
19. **d (Objective 3)**
20. **b** Thermal burns are the most common type of burns. **(Objective 1)**
21. **b (Objective 6)**
22. **c (Objective 4)**
23. **e (Objective 3)**
24. **e (Objective 1)**
25. **d (Objective 4)**
26. **c (Objective 1)**
27. **b (Objective 7)**
28. **(a)** Depth: third degree
    Extent: 18%
    Severity: major
    Referral: yes
    (b) Depth: first degree
    Extent: 4.5%
    Severity: major
    Referral: yes
    (c) Depth: third degree
    Extent: 46%
    Severity: major
    Referral: yes
    (Objective 4)

Chapter 50: General Principles of Rescue

1. **a** After you have called for expert assistance, power interruption should be assessed for scene safety. Once this has been determined, a danger zone should be established. Patient rescue should not begin until the scene is safe. **(Objectives 1 and 2)**
2. You should instruct the driver to remain in the vehicle and to touch nothing that is outside of the car. Whenever power has been interrupted, all wires, utility poles, support structures, and surrounding structures (e.g., fences) should be considered electrically energized until an appropriately trained person verifies otherwise. **(Objective 2)**
3. Protective gear is needed for yourself, and also for the patient, if available. Make sure fire suppression support is available at the scene and that there is a water supply for washdown. **(Objectives 1 and 2)**
4. **a, b,** and **d** The side window may provide the quickest access; however, shattered glass and the smaller opening surrounded by glass fragments may injure the patient further. **(Objective 4)**
5. With two critical patients, getting additional help mobilized is the immediate priority. **(Prerequisite Chapter Objective)**

6. Provide critical field interventions and transport the patient as quickly as possible to an appropriate hospital. **(Objective 5)**

7. Starting one or two IVs; providing respiratory support for possible flail chest; assisting ventilation for potential head injury; checking the ECG; and continuing assessment. **(Prerequisite Chapter Objective)**

8. Noxious gases, cave-ins, equipment injuries, and explosions. These are very dangerous situations for the patient and for rescuers. **(Objective 6)**

9. **c** In such dangerous environments, specially trained personnel should attempt rescue, if they are available. **(Objective 6)**

10. _5_ Stabilize the femoral fractures.

    _2_ Provide C spine stabilization.

    _4_ Start two IV lines of Ringer's lactate.

    _1_ Assist ventilations and give oxygen.

    _6_ Apply dressings to the burns.

    _3_ Call for air medical transport.   **(Objective 6)**

11. The patient shows signs of severe hypovolemic shock. Keeping him warm is a basic principle in the management of any patient who is in shock; it also will lessen or prevent hypothermia. **(Prerequisite Chapter Objective)**

12. Acknowledge his fears. Explain that his condition is serious, but that he is stable now and that you are doing all you can to take care of him. Tell him that it is very important to get to the hospital as quickly as possible and that efforts to that end are in progress. **(Prerequisite Chapter Objective)**

13. **d** With severe crush injuries, sudden cardiac arrest may occur after the debris is removed, secondary to acidosis and hyperkalemia. **(Objective 6)**

14. Stabilize the C-spine; provide ventilation support; administer oxygen; and keep the patient warm. IV(s) should be started, and use of PASG should be considered. **(Objective 6)**

15. Sodium bicarbonate may be given to prevent potential acidosis. When certain areas of the body are compressed and are not perfused properly, lactic acid builds up in response to compromised or absent circulation. This medication is used for protection from the sudden release of these acids, which can be very harmful. **(Objective 6)**

16. **False.** Protective gear is particularly important in enhancing rescuer safety in these potentially hazardous situations. Its use is standard during the initial scene survey. **(Objective 2)**

17. **True.** The hydraulic cylinder can be pushed back and left in a "loaded" mode. If the pressure is released, the bumper is violently rammed back to its original position. If the patient or rescuer is in contact with the bumper at this point, serious injury can result. **(Objective 2)**

18. **True.** This is an urgent circumstance that would permit a shift in priorities, related to patient and rescuer safety. **(Objective 6)**

19. **True.** Confined spaces present a potential hazard caused by the limited space and the poorly ventilated entrances/openings. **(Objective 6)**

20. **True.** When unsupported trench walls collapse, tons of earth and stone can bury a worker. Severe crush injuries can easily result. **(Objective 6)**

21. **(a)** Patient access

    (b) Initial patient care

    (c) Patient extrication and removal

    (Objective 3)

22. **c** Aspects of the terrain, access, and environment make this a particular challenge, and it is imperative that patients be immobilized properly. Managing the airway, starting the IV, and performing a continued assessment are general aspects of any rescue situation. **(Objective 6)**

23. **a, c,** and **d**   CPR in the water is an unproven procedure. Chest compressions should be deferred until the patient is on a stable surface. **(Objective 6)**

24. **Yes.** This situation is analogous to sudden deflation of PASG; it causes a sudden release in peripheral vascular resistance. When the pressure on the torso is released, you should be prepared for the patient's circulatory collapse, as well as potential deterioration in the patient's condition. **(Objective 6)**

25. Silos, storage tanks, mines, trenches, septic tanks, sewers. **(Objective 6)**

Chapter 51: Multiple-Casualty Incidents and Disasters

1. **e** Preplanning for an MCI is the key factor, so mentally reviewing the plan, as well as triage principles, is important. The EMT could be used to begin triage of patients. **(Objectives 1, 2, 3, and 4)**

2. **a, b, c,** and **d** All are important and appropriate aspects of the assessment phase. **(Objectives 2, 3, 4)**

3. Stop and intervene with each patient. The goal of triage (greatest good for the greatest number) will be defeated if you stop and take care of each patient. **(Objectives 2, 3, 4, and 5)**

4. Mobilize other units and personnel that are needed. The "initial" size-up may not determine all that is needed, but it can be an important step toward getting assistance. **(Objectives 2, 3, and 4)**

5. **e** The EMT can tag patients as you determine the appropriate categories, while also helping to direct incoming units. The EMT should not start CPR on patients in the "dead" category, nor start IVs. **(Objectives 2, 3, 4)**

6. **(a)** Dead — No pulse or respirations
   (b) Delayed — No life-threatening injury; treatment delay is acceptable.
   (c) Urgent — Condition is serious and could deteriorate rapidly, although it is stable now.
   (d) Critical — Patient is unconscious, and condition is unstable. The patient could be salvageable with timely intervention.
   (e) Dead — No vital signs
   (f) Critical — Airway compromise is severe and acute. The patient is potentially salvageable with timely intervention.
   (g) Delayed — Injury is not immediately life-threatening; patient's condition is stable. Treatment delay is reasonable.
   (h) Delayed — Injury is not immediately life-threatening; the patient is conscious and alert. ("Walking wounded.")
   (i) Critical — Unconscious with airway compromise and a weak pulse; potentially salvageable with timely intervention. **(Objective 6)**

7. **d, f,** and **i** The three patients whose condition is critical should be transported after triage is completed. **(Objective 6)**

8. **d** All of these should be considered initially at the scene in this type of incident. **(Prerequisite Chapter Objective)**

9. To determine (1) the total number of victims involved; (2) the severity of their injuries and how many are in each category; and (3) what additional resources and personnel are needed to handle the incident. **(Objective 2)**

10. **d** The goal and definition of triage is just that: to provide the most benefit to the greatest number. Other tasks may be performed as the situation evolves, but they are *not* the initial priorities. **(Objectives 2 and 5)**

11. **e** Individuals responding to the scene of an MCI should be informed about the plan and requested to report to the command center to receive their assignments. "Doing their own thing" leads only to confusion and further chaos. **(Objective 4)**

12. **b** With the situation relatively under control, the most important task now is getting patients to the appropriate hospital. A knowledgeable physician could help most at this point by assisting this effort. **(Objectives 4 and 9)**

13. Participating in such a tragic event can leave emotional wounds on the caregivers. Frequently, the impact on an individual(s) is not realized until much later. A formal system (CISD) allows these individuals to "debrief" and discuss their feelings. Families of rescuers and victims can be included. Supervisors should recognize this as an important matter to be dealt with and should provide appropriate mechanisms for handling it. **(Objective 11)**

14. **(a)** Victims

    (b) Medical personnel who are immediately available to handle victims' needs.

    (Objective 1)

15. **(1)** e

    (2) a

    (3) c

    (4) b

    (5) d

    (6) g

    (7) f

    When these steps are followed, in order, they provide a baseline "protocol" for any MCI. Even in situations that are variable, they should generally be followed. **(Objective 2)**

16. **d** Although it is not a necessity, these centers are often combined, thus allowing efforts to be unified. This often helps to minimize confusion and mobilize resources. Each center should have an incident commander. **(Objectives 2 and 4)**

17. **c** The incident commander can come from multiple sources (e.g., fire department, EMS, or hospital). However, with an organized disaster plan, a key to success is establishing this ahead of time. **(Objectives 2, 4, and 10)**

18. **(a)** Airway

    (b) Breathing

    (c) Circulation

    (Objective 7)

19. **(a)** Ability to walk

    (b) Breathing and rate

    (c) Perfusion

    (d) Mental status

    (Objective 7)

20. **e** Once treatment has started, one medical person oversees this effort. Priority setting is paramount to the process. The treatment officer also determines if additional resources are needed. **(Objective 4)**

21. Assist you and other patients. With many tasks at hand, these patients can be employed as manpower, and often they wish to "help." **(Objective 6)**

22. **a, b, c,** and **d** All aspects of preplanning for an MCI are important, as are debriefing and discussing how to better manage MCIs in the future. **(Objective 10)**

23. **e** Transport categories are the virtually same as those used in triage: critical, urgent, and delayed. However, the availability and capability of local hospitals also should be considered in these decisions. These decisions are not crucial initially because patients are still being evaluated. **(Objectives 8 and 9)**

24. **d** All of these aspects are important in evaluating the overall effectiveness of the emergency response and in discussing problems encountered during management of the incident. **(Objectives 10 and 11)**

25. **(a)** Critical

    (b) Urgent

    (c) Delayed

    (d) Dead

    (Objective 6)

CHAPTER 52
Hazardous Materials and Radiation Incidents

1. **a** When responding to an accident involving a cargo truck, you should remember that hazardous materials are often transported by truck. **(Objective 2)**
2. **b** If you suspect that the scene involves a hazardous material, you should not put yourself at risk for exposure; wait until you have determined that it is safe to approach victims to render aid. **(Objective 3)**
3. *Emergency Response Guidebook* **(Objective 8)**
4. A listing of actions to be taken at the scene; possible health hazards; suggested first aid measures. **(Objective 8)**
5. **a** This is your safest action, considering that the hazardous material is loose from its container and remains unidentified at this time. **(Objectives 3 and 9)**
6. **d** These actions may be lifesaving. **(Objective 7)**
7. You should wear chemical protective clothing (CPC) in conjunction with eye, nose, and mouth protection. CPC is designed to protect emergency medical personnel from hazardous materials that can affect the body through inhalation, ingestion, or direct contact. **(Objective 5)**
8. **(a)** Cut away and/or remove all suspected contaminated clothing, including jewelry and watches.
   (b) Brush and wipe off any obvious contamination.
   (c) Protect any open wounds from contamination.
   (d) Make every attempt to avoid contact with potentially hazardous material.
   (Objective 7)
9. To protect staff members and other patients from contamination, and to limit the exposure of hospital facilities. **(Objective 7)**
10. Any equipment that is suspected of being contaminated should be kept sealed until the incident commander or his designee gives further instructions. **(Objective 6)**
11. When faced with a patient who is in a situation in which there is evidence of an unknown radioactive material being out of its container (and the amount and type of radiation that is being given off by this material are not known), the paramedic should not enter the scene until personnel are available for proper monitoring of the area. **(Objectives 10 and 11)**
12. The patient should be moved away from areas of potential radiation exposure or contamination, making use of the principles of time, distance, and shielding to lessen the radiation exposure to you, your partner, and the victim. **(Objectives 10 and 11)**
13. Remove the patient's contaminated clothing, and seal it in a labeled plastic bag to be left at the scene. Brush off any radioactive material from the skin into a plastic bag, exercising caution not to contaminate the patient's nose, mouth, eyes, ears, and wounds. **(Objective 11)**
14. The stretcher must be covered with a sheet, which should be placed on the contaminated side of the control line that separates the contaminated from the noncontaminated area. The patient is then transferred to the covered stretcher, and the sheet is folded to securely package the patient. Isolate any contaminated substance within a package. **(Objective 11)**
15. **c** **(Objective 9)**
16. **d** Bradycardia, hypersalivation, constricted pupils, and profuse sweating all are signs and symptoms of organophosphate exposure. **(Objective 6)**
17. Atropine is used as the antidote for organophosphate poisoning and should be administered as soon as possible, even before you have finished decontamination procedures. **(Prerequisite Chapter Objective)**
18. Wear chemical protective clothing; remove the patient's clothing and bag it; try to find a water source and wash down the patient. **(Objective 7)**

19. One of the side effects of chemical exposure is irritability of the conduction system of the heart, which leads to cardiac dysrhythmia. Thus, every chemically contaminated patient must be monitored for dysrhythmia and ectopic beats. **(Objectives 6 and 7)**

20. Wind direction; drainage. **(Objective 9)**

21. **(a)** Identity of the relevant hazardous materials

    (b) Routes by which rescue personnel may enter the area

    (c) The degree of contact with the hazardous material or the contaminated victim

    (d) The specific task assigned to the user

    (Objective 5)

22. **(a)** Do not allow wash water or chemical agents on the skin to enter the eyes, nose, or mouth of the patient.

    (b) Do not be so vigorous with the cleansing that the fluids are splashed on EMS personnel or about the area.

    (c) Do not neglect the hidden areas of the body, such as the armpits, the groin, and the crease in the buttocks. **(Objective 7)**

23. Dry decontamination, which is the use of disposable outer protective clothing. **(Objective 5)**

24. **(a)** Do not enter the scene; withdraw to a safe place while considering wind direction and possible liquid runoff.

    (b) Call for the hazardous materials team to evaluate and manage the problem.

    (Objective 9)

25. **False.** A hazardous material is any substance that is capable of posing an unreasonable risk to health, safety, and property. **(Objective 1)**

26. **False.** For the most dangerous hazardous materials, regardless of their amount, the shipping container and the vehicular means (truck/tank car) by which they are being transported must bear a placard. Hazardous materials that are considered less dangerous require placards only if more than a thousand pounds is on board. **(Objective 2)**

27. **False.** This must be accomplished by trained teams with special equipment. **(Objective 3)**

28. **False.** The nature of many hazardous materials scenes is that they are dangerous zones as long as the hazardous material is present, even if it remains within its shipping container. **(Objective 2)**

29. **True.** **(Objective 7)**

30. **(a)** Hot zone — includes all areas or locations in which hazardous materials either have spilled or may spill if a container is breeched

    (b) Warm zone — area to which rescue personnel and/or hazardous materials team members take patients for decontamination, evaluation, and treatment

    (c) Support zone — location of the incident commander with his command post and any needed support personnel and equipment **(Objective 4)**

Chapter 53 Air Medical Services

1. (a) Lengthy extrication
   (b) Extended ground transport time
   When one or more of the following conditions exist, helicopter transport should be seriously considered: lengthy extrication of a critically injured patient, especially if the aircraft can arrive at the scene before extrication is completed; lengthy manual transport of the patient out of a remote area so that motorized transport can be accessed; or the need for extended ground transport time to get the patient to an appropriate medical facility. **(Objective 2)**

2. Spilled gasoline **(Prerequisite Chapter Objective)**

3. (a) Gloves
   (b) Goggles
   (c) Helmet
   (Prerequisite Chapter Objective)

4. Tension pneumothorax **(Prerequisite Chapter Objective)**

5. Chest decompression **(Prerequisite Chapter Objective)**

6. A tension pneumothorax that is already life-threatening worsens dramatically without decompression because of gas expansion that occurs during air transport. **(Objective 8)**

7. a Typically, the helicopter requires a square area that is at least 100 feet by 100 feet. **(Objective 7)**

8. (a) Do not run or smoke within 50 feet of the aircraft.
   (b) Remove all hats, loose clothing, and other items that can be blown away by air turbulence that is created by the aircraft rotors.
   (c) Always approach the aircraft directly from the front, never from the side or rear.
   (d) No objects should be carried higher than your head.
   (e) Do not open or close the doors of the aircraft.
   (Objective 6)

9. (a) Effect: Gas expands as the aircraft ascends.
      Compensation: Oxygen flow rates must be increased.
   (b) Effect: Gas bubbles expand in IV fluids as altitude increases.
      Compensation: A pressure infuser must be used on the plastic IV bag.
   (c) Effect: The endotracheal cuff overexpands or underexpands.
      Compensation: There must always be a slight air leak around the cuff.
   (Objective 4)

10. (a) Air medical crews are unable to hear normal breath sounds during helicopter flight because of the noise of the helicopter.
    (b) There may be a substantial decrease in the ability to detect carotid pulses during flight. **(Objective 3)**

11. The air medical communication specialist should receive and coordinate all requests for air medical services; this person must also interact on a regular basis with the ground-based emergency medical dispatch center and with the receiving facility. **(Objective 5)**

12. Probably the most vital component of the communications center is its radio communication capabilities. **(Objective 5)**

13. **(a)** Transportation time to the trauma center by ground ambulance is longer than 15 minutes.

    (b) Transport time to the local hospital by ground is longer than transport time to the trauma center by helicopter.

    (c) Patient extrication time is longer than 20 minutes.

    (d) Use of the local ground ambulance leaves the local community without ground ambulance coverage.

    (Objective 2)

CHAPTER 54 Rural EMS

1. **Yes.** Air medical transport offers an advanced level of care for this patient whose condition is potentially unstable. The availability of a heart monitor and defibrillator could be crucial to this patient's outcome. **(Objective 7)**

2. **c** With your limited resources, this patient requires rapid transport to the hospital. Additional medical history information can be obtained while en route, or by calling her physician. It would be inappropriate for the patient to be transported in a private vehicle. **(Objectives 1 and 3)**

3. **Yes.** If the physician is available and agrees, this medication could help to alleviate some of her pain during the long transport. It could also help to get more oxygen to the heart muscle. **(Objectives 3 and 6)**

4. **d** Because of the long transport time remaining before arrival at the hospital, it is in the patient's best interest that you manage ABCs in the most effective manner (i.e., endotracheal intubation and automatic CPR device). A single EMS provider most likely would fatigue from performing one-man CPR and assisting respirations with a bag-valve mask. **(Objectives 3 and 6)**

5. **Yes.** Epinephrine is the first drug to be administered in any type of cardiac arrest, regardless of the rhythm. **(Prerequisite Chapter Objective)**

6. **c** Dopamine is indicated secondary to low blood pressure when the heart rate and rhythm are adequate. Adenosine would be indicated for PSVT, and lidocaine and bretylium for rhythm of ventricular origin. **(Prerequisite Chapter Objective)**

7. **d** Patient extrication is the next priority. The appropriateness of administering pain medication is determined by local protocol, but it is still a secondary priority, along with bandaging and the use of PASG. **(Prerequisite Chapter Objective)**

8. You should activate air medical transport. The patient's condition is critical, and rapid transport to a trauma facility is essential. Air medical transport could best facilitate this goal. **(Objective 7)**

9. If you are waiting to rendezvous with the helicopter, you should start an IV at the scene. If air medical transport is on the scene, an IV can be started by the air transport crew while en route. **(Objective 6)**

10. **(a)** Absence of strong medical direction

    (b) Extended response times

    (c) Inadequate funding and public access to the EMS system

    (d) Limited personnel training opportunities

    (e) A shortage of volunteer personnel

    (Objective 1)

11. **False.** According to the Department of Transportation, over one half of fatal traffic accidents in the United States occur in rural areas. **(Objective 5)**

12. **True. (Objective 5)**

13. **True.** Boating, fishing, camping, skiing, hiking, and hunting often take place in locations where only limited medical resources are available. **(Objective 5)**
14. **False.** Because call volume is lower in rural areas, there is limited exposure to clinical cases. Because of the limited exposure to clinical cases, skill and knowledge deterioration can also be a problem. **(Objective 1)**
15. **True.** Because of the inherent variables that make system setup difficult, community support is extremely important. **(Objective 1)**
16. **True.** This is probably the single most significant factor affecting rural health care delivery. **(Objective 3)**
17. **False.** Communication with on-line medical direction may be difficult or unavailable for rural EMS personnel. Therefore, standing orders that enable trained personnel to perform lifesaving procedures without direct contact with a physician are indicated. **(Objective 2)**
18. **True.** This can affect providers' knowledge and skills retention; it can also impose difficulty in terms of recertification. **(Objective 1)**
19. Many communities do not have 9-1-1 or enhanced 9-1-1; emergency numbers may be different for each county or fire district; numbers are not posted on public phones; there may be limited number of public telephones, or there may be residents who do not have telephones; terrain can affect communication signals (e.g., may block transmission signals); equipment may be outdated or inadequate; it may be difficult to get on-line medical directions at times. **(Objective 2)**
20. **a, b,** and **d** All-terrain vehicles and four-wheel drive vehicles have better access capability than do ambulances in some rural settings. Therefore, response times may be improved by using them, not just ambulances. **(Objectives 3 and 4)**
21. (a) Because of extended transport times, EMS personnel may be permitted to use medical criteria to determine when it is appropriate to discontinue CPR in the field. **(Objective 6)**

    (b) Starting IVs while en route with a critical trauma patient is the standard of care. However, in certain cases (e.g., long transport times and rough road conditions that make it difficult to start an IV while en route), it may be appropriate to take time to start an IV on the patient at the scene. Transport time also affects decisions regarding airway management techniques. Advanced airway techniques (e.g., endotracheal intubation) may be more appropriate than use of a BVM. **(Objective 6)**

    (c) With limited services, individuals with "first aid" types of injuries may be treated at the scene and not transported. In some cases, it may be appropriate to transport a patient to a local physician's office rather than to a hospital. Additionally, there may be times when releasing a patient from EMS care to be transported by the family is an appropriate choice. **(Objective 6)**

    (d) Air medical transport offers an advanced level of care and more expeditious transport times. This not only benefits the patient being treated, but it allows the rural unit to return more quickly to be available for service in its area. **(Objectives 6 and 7)**

CHAPTER 55 Specialized Adjuncts for Therapy

1. Dizziness caused by rising from a recumbent to a sitting position may indicate excessive fluid loss. This patient most likely has fluid depletion that is the result of vomiting for three days. **(Prerequisite Chapter Objective)**
2. In critical situations, a VAD may provide immediate and lifesaving venous access. This patient could be considered critical based on her presentation. **(Objective 2)**
3. (a) Aspirate slowly for a blood return.

    (b) Flush the line with solution.

    (Objective 4)

4. **d** Despite proper care, clots may form in the catheter, thus disrupting the flow of solutions. Never attempt to force or dislodge the clot. The patient may require medical intervention with thrombolytics to declot the catheter, or complete replacement of the catheter may be needed. **(Objective 3)**

5. **b** Respirations of 6 per minute are inadequate for proper ventilation and require assistance. **(Prerequisite Chapter Objective)**

6. The left arm should be used. You should avoid taking blood pressure readings in the extremity with a shunt because this disrupts blood flow. **(Objective 5)**

7. You should first attempt to establish a peripheral or external jugular line. The decision to use a dialysis access device in the prehospital setting must be carefully considered before insertion of any needle because of the high incidence of infection that is associated with poor technique. If appropriate, endotracheal or intraosseous routes may also be considered for the administration of medications. **(Objective 6)**

8. Normal saline is the crystalloid of choice for fluid resuscitation; lactated Ringer's should be avoided because of its higher concentration of potassium. **(Objective 5)**

9. This patient's unconsciousness probably resulted from hypotension and hypovolemia, which most likely were caused by rapid removal of fluid from the intravascular space during dialysis. **(Objective 5)**

10. **Yes.** This patient has early signs and symptoms of increasing intracranial pressure (ICP). An occlusion in her ventricular shunt is causing cerebral spinal fluid to build up in the ventricle, thus increasing ICP. Increasing ICP is a true medical emergency that requires rapid intervention to prevent brainstem herniation. **(Objectives 10 and 11)**

11. Caution is necessary to avoid inadvertently overloading (overhydrating) the patient and worsening the increasing ICP. **(Objective 11)**

12. **(a)** Vomiting

    (b) Irritability

    (c) Visual disturbances

    (d) Rising systolic blood pressure

    (e) Widening pulse pressure

    (f) Bradycardia

    (Objective 11)

13. Patients with chronic illnesses, such as acquired immunodeficiency syndrome (AIDS) or sickle cell disease, that require prolonged and frequent access to venous circulation for administration of fluid, medications, parenteral nutrition, and/or blood transfusions. **(Objective 1)**

14. **(a)** Peripheral inserted central catheters

    (b) Implanted ports

    (c) Central venous catheters

    (Objective 2)

15. **(1)** b

    (2) e

    (3) g

    (4) a

    (5) f

    (6) h

    (7) c

    (8) d

    (Objective 6)

16. Dialysate may fail to drain from the peritoneal cavity if the catheter is closed, or if the tip is lodged against the abdominal wall. Occasionally, turning the patient from side to side and/or gentle pressure on the abdomen may alleviate the fluid accumulation. **(Objective 5)**

17. Select an endotracheal tube that will easily pass through the stoma; however, remember that the tube must be large enough to allow for suctioning and adequate ventilation. **(Objective 8)**

18. **(a)** Complication: respiratory distress

    Signs & Symptoms: shortness of breath, dyspnea, stridor, congestion

    (b) Complication: sepsis

    Signs & Symptoms: dyspnea, tachycardia, hypotension

    (c) Complication: site infection

    Signs & Symptoms: swelling, drainage

    (Objective 8)

19. Maintaining an open airway and providing adequate oxygen exchange. **(Objective 8)**

20. **(a)** Recurrent ventricular tachycardia

    (b) Ventricular fibrillation

    (Objective 12)

21. **False.** Because the patient has already received internal countershocks that were unsuccessful, external shocks are indicated. **(Objective 12)**

22. **False.** Direct pressure with a sterile dressing should be applied; careful assessment should be performed to check for any other complications. **(Objective 9)**

23. **True.** A single tube has a built-in tracheal cuff, and an obturator or stylet is used for insertion. A double tube has a similar attached cuff, but it also has an inner cannula that is designed to be removed easily. **(Objective 7)**

24. **False.** Because it is impossible to know the specific details of each ventilator, it is also impractical to troubleshoot the alarms or to adjust settings. Treat the patient, not the alarms. **(Objective 8)**

CHAPTER 56: Issues of Personal Violence

1. Paramedics are often dispatched to violent scenes at which the perpetrator is still present. Because the potential for injury exists, you should wait for police assistance to ensure that the scene is safe. Do not argue with violent people. A means of escape should always be accessible; therefore, do not let a threatening person block an exit. **(Prerequisite Chapter Objective and Objective 1)**

2. She needs to be convinced that she is safe and that any disclosure is private. Supportive, nonjudgmental, nonthreatening questions are reassuring. **(Objective 6)**

3. **Yes.** Typically, there is a cyclic pattern to spousal abuse. It is common for the abused spouse to remain in the abusive relationship. The primary reason for this is fear of the abuser's retaliation. Also, women who are abused are usually economically dependent on the abuser and wish to maintain their commitment to the relationship. **(Objective 5)**

4. **a, c, d,** and **e** The patient exhibits signs of a possible head injury; therefore, an IV, oxygen, and ventilation assistance are all appropriate. Typically, dopamine is used to raise blood pressure in patients with shock that is unrelated to trauma. **(Prerequisite Chapter Objective)**

5. Yes, this is typical behavior. The cycle begins with a tension-building phase marked by arguments and fights. Often, the woman accepts this behavior to avoid a more severe beating. Because she is unable to control events, the man ultimately loses his temper, and the second phase of the acute battering episode begins, usually accompanied by a beating. Following this, the man typically becomes remorseful, which leads to the final phase. She is soothed by the tender, caring, and now loving male, and in fact experiences more nurturing and attention than during any other part of the relationship. The cycle and the victimization are complete, and she remains in the relationship. **(Objective 3)**

6. Treating her with respect, dignity, and compassion throughout the time you are with her increases her feeling of well-being. Encourage her to disclose information for her own safety and well-being. Encourage her to talk to a social worker, a crisis shelter worker, or a friend. Her disclosure of information about the abuse increases the likelihood that she will leave the abusive situation. **(Objectives 6 and 8)**

7. State laws vary in regard to reporting adult abuse. When it is suspected, paramedics should inform the police, emergency department personnel, and, if appropriate, social services. Careful documentation is especially important for continuity of patient care. **(Objective 8)**

8. Let her know that you are there to help and will take very good care of her and her sister. A calm, supportive approach is particularly important. **(Objective 6)**

9. Tell her that you would like to take her and her sister to the hospital. Acknowledge any fears that she may have, and reassure her that she will be safe and protected, both in your care and after she reaches the hospital. **(Objectives 4, 5, and 6)**

10. **Yes.** An emergency court order can be obtained in cases of suspected child abuse. The most important and dynamic historical finding for verification of sexual child abuse is the child's actual report of the sexual activity to an outsider. A paramedic's identification of child abuse is important because of the significant mortality and morbidity associated with it, and because of the potential for effective remedial action and prevention. **(Prerequisite Chapter Objective and Objective 8)**

11. All states require that suspected child abuse cases be reported to a child welfare agency or the District Attorney's office. This applies to cases in which there is reasonable cause to suspect child abuse and neglect, as well as to confirmed cases. Paramedics should use the emergency department to coordinate the appropriate reporting materials and procedures. **(Objective 8)**

12. **No.** Most states provide protection from liability for the individual who makes a report of suspected child abuse in good faith. **(Objective 8)**

13. This patient is in a very undesirable and unhealthy environment; she is in need of immediate assistance. Social services may be required to evaluate her situation and to secure some type of ongoing care. **(Objective 3)**

14. Have you eaten today?

    How is your diabetes controlled?

    What medications, if any, do you take for your medical problems?

    Have you been taking your medications regularly?

    How long has your stomach been hurting?

    Have you had any associated symptoms such as vomiting or diarrhea?

    What does your daughter do for you?

    Has your daughter ever hurt you?

    Does anyone prevent you from maintaining social contacts outside the home?

    (Prerequisite Chapter Objective and Objectives 3, 4, and 6)

15. Companions or caretakers who deny an elder the chance to interact privately with any health care provider should be considered suspect for elderly abuse. Tactfully explain to the daughter that her mother has summoned your help and that you are obligated to provide it. Explain that you are very concerned about her mother's slurred speech and disorientation. Also, explain that the unsanitary environment can complicate her medical problems. **(Objectives 3 and 6)**

16. Proper documentation in these cases is essential. Observable behavior of the patient and family should be recorded. Judgmental statements should be avoided. If the patient confirms abuse, you should note the following information: length of time the abuse has gone on; the number of incidents; the seriousness and consequences of the abuse; and whether she has received any help for this problem. Physical signs that you observe should be noted, as well as information about the environment in which you found the patient. (Because determination of elder abuse is a legal matter, it should be qualified in your report as an allegation made by the patient.) **(Objective 8)**

17. Young males. Their violent behavior is often a manifestation of feelings of anger, guilt, agitation, helplessness, and hopelessness. A threatening mannerism, a loud and forceful voice, confusion or delirium, and anxious pacing can forewarn of violent behavior. Drug-induced behavior, concealing a weapon, and threatening to hurt someone are also clues. **(Objective 1)**

18. Hypoglycemia; hypoxia; drug ingestion; head trauma; intracranial bleeding. **(Prerequisite Chapter Objective)**

19. Scene safety is important. You should establish yourself as an authority figure and engage in active listening. In some cases, restraining the patient may be necessary. If this is the case, be sure that adequate help is available. Secure the patient's trunk at a bony prominence (e.g., extremities, pelvis, shoulder). Do not apply pressure to the chest, throat, or neck. The goal is to restrain, not to injure. Intoxicated patients are particularly prone to aspiration, especially if transported in a supine position. A particular issue that can arise is "the duty to protect" a potential victim. Specific threats made to the paramedics or other individuals must be seriously considered. **(Objectives 1 and 2)**

20. **(a)** The patient has a medical or psychiatric condition that requires immediate transport, and the patient is demonstrating behavior that may harm himself or others.

    (b) A serious medical condition exists that may threaten the patient's life if there is a delay in treatment or transportation, and there is no reasonable way to obtain consent to provide treatment or to accept an informed refusal of care

    (c) You are directed by appropriate authorities to transport a patient on the basis of a mental health hold or police custody.

    (Objective 2)

21. Typically, abusive parents are experiencing a number of life crises and have limited resources to deal with them. Drug or alcohol abuse in the family, chronically ill children, single-parent families, frequent absence of a parent from the family, and social isolation of families all are contributing risk factors. Often, these parents have been victims of abuse themselves. They delay or avoid seeking care for their children; the children who are abused are often those from unwanted or accidental pregnancies. **(Objective 3)**

22. **c** In most cases, young children are scalded by immersion, and older children by having liquid thrown or poured on them. **(Objective 4)**

23. This syndrome results from holding and violently shaking a child. It is most commonly seen in infants. Hyperflexion and avulsion fractures of the thorax and lumbar vertebrae may be the resulting injuries. Intracranial injury also is associated with this syndrome, which results in a mortality of approximately 15%; 50% of survivors have significant neurologic deficits. **(Objective 4)**

24. **d** All other injuries and conditions listed here do occur, but they are not as frequent as fatal neurologic injury. **(Objective 4)**

25. Characteristics include social isolation and stress; as with child abuse, the "abuser" often has been a victim of child abuse. Abusers usually hold a traditional view of marriage in which the man is "king of the castle." Both the men and women in abusive relationships may have witnessed their fathers abusing their mothers. A family history of alcoholism or drug use is also a risk factor. Abuse usually occurs inside the home during times of intense interpersonal interaction; it is rarely witnessed by outsiders. **(Objective 3)**

26. Victims should be encouraged not to wash, change their clothing, eat or drink, go to the bathroom, douche, bathe, shower, take any medication or alcohol, gargle or brush teeth, or delay in getting to the emergency department. Police should be notified immediately, and the scene should not be disturbed. If the victim has already changed clothes, advise her or him to place the discarded clothing in a paper bag and take it to the hospital. (Plastic bags can affect the integrity of the evidence.) Documentation must be made of each person who takes possession of the evidence so that the chain of custody can be preserved. **(Objective 7)**

Chapter 57: Death and Dying

1. **a** Your own safety in a potentially dangerous situation is of utmost importance. An injured rescuer is of no benefit to an injured patient. Checking the patient and performing any other resuscitation measures are secondary to scene assessment. **(Prerequisite Chapter Objective)**

2. **d** Continuing CPR, providing defibrillation, initiating an IV, and securing the airway are standard procedures for a patient in ventricular fibrillation. An external pacemaker is not indicated. **(Prerequisite Chapter Objective)**

3. **e** Resuscitation efforts must continue, but at the same time, someone should speak with the family. It is not appropriate for the family to be ignored; however, your primary focus is patient care. Other personnel should be asked to communicate with the family. **(Objective 6)**

4. **d** Communication with the family at the scene may assist them in "acute grief preparation." It does *not* eliminate the grief or shock response to loss, but it may assist the family in the first critical minutes after they receive such devastating news. An example of an appropriate response is: "We are doing everything possible to help him, but his condition is critical." **(Objectives 3, 5, and 6)**

5. You might encourage her to have a neighbor or friend drive her to the hospital, but do allow her to accompany her husband if she insists. To deny her request may cause additional stress, as well as problems for her later on. For example, "Mrs. G., you are welcome to ride with us, if you wish; however, you might be more comfortable going with your neighbor, Mr. Jones." **(Objectives 3, 5, and 6)**

6. **c** A tactful but honest approach is usually best. Words such as "passed on" or "gone" could be misinterpreted. Positioning yourself at eye level, identifying who is present, and exhibiting compassion all are helpful measures in such a delicate situation for the family. **(Objectives 3, 5, and 6)**

7. **d** The length of time that grief and mourning will last is highly individualized. Therefore, it is neither necessary nor appropriate for the paramedic to suggest such a time frame for the survivors. **(Objectives 5 and 6)**

8. **a, b,** and **d** How you will mobilize the engine crew, what equipment you will need, and review of local protocols for managing cardiac arrest should all be considered while en route. The decision not to resuscitate a patient is based on local medical protocols and generally is considered to be a medical/legal decision, not an ethical one (i.e., the patient is "terminal"). **(Objective 10)**

9. Acknowledge that *any* response to this news is *acceptable*, even when the death is expected. Tactfully and compassionately express your sympathy, but honestly explain that resuscitation measures are not indicated by the physical findings of the patient. An appropriate response may be to ask if there is someone you can call who will come and be with the bereaved family member. **(Objectives 5 and 6)**

10. **e** Viewing a body at the time of death is a personal choice, and it is not one that you or anyone else should make for another individual. In fact, this experience may help the family member begin to acknowledge that death has occurred. **(Objectives 5 and 6)**

11. Communicate this information to the receiving faculty and/or medical examiner's office. Helping the family initially to support their lost loved one's wishes is also important. **(Objective 7)**

12. **d**
13. **a**
14. **b**
15. **c**

    (Answers 12 to 15: Objective 2)

16. **e** Every paramedic will be faced with this situation at some point, so an awareness of these influences is important. **(Objective 1)**

17. **(a)** *Psychic pain spike:* This refers to the first 5 to 15 minutes after hearing the news that a loved one has died. It is a paralyzing feeling. All types of emotional and physical responses are plausible.

    (b) *Feelings phase:* An intense longing for the lost loved one exists for approximately 4 to 8 weeks. Sadness, depression, anger, guilt, and anxiety are common feelings during this phase. The closer the relationship is, the more intense the feelings are.

    (c) *Recovery:* Absorption and preoccupation with the loss diminishes, and reconstruction of life begins. The length of the process varies.

    Times mentioned in all phases are not prescribed, but rather they are estimated. Each can be shorter, or much longer. **(Objective 3)**

18. **d** Because you are an active participant in those first moments after shocking news, it is important to have a sensitive but honest approach. Euphemisms such as "passed on," "gone," or "this was God's will" should be avoided. These can be misinterpreted or resented by the family. **(Objectives 5 and 6)**

19. To "err on the side of the patient" and to resuscitate. Omission of such efforts could present subsequent legal problems. Also, familiarization with your local DNR protocols should verify the appropriate response. **(Objective 10)**

20. **(a) False.** How each system responds to DNR orders depends on the local medical protocols. Issues of malpractice liability and practitioner immunity must be considered. **(Objective 10)**

    (b) False. Local medical protocols, not the patient's family, dictate when patients are or are not resuscitated. **(Objective 10)**

    (c) True. The paramedic has a unique opportunity to significantly impact these situations. Part of that responsibility includes remaining compassionate and responding appropriately during a very personal moment of a family's life. **(Objective 5)**

21. Critical incident stress debriefing can be indicated for the prehospital care provider in a variety of situations, many of which involve death or dying. The emotional and physical health of an EMS provider can suffer if such intervention does not occur when necessary. The formal debriefing process is a widely accepted practice in EMS. **(Objective 4)**

22. | **Sudden death** | **Anticipated death** |
    |---|---|
    | • No warning... shock/denial. | • Survivors may become "new" patients. |
    | • Guilt and resentment possible. | • Reactions vary; may still be in denial. |
    | • Unresolved relationships may create problems. | • Although the death was expected, family still may not be ready. |
    | **What to do:** | **What to do:** |
    | • If resuscitation efforts have been begun, honestly tell the family of potential severity. | • Be at eye level; position close. |
    | | • Introduce yourself, identify the relationships of those present. |
    | • Keep the family informed. | • Be honest, yet compassionate; use appropriate terms (e.g., "dead," and not "gone" or "passed on"). |
    | • Be honest. | |
    | • Call someone to be with them. | • Call someone to be with them. |

    (Objective 5)

23. Denial, anger, bargaining, depression, and acceptance. A patient's progression and the family's reaction to this are quite variable. **(Objective 8)**

24. The goal of hospice is to provide a dignified and caring environment for dying people, typically in their homes. Hospice provides professional and medical assistance for both the patient and the family as they cope with the process. Hospice tries to minimize unnecessary calls made to the EMS; however, if the paramedic is called to a scene for a hospice patient, he or she is obligated to respond according to local protocol. **(Objective 9)**

58 Stress and Stress Management

1. **a** Establishing an airway is the first priority. Breathing for the victim and starting cardiac compressions would be next in importance. **(Prerequisite Chapter Objective)**

2. Acute. The situation that you have just experienced has triggered a normal initial response in this situation. Frequently, EMS providers feel as though they could have "done more," or something else, to save a victim. Also, pediatric calls typically are more stressful. **(Objective 6)**

3. **Yes.** Sometimes a single event triggers a response to previous events that were not dealt with at the time, or it may be related to concurrent stressors in a person's life. **(Objective 6)**

4. Your acknowledgment that the feelings exist is essential. Discussing your reactions with a spouse or friend, writing your reactions to the incident in a journal, and participating in strenuous physical exercise all are *healthy* methods for dealing with your feelings. Avoiding the pain, or using drugs or alcohol to "numb the pain" only serves to delay the need for emotional release. **(Objectives 6 and 11)**

5. **a, b, c, d,** and **e** All are physiologic and emotional responses that are common to an acute stress reaction. **(Objectives 5 and 6)**

6. Cumulative **(Objective 6)**

7. **d** All are signs and symptoms of cumulative stress. Hostile behavior, increased absence from work, and a negative attitude are common manifestations of this problem. **(Objectives 4, 5, and 6)**

8. Do not. These individuals often feel that they are reacting appropriately to things that "keep happening to them" (i.e., they take no responsibility for their actions). They often withdraw from family and friends and may be physically exhausted. This often results in a decline in job performance. **(Objectives 5 and 6)**

9. Personal difficulties at home often can have a compounding effect in the work setting. "Stressors" in our lives may come from several sources, thus combining to contribute to the behavior demonstrated. **(Objectives 5 and 6)**

10. **True.** A disaster of this magnitude that results in many horrifying injuries and loss of life clearly is classified as a critical incident. **(Objective 9)**

11. **True.** Emergency personnel are "lifesavers". Therefore, the innate desire to "carry on" is typical. Also, this is an example of "eustress," or good stress, which mobilizes one to act when an emergency calls for quick action and reactions. **(Objectives 9 and 10)**

12. **True.** Acute or delayed reactions may occur, and both must be managed effectively. **(Objectives 9 and 10)**

13. **True.** Following such a dramatic event, the caregiver needs a respite. The officer's actions are entirely appropriate in this case. **(Objectives 9 and 10)**

14. **True.** Critical incident stress debriefing is very appropriate. This event involved many people; the sooner debriefing begins, the healthier the outcome will be for those involved. **(Objectives 9 and 10)**

15. Eustress is a positive, creativity-producing stress. It usually increases productivity, enthusiasm, and a desire to excel. Examples include: (1) responding to a cardiac arrest call that went well and the patient survived; (2) being assigned a specific project that you can control, organize, and execute; 3) having a deadline that is *reachable*; you do a good job with good results. **(Objective 1)**

16. **e** All of these are involved physiologic responses to stressors. The body senses the "distress" and mobilizes forces to deal with it. **(Objective 2)**

17. **(a)** Alarm — increased sympathetic response; "fight or flight" response; most organ and body systems are affected.

    (b) Resistance — arousal of the stress response is targeted to one or more target organ systems that are capable of handling it. This works for the short-term response.

    (c) Exhaustion — results from prolonged stress; organs are energy depleted. It may result in stress-related diseases.

    (Objective 3)

18. **a, b, c,** and **d** All of these listed can cause stress. Stress can occur as a result of psychosocial, bioecological, and personality causes. **(Objective 4)**
19. The suddenness of the incident or event; the intensity of the stressor; whether or not the provider knew the victim; the provider's previous experience in handling similar situations. All of these may have an effect on the magnitude of a response. **(Objective 5)**
20. **True.** Delayed stress can occur at any time subsequent to a single event, or series of events. **(Objective 6)**
21. **True.** Sleep disturbances are the most common sign of delayed stress. **(Objectives 7 and 8)**
22. **False.** Paramedic school demands an additional sphere of time constraints and pressure in the lives of most individuals. **(Objectives 7 and 8)**
23. **True.** Typically they have a high need for stimulation and challenge, thereby exhibiting these characteristics. **(Objectives 7 and 8)**
24. **False.** The opposite is true. This may be an inherent, learned, or protective mechanism. **(Objectives 7 and 8)**
25. Certain events are classified as critical incidents that require critical incident stress management (CISM) intervention. These include:
    - Death of an emergency worker in the line of duty
    - Serious injury to an emergency worker in the line of duty
    - Mass-casualty incidents resulting in serious injury or death
    - Suicide of an emergency service worker
    - Death of a civilian as a result of emergency service or law enforcement operations

    Other incidents that may precipitate critical incident stress reactions include:
    - Death or serious injury of a child
    - Response to a call for a victim who is known to the emergency worker
    - Threat to the safety of the responders (i.e., hostage or sniper situation, hazardous materials, other threat to personal safety)
    - Situations associated with excessive media interest or criticism
    - Loss of a patient following prolonged effort
    - Personal identification with the victim or circumstances
    - Incident in which the sights and sounds are particularly distressing

    (Objective 10)
26. Death. Forty percent of such calls involve the death of a child or adolescent; 26% the death of adult; 7% the death of emergency personnel. Ten percent are suicides. **(Objective 10)**
27. **a, b, c, d,** and **e** All are characteristics that contribute to an incident becoming a critical one for most caregivers. **(Objective 10)**

ILLUSTRATION CREDITS

CHAPTER 6
6-1 A-F From American College of Emergency Physicians: Paramedic field care—a complaint-based approach, ed 1, St. Louis, 1997, Mosby–Year Book.

CHAPTER 7
7-1, 7-2 From American College of Emergency Physicians: Paramedic field care—a complaint-based approach, ed 1, St. Louis, 1997, Mosby–Year Book.

CHAPTER 12
12-2, 12-2, 12-4, 12-5, 12-8, 12-9, 12-11, 12-13, UN 12-1 From Aehlert B: ACLS quick review study guide, ed 1, St. Louis, 1994, Mosby–Year Book; **12-3, 12-6, 12-7, 12-10, 12-14** From Huszar R: Basic dysrhythmias: interpretation and management, ed 2, St. Louis, 1994, Mosby–Year Book.

CHAPTER 17
17-1 From Aehlert B: ECGs made easy, ed 1, St. Louis, 1995, Mosby–Year Book.

CHAPTER 18
18-1 From American College of Emergency Physicians: Paramedic field care—a complaint-based approach, ed 1, St. Louis, 1997, Mosby–Year Book.

CHAPTER 19
19-1 From Aehlert B: ACLS quick review study guide, ed 1, St. Louis, 1994, Mosby–Year Book; **19-2** From Cummins R, Graves J: ACLS scenarios: core concepts for case-based learning, ed 1, 1996, Mosby–Year Book; **19-3, 19-4** From Huszar R: Basic dysrhythmias: interpretation and management, ed 2, St. Louis, 1994, Mosby–Year Book.

CHAPTER 21
21-1 From Huszar R: Basic dysrhythmias: interpretation and management, ed 2, St. Louis, 1994, Mosby–Year Book.

CHAPTER 22
22-1 From Huszar R: Basic dysrhythmias: interpretation and management, ed 2, St. Louis, 1994, Mosby–Year Book.

CHAPTER 29
29-1 From Aehlert B: ECGs made easy, ed 1, St. Louis, 1995, Mosby–Year Book.

CHAPTER 31
31-1 From Huszar R: Basic dysrhythmias: interpretation and management, ed 2, St. Louis, 1994, Mosby–Year Book; **31-2** From Aehlert B: ECGs made easy, ed 1, St. Louis, 1995, Mosby–Year Book.

CHAPTER 32
32-1 From Huszar R: Basic dysrhythmias: interpretation and management, ed 2, St. Louis, 1994, Mosby–Year Book; **32-2** From Conover M: Understanding electrocardiography, ed 7, St. Louis, 1996, Mosby–Year Book.

CHAPTER 33
33-1 From Aehlert B: ACLS quick review study guide, ed 1, St. Louis, 1994, Mosby–Year Book.

CHAPTER 34
34-1 From Huszar R: Basic dysrhythmias: interpretation and management, ed 2, St. Louis, 1994, Mosby–Year Book.

CHAPTER 47
47-1 From McSwain, White, Paturas, Metcalf: EMT-B: the basic EMT comprehensive prehospital patient care, ed 1, St. Louis, 1997, Mosby–Year Book; **47-2, 47-3** From American College of Emergency Physicians: Paramedic field care—a complaint-based approach, ed 1, St. Louis, 1997, Mosby–Year Book.

CHAPTER 52
52-1 From American College of Emergency Physicians: Paramedic field care—a complaint-based approach, ed 1, St. Louis, 1997, Mosby–Year Book.